COPYRIGHT

Graphic design, cover and photographs:

Promonet Publishing

Email: healthyebookblog@gmail.com

Registered copyrights: United States of America

1. Aesthetics and dermatology. 2. Nutrition: Skin care and aging l. Title.

Second printed and digital reissue: September, 2023. Improved and augmented content, with full color and new features.

Visit official Publishers website: https://healthyebookblog.wordpress.com

Contact email: healthyebookblog@gmail.com

AF703652

BODY, SKIN AND BEAUTY

Table of contents

Foreword

CHAPTER 1: AESTHETICS

Contemporary aesthetics

Physical appearance and beauty

The Egyptian legacy

Aging and biological clock

Famous Video and its aesthetics

Key Ideas and Activities

CHAPTER 2: AESTHETIC SUBSPECIALTIES

Classification of aesthetic sub-specialties

Dermatology

Spa: definition and benefits

Types of spa Aesthetic clinics

Beauty salon

Barbershop

Tattoos and care

Plastic surgeries

Biopolymers risks

Types and techniques of epidermal grafts

Key Ideas and Activities

CHAPTER 3: COSMETOLOGY AND PRODUCTS

Introduction to cosmetology

Typology and skin care

Makeup Cosmetic products

International Nomenclature of Cosmetic Ingredients

Microdermabrasion

Wrinkles and botox

Video Cellulite.

Key ideas and activities

CHAPTER 4: BODY THERAPIES

Body treatments

Facial massage protocol

Anticellulite and reducing cosmetics

Body Massage Protocol

Radio frequency protocol

Cavitation Protocol

Reducing massage protocol

Thermotherapy

Vaccination therapy

Filling Forms for professional estheticians

Key ideas and activities

CHAPTER 5: HAIR REMOVAL TECHNIQUES

Hair characteristics

Hair removal areas of the body

Depilatory techniques classes

Depilatory selection criteria

Hair removal protocol

Key ideas and activities

CHAPTER 6: ANATOMY

Skin organ

Treatable diseases

Circulatory system

Lymphatic system

Locomotor apparatus

Key ideas and activities

CHAPTER 7: NUTRITION

Three eating practices

Vegetables

The fruits

The grains

The meats

Spices and seasonings

Medicinal plants

Obesity and calories

Diet flow charts

The digestive system

Sex and nutrition

Healthy recipes

Nutrition Articles

Key ideas and activities

CHAPTER 8: PROTOCOL AND ETIQUETE

Protocol and ceremonial

Origin of the label

Social and business etiquette

Dress: from formal to informal

Customs at cultural level

Label on the Table

Artistic projection

Key ideas and activities

CHAPTER 9: BIOSAFETY

Scientific bases of biosafety

Safety rules Professional ethics of the esthetician

Key ideas and activities

CHAPTER 10: RELAXATION THERAPIES

THE ESTHETICIAN BOOK

Charts

CHAPTER 1

BODY MORPHOTYPE

CHAPTER 2

SPECIALTIES AND SUBSPECIALTIES of HEALTH SCIENCE

DERMATOLOGICAL PATHOLOGIES

BEAUTY SALON GADGETS

HAIR EXTESIONS

CHAPTER 3

SKIN TYPES PRODUCTS

INCI INGREDIENTS LIST

ACNE GRADES

CHAPTER

4 MASSAGE POSITION

FORMS FOR ESTHETICIANS

CHAPTER 5

HAIR REMOVAL BY SEX

NAILS DISEASE

HANDS AND FEET

CHAPTER 6

10 SKIN DISEASES

LYMPH NODES

LYMPHATIC ORGANS

MUSCLES of THE HEAD

BODY MUSCLES

CHAPTER 7

CALORIES BY ACTIVITY LEVEL

CALORIES BY SEX

FOOD PORTIONS

BODY MASS INDEX

DIET FLOW CHARTS

SEX FRECUENCY

BABIES FEEDING

CHAPTER 8

TYPES of PROTOCOL & LABEL CUTTERY AND LABEL

CHAPTER 9

BIOSAFETY LEVELS

CHAPTER 10

AROMATERAPHY

PERFUMERY

WINE AND CHOCO THERAPHY

CONTRAINDICATIONS IN THERAPIES 10

BODY, SKIN AND BEAUTY

Foreword

Dave Rivers - Writer

Seeing ourselves better enhances our self-esteem, at a level of personal that projection allows us to reach the attention of others and communicate effectively. That is the purpose of aesthetics. In May 2017 we published the first edition of this aesthetics manual, which in these three years of continuous promotion has received a great acceptance from the public of Spanish and English speakers' readers and translated into six other languages from the continents of Europe and Asia. We consider that the health and wellbeing of our dear readers is a sensitive and very important topic, so we decided to review its content to improve it with 24 additional topics that had not been included before, more graphics, in addition to adding an additional chapter at the end with relaxation therapies that summarizes in a concise and enjoyable way those concepts that complete a work in this field of beauty science. Another innovation that we apply in this version are the sections of "Key ideas and suggested activities" for instructors and students of aesthetics of specialized schools. Here the reader will find videos and audiobooks as exclusive teaching material, with topics that are included in this edition to strengthen the learning process.

For all these reasons we celebrate this second edition with great pride and satisfaction. For this reason, this book was published for all those who see in the art of body aesthetics a way to use their time profitably. And like the female and male figures, they are part of self-esteem, which is the factor most related to mental health, personal fulfillment and happiness, it has several chapters that illustrate, define and explain many of the concepts and procedures which are necessary to work within an aesthetic clinic, or even manage it as your own business.

The bibliography available on the Internet on the techniques and protocols of beauty most accepted at present, has been updated with this Manual that left nothing pending because all the topics and subtopics have been included that Will complete any questions that may be had and are related to this field so recommended in our days. Starting with chapter one where we address the origin and theory of Aesthetics from ancient Greece and compare it with contemporary rethinking. In the second entitled "Aesthetic sub specialties" we define its concept, intermediate relationships, its types and we highlight the healthy benefits that can be obtained from various types of therapies that combine natural and ancient techniques. And we Will see how aesthetics also help people in more serious cases where facial trauma suffered by some accidents that disfigure our face with more invasive scientific methods.

"Cosmetology and products" is the title of the third chapter that describes the protocols with the detailed steps of a massage for facial discomfort and presents the skin typology. We also find here a more extensive introduction to cosmetology. Below we extensively address nine of the body treatments most used in clinics by beauticians who will also warn us when they are applicable to patients and to whom they are contraindicated. In some this chapter you Will also find the examples of the medical documents for the cosmetic clinic patient file as they must be filled out and filed for excellent service.

Specialized hair removal is another chapter of this topic that we develop from the characteristics of the hair, selection criteria for the depilatory technique, classes of techniques and, of course, their protocols when applying them. Another topic that we have not left out of this book is Anatomy, encompassing three of the body systems and devices most directly associated with aesthetic treatments and therapies available to beauty clinics.

Chapter seven is about nutrition that in its nine previous subtitles adds dietary practices, health articles and healthy recipes, so in this reissue it reproduces some chapters of the book "12 Diets of Fullness" where, among Other options, you can determine the body mass index. In the eighth chapter we will know how and etiquette terminologies differ, their historical origins and evolution until our days when postmodernism introduces subconscious norms or rules in the members of society on how to project their career in the artistic environment, among many other tips on dress styles for both ladies and gentlemen.

Cultural etiquette is also another interesting topic that we have wanted to present exhaustively in this section. The penultimate chapter is for aesthetic professionals and ends with the details and knowledge that every esthetician should know, and finally the new tenth chapter of this reissue that compiles 4 of the relaxation therapies previously discussed along with six other new therapies that thus expand the themes of this 2023 reissue.

It is a pleasure for us to share with you, friends and readers, the most important data on aesthetics and beauty that you have been able to compile so far for this manual or guide, which becomes more extensive. We hope that you will not be forgotten and that you can take advantage of this knowledge for your profession, your family and personal well being.

Yours,

the authors

CHAPTER 1 AESTHETICS

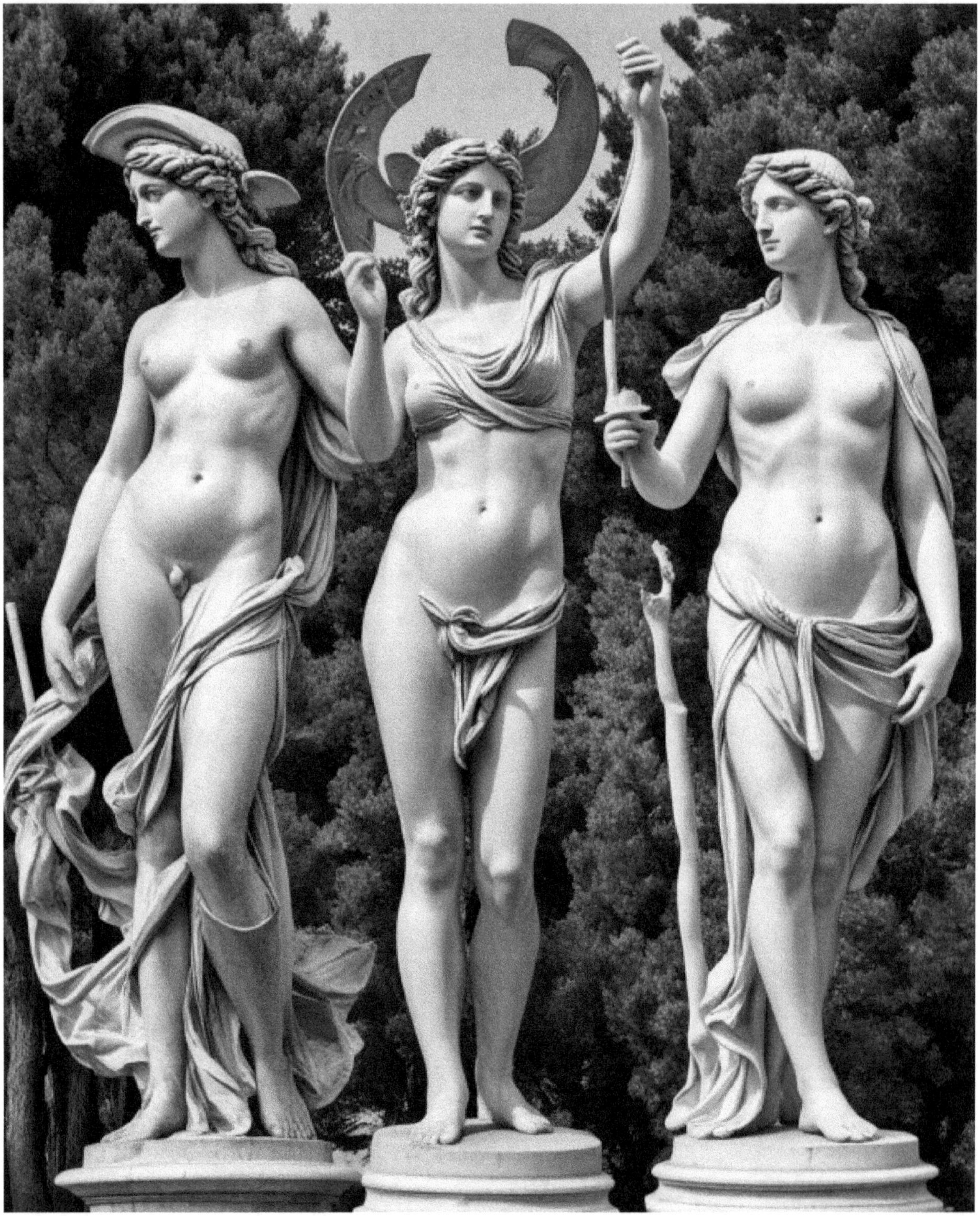

We recognize that the physical appearance, dress and manners of our behavior are signs of education or academic preparation, as well as social status, but physical attractiveness also arises if there is a difference between the beautiful and the sublime. On the one hand we find the factors inherent in the personality and experience of each person such as 'Vanity' which is defined as a quality of conceit and presumption for what is displayed or demonstrated. At the same time, the sense of personal taste" differs in each individual or group of influence, between the evolution of social fashions, we can point out that submitting to the discretion of the jury after preparing and instructing ourselves in the area of communication, audiovisual media, modeling, advertising and Other similar fields; It requires a prior process of adaptation to criticism by not falling in grace and dreaming of a goal for the sake of pleasure. Another aspect of aesthetics that should not embarrass or inhibit us at all times is the sense of belonging to a racer a term used to classify humanity according to physical and genetic characteristics.

Historically, physical anthropologists had divided humanity, according to its morphological features, into three major subdivisions or races: Negroid, Mongoloid, and Caucasian. Some scientists went further by adding Amerindian and Oceanic. As a biological concept, race was more evident when the differences made reference to morphological traits, such as skin pigmentation, hair color, shape and thickness, nose shape or body structure. The appearance of genetic analysis came to refute this idea. Before this definition, breed classification depended on a combination of geographic, ecological, and morphological factors. However, the term race is controversial because of the implicit notions of superiority and inferiority. The concept of race is not particularly useful from a biological or sociological point of view, since all races belong to a single biological species, Homo sapiens, and show only small genetic variations. Culture is a much more important factor in determining the behavior and lifestyle of different human groups. Race was the justification for it establishing the state of slavery, the persecution of minorities and other social groups, such as the Jewish people during Nazi Germany, or the apartheid system in South Africa.

Medicine, and the psychology of art, although independent disciplines, are related to aesthetics. The psychology of art is related to elements of this discipline such as human responses to color, sound, line, shape and words, and to the ways in which emotions condition such responses. In medicine, surgeries are the treatment of a disease or correction of a deformity or defect, by manual or operative procedures, with or without the use of medications.

This branch of medicine is subdivided according to the nature of the procedure used in: general surgery, which treats all types of injuries; orthopedic surgery (of the musculoskeletal system) that is responsible for correcting deformities; plastic surgery, which tries to rebuild tissues and repair tissue loss, especially through tissue transfer. Surgery is also subdivided according to the region concerned into: neurosurgery (central nervous system and spinal cord); ENT surgery (ear, nose, throat); cardiac (heart) surgery; vascular surgery (arterial, venous and lymphatic systems); thoracic surgery (chest and lungs); digestive surgery (abdominal and pelvic organs); urological surgery (kidneys, excretory system and genitalia) and gynecological surgery (female reproductive system).

ORIGIN & THEORY

Like many of the philosophical branches, aesthetics originated in Greece alongside philosophy. In this evolution, among the legends of the various Greek gods the values of male and female ugliness and beauty are personified, we find some of the most revealing myths of human feelings. By the personification of feminine beauty, Aphrodite is pointed out, goddess of love and beauty, equivalent to the Roman Venus. In Homer's Iliad she appears as the daughter of Zeus and Dione, one of her consorts, but in later legends she is described as sprouting from the foam of the sea and her name can be translated as 'born of foam'.

In Homeric legend, Aphrodite is the wife of Hephaestus, the ugly and lame god of fire. Among her lovers is Ares, the god of war who in later mythology appears as her husband. She was the rival of Persephone, queen of the underworld, with whom she fought for the love of the beautiful young Greek Adonis. While the beautiful young Adonis, loved by the goddesses Aphrodite and Persephone is the male personification. Born of the incestuous union of King Cyniras of Cyprus and his daughter, Adonis was placed in the custody of Persephone, queen of the underworld. When Adonis died from being attacked by a wild boar he was hunting, Aphrodite implored the god Zeus to return him. Zeus decreed that Adonis would spend the winter months with Persephone in Hades and the summers with Aphrodite. The story of his death and resurrection is symbolic of the natural cycle of death and rebirth. The pagan incarnation of ugliness is Pan, who in Greek mythology is the god of forests, fields and fertility, son of Hermes, messenger of the gods, and of a nymph. Part animal, with the horns, legs and ears of a goat, he was a robust deity, god of shepherds and goatherds. A magnificent musician, with his reed or reed flute, he accompanied the nymphs of the forest as they danced. His favorite places were mountains, caves and wild places, but his favorite was Arcadia, where he was born. He invented this flute when he was chasing the nymph Syringa and locked her in a bed of reeds so that she could not escape from it; Pan then took reeds of unequal length and played with them. The god always wooed the nymphs by playing the instrument, but they all rejected it for its ugliness.

The word panic is supposed to derive from the fear that travelers felt when they heard the sound of their flute in the solitude of night. Regarding the first aesthetic theory of any scope, it was the one formulated by Plato, who considered that reality is composed of forms that are beyond the limits of human sensation and that they are the models of all things that exist for human experience. The objects that humans can experience are examples or imitations of those forms. The work of the philosopher, therefore, consists of understanding from the experienced or perceived object, the reality that it imitates, while the artist copies the experienced objects or uses it as a model for his work. Thus, the artist's work is an imitation of what is itself an imitation.

In his dialogue, The Banquet, he indicated the difference between contemplating the appearance of beauty and reaching one's own ideal of beauty. Platonic thought had a marked ascetic tendency. In another of his most famous dialogues, La República, he went even further by repudiating some types of artists from his ideal society because he believed that their works stimulated immorality or represented despicable characters and that certain musical compositions caused laziness and incited individuals to perform actions that were not subject to any notion of measurement.

Oneself could imitate "things as they should be," he wrote, adding that "art complements to some extent what nature cannot bring to an end." Aristotle also spoke of art as imitation, but not in the Platonic sense. The artist separates the form from the matter of some objects of experience, such as the human body or a tree, and imposes the form on another matter, such as a canvas or marble.

Thus, imitation does not consist only in copying an original model, but in conceiving a symbol of the original; rather, it is the concrete representation of one aspect of a thing, and each work is an imitation of a universal whole. The way of administration was considered an art when quoting Aristotle and Plato, aesthetics were inseparable from morals and politics. The first, when dealing with music in his Politics, maintained that art affects the human character and, therefore, the social order. Since Aristotle held that happiness is the destiny of life, he believed that the main function of art is to provide satisfaction to men. In his great work on the principles of artistic creation, Poetics, he reasoned that tragedy stimulates the emotions of compassion and fear, which he considered pessimistic and insane, to such an extent that at the end of the performance the viewer is purged of all this. This catharsis makes the audience healthier psychologically and thus more capable of achieving happiness. From the seventeenth century, the neoclassical drama was greatly influenced by the Aristotelian Poetics.

The works of the French playwrights Jean Baptiste Racine, Pierre Corneille and Moliére, in particular, embraced the guiding principles of the doctrine of the three units: time, place and action. This concept dominated literary theories until the 19th century. Finally, a modern situation would be the provocation of the compliment or compliment that is given when seeing someone of the opposite sex pass. How to say The aesthetic experience is very close to the mystical experience, since it generates an earthly abandonment while contemplating the aesthetic object. During the Middle Ages, art was at the service of religious expression and its aesthetic principles were based primarily on Neoplatonism.

Throughout the Renaissance, in the 15th and 16th centuries, art underwent a process of secularization and classical aesthetics covered more fields than the merely religious one. Although linked to Neoplatonism, the 3rd century philosopher Plotinus attached greater importance to art than Plato himself. In his theses, he stated that art revealed the shape of an object more clearly than normal experience and leads the soul to contemplate the universal. According to Plotinus, the highest moments of life are mystical states, which implied that the soul is united, in the world of forms, to the divine, which he conceptualized as "the Onen.

CONTEMPORARY AESTHETICS

Aesthetics as exogenous therapeutic treatments are a term that is used as a "neologism", however modernity brought us the contributions of four philosophers from the late 19th and early 20th centuries with their respective thoughts on the main contemporary aesthetic influences. In France, Henri Bergson defined science as the use of intelligence to create a system of symbols that describes reality even though in the real world it falsifies it. Art, however, is based on intuitions, which is a direct apprehension of reality not interfered with by thought. Thus, art makes its way through conventional symbols and beliefs about man, life and society and confronts the individual with reality itself.

In Italy, the philosopher and historian Benedetto Croce also exalted intuition, considering that it was the immediate awareness of an object that in some way represents the shape of that object, that is, the apprehension of things instead of what one reflects from they. Works of art are the expression, in material form, of such intuitions; Beauty and ugliness, however, are not traits of works of art but qualities of the spirit expressed intuitively in that same work of art.

The Spanish born philosopher Jorge Ruiz de Santayana reasoned that when one derives pleasure from a thing, the pleasure can be considered as a quality of the thing itself, rather than as a subjective response from it. No human act can be characterized as good in itself, nor can it be called good just because it is socially approved, nor can it be said that any object is beautiful, because its color or shape leads to calling it beautiful. In his essay The Sense of Beauty (1896) he proposed novel arguments for a well-founded consideration of the aesthetic phenomenon. The American pedagogue and philosopher John Dewey viewed human experience as disjointed, fragmentary, full of principles without conclusions, or as experiences clearly manipulated as means to achieve specific ends.

Those exceptional experiences, which flow from their origins to their consummation, are aesthetic. The aesthetic experience is pleasure for its own interest, it is complete and independent and it is final, it is not limited to being instrumental or fulfilling a specific purpose.

PHYSICAL APPEARANCE AND BEAUTY

We can emphasize here that being physical appearance the way in which people perceive other individuals, genetic inheritance is also a factor of interest in determining the physical characteristics acceptable to most people, such as attributes of natural beauty. This scientific study of how parents transmit their physical, biochemical and social behavioral traits to their children is known as genetics.

The hereditary genes or human chromosomes contain the information of the parents, grandparents, great-grandparents and Other ancestry as well as the result of crosses foreigner and ancestral races. The morphotype, also known as biotype, is defined as the category in which the individual is classified according to their morphological forms or frontal body density, in addition to the loco-motor. It is then based on hereditary genes

There are three types of human physique or morphotypes:

Endomorph: soft, round, fat.

Endomorphy is the predominance of soft forms and there is a predisposition to fat. Mesomorph: robust, muscular, athletic. In mesomorphy, there is a predominance of muscle and bone masses.

Ectomorph: tall, thin, fragile. The ectomorphy is the predominance of linear forms, generally they are thin and narrow people. Although there is an individual classification, people not only fall into a single pattern, they are generally combinations of these, which are genetically determined.

These morphotypes of male examples can also occur in the female gender.

Similarly, beauty is the abstract notion of the viewer that is conceived from numerous aspects of human existence such as philosophy, symmetry in the arts, beauty contests, even narrative expression in literature. A postmodern neologism that has been consolidated in the last decade is 'body transformation" and refers to voluntary submission during challenges of 3, 6 and up to 9 months as periods of strict monitoring and is through a set of physical calisthenics exercises and a ketogenic diet.

THE EGYPTIAN LEGACY

Egyptian mythology found its own explanation for the emergence of cosmetology in the myth of the creation of the incarnate good in Horus; god of sky, a mythological being with the head of a hawk and the body of a man, which represented light and goodness. This myth tells that Osiris, god of the underworld, and his wife Isis, goddess of nature, conceived a son they named Horus. But she had a brother named Set, god of darkness and evil who murdered her husband Osiris, perhaps out of incestuous jealousy. Horus decided to avenge his father's death and waged a fight against his Uncle Set. During the combat Set wounded the eye of Horus, thus losing the battle.

Horus looked worriedly at his reflection on the river water and thought about covering that defect of his mutilated face and drew the shape of his eye taken from the tip of his finger the Clay sediments of nature, thus inventing makeup. This fact later influenced the Egyptians who highly revered these mythological gods. The term cosmetic comes from the Greek "kosmos" which means decoration or ornament. Thus we also see that religion and the event of death represented for the Egyptian culture a challenge that sought with alchemy or magical and medicinal preparations to extend life indefinitely. Although some of these procedures were doubtful, there are methods that were accepted and transferred to Other parts of the Mediterranean region to adorn kings and their courts throughout the centuries and have allowed their therapeutic and aesthetic uses to be appreciated today. Among the sculptural pieces that became icons of Egyptian beauty, we mention Nefertiti, the great main consort of the retinue of Pharaoh Akhenaten, who reigned in the 18th dynasty of Egypt. His bust, found in 1912 by the German archaeologist Lwdwig Borchardt, was created in a workshop in Armana that is believed to have been used for teaching artists.

This piece is a faithful example of the cosmetic customs of the ancient Egyptians and it is made of limestone with stucco and was made by Tutmose; a sculptor from 1330 BC They made polished bronze mirrors when mirrors didn't exist. Some types of makeup were used for both sexes of members of the royal caste and had a religious symbolism, in addition to being used against diseases, insects and the harshness of the arid desert climate. At least 160 recipes for these cosmetic compounds have been translated, describing their use on solemn occasions for marriage or funeral services. For example we define the following:

• Mesdemet: It was what they called the eyeliner recognized as a carbon black line that borders the contour of the eyes that is believed to prevent the contagion of conjunctivitis due to its disinfecting properties of chlorine and lead. It is known in Arabic as kohl.

• White lead: it is the White powder base used to whiten the skin of theface.

• Myrrh: It was used as a cosmetic against wrinkles.

• Carmine: a lip tincture made from poppy flowers.

• Ouadjou: shades of green tones that were used on the eyelids to evoke the god Hathor, Egyptian goddess of festivities.

• Kiphi: Egypt's most popular perfume was made with 27 ingredients and was believed to ward off evil spirits.

• Henna: A natural sediment dye that is Still used for nails and to temporarily tattoo marks on the skin.

• Aromatic oils: they restore the elasticity of the skin of the whole body.

• Fragrant tallow: Also known as a cone of animal fat, it is believed that its use was in occasional cases and conformed to the crown of the wigs of the servants used in the funeral procession and provided an effect of communion with the deceased.

All these cosmetics were preserved in a toiletry bag or wicker basket that was placed next to the corpse, according to the belief that on his journey to the afterlife, he would use them to make up the passage of time on his limbs.

AGING AND BIOLOGICAL CLOCK

Wrinkles, gray hair, physical decay and loss of senses have always been an enigma for humanity that resigns itself to the passage of time with its inexorable power.

Aging is defined in biology as the set of inevitable and irreversible changes that occur in an organism over time, and that ultimately lead to death. Such changes vary considerably, in the time and severity of events, according to the different species, and from one organism to another. In man, these changes include a reduction in the flexibility of tissues, the loss of some nerve cells, the hardening of blood vessels, and a general decrease in body tones Biologists interested in aging investigate such changes or focus on bodily deficits and disabilities that accumulate with age, although these appear to be a more direct result of disease, stress, or environmental factors.

Although research on biological aging is not based on any universally accepted theory, genetic, cellular, and physiological studies have raised several hypotheses. One of the most important genetic concepts, the so-called error theory, assumes that age-related alterations are due to the accumulation of random genetic errors, or to small errors in the transmission of genetic information (see Genetics). These damages or errors reduce or prevent the proper functioning of the cells. In cell studies, the best-known theory of aging is based on the so. called Hayflick effect, which was named after the American microbiologist Leonard Hayflick. He observed in cell culture that certain human cells underwent only a limited number of cell divisions before dying.

This finding suggests that aging is programmed inside cells, and could explain the differences that exist in the lifespan of different animal species, as well as the unequal longevity of the different sexes in the same species. For example, in the human species, women usually live an average of eight years longer than men. Physiological theories of aging focus on organ systems and their interrelationships. For example, one of the areas most investigated today is the immune system that protects our body from foreign cells. A characteristic of mammals is that their immune system gradually loses its ability to cope with infections and Other situations such as aging. As a result, the antibodies produced by the body are unable to distinguish between "friendly" or "self' cells and "enemy" or "non-self' cells.

Currently, most experts consider that aging is not the result of an isolated mechanism but comprises a set of phenomena that act in concert. Some researchers also ask a large number of questions about how social changes, changes in smoking habits, exercise, dietary habits, economic fluctuations, political reforms and new technologies can affect the aging process. In addition to the scientific interest itself, knowledge of biological clocks could be important in many ways. There is, for example, a theory of aging based on the fact that during Old age the great number of clocks in the body subordinate to the brain, for some reason, adjust less to it. This lack of synchronization can contribute to exacerbating many of the problems associated with aging.

REGENERATIVE MEDICINE

Body Rejuvenator: A Look at Regenerative Medicine

The human body possesses a remarkable ability to heal itself, from minor cuts to broken bones. However, as we age or encounter debilitating injuries, this natural healing capacity diminishes. Regenerative medicine is emerging as a revolutionary field that aims to address this limitation by promoting the body's inherent regenerative abilities or introducing new cells to repair or replace damaged tissues and organs.

* Understanding the Basic Principles: Regenerative medicine is based on three fundamental pillars:

* Stem cells: These are the body's master cells, which have the potential to develop into various specialized cell types such as muscle, bone, or nerve cells. They play a crucial role in tissue repair and regeneration.

* Biomaterials: These are natural or synthetic materials used to create scaffolds or support structures that guide tissue growth and function. They can mimic the extracellular matrix (ECM), the natural environment that surrounds cells, providing them with signals to differentiate and organize.

* Growth factors: These are signaling molecules that stimulate stem cell proliferation, differentiation, and cell migration into areas of damage.

Exploring different approaches:

There are several exciting approaches within regenerative medicine, each offering unique strategies for tissue repair and regeneration:

* Cell therapy: This approach involves introducing healthy cells directly into a damaged area. These cells can be a patient's own stem cells, collected from bone marrow, fat, or blood, or donor-derived stem cells. Depending on the specific application, the cells can be manipulated or expanded in a laboratory before transplantation.

* Autologous cell therapy: This involves the use of a patient's own stem cells, minimizing the risk of rejection. It is a promising approach for treating conditions such as cartilage damage, heart disease, and certain types of cancer. * Allogeneic cell therapy: This approach uses stem cells from a donor, offering a readily available source of cells. However, there is a higher risk of rejection, requiring careful matching between donor and recipient.

* Tissue engineering: This technique involves creating functional tissues by combining stem cells and biomaterials. Scaffolds are seeded with stem cells and growth factors, stimulating the cells to differentiate and form new tissues in a controlled environment. Tissue-engineered constructs are

then implanted into the body to promote tissue regeneration. This approach shows promise for treating conditions such as burns, skin grafts, and bone defects.

* Gene therapy: This approach focuses on correcting faulty genes that contribute to disease. By introducing healthy copies of genes into damaged cells, gene therapy aims to restore normal cell function and promote tissue regeneration. Applications are being explored for conditions such as cystic fibrosis, hemophilia, and certain neurological disorders. * Exosomes: These are tiny membrane vesicles released by cells that contain various molecules such as proteins, RNA, and lipids. Exosomes can act as messengers, influencing the behavior of other cells. Researchers are exploring the potential of exosomes as a cell-free therapy for regenerative medicine. Exosomes derived from healthy cells may promote tissue repair and regeneration by delivering beneficial molecules to damaged areas.

* The Application Process: Regenerative medicine therapies are still in their early stages of development, but ongoing research promises exciting possibilities for treating a wide range of conditions. The application process typically involves several steps:

* Diagnosis and Evaluation: A physician first diagnoses the underlying condition and assesses whether regenerative medicine is a suitable treatment option.

* Patient Selection: Candidates for regenerative medicine therapies are carefully selected based on several factors such as age, overall health, and the severity of the condition. * Cell collection or biomaterial design: Depending on the specific treatment, this may involve collecting stem cells from the patient, selecting donor cells, or designing suitable biomaterials.

* Cell preparation or scaffold manufacturing: Cells can be expanded or manipulated in a laboratory setting, and biomaterials are formed into appropriate scaffolds.

* Delivery and implantation: The prepared cells or biomaterials are then delivered to the target site in the body using minimally invasive procedures such as injections or surgery.

* Monitoring and follow-up: After the procedure, patients are closely monitored to track the progress of regeneration and address any potential complications.

* Ethical considerations: As a rapidly evolving field, regenerative medicine raises important ethical considerations:

* Informed consent: Patients must be fully informed about the potential benefits and risks associated with these new therapies before giving their consent.

* Stem cell sources: Ethical concerns surround the use of embryonic stem cells due to the destruction of embryos. Adult and induced pluripotent stem cells (IPSCs) offer alternative sources with fewer ethical concerns.

* Intellectual property rights: The development of new cell therapies and biomaterials involves significant research and development costs. It is crucial to balance research incentives with patient affordability.

* Regulation and Oversight: Ensuring the safety and efficacy of these therapies requires robust regulatory frameworks and oversight mechanisms.

* The Future of Regenerative Medicine: Regenerative medicine has immense potential thanks to recent and ongoing advances.

CHAPTER 2 AESTHETIC SUBESPECIALITIES

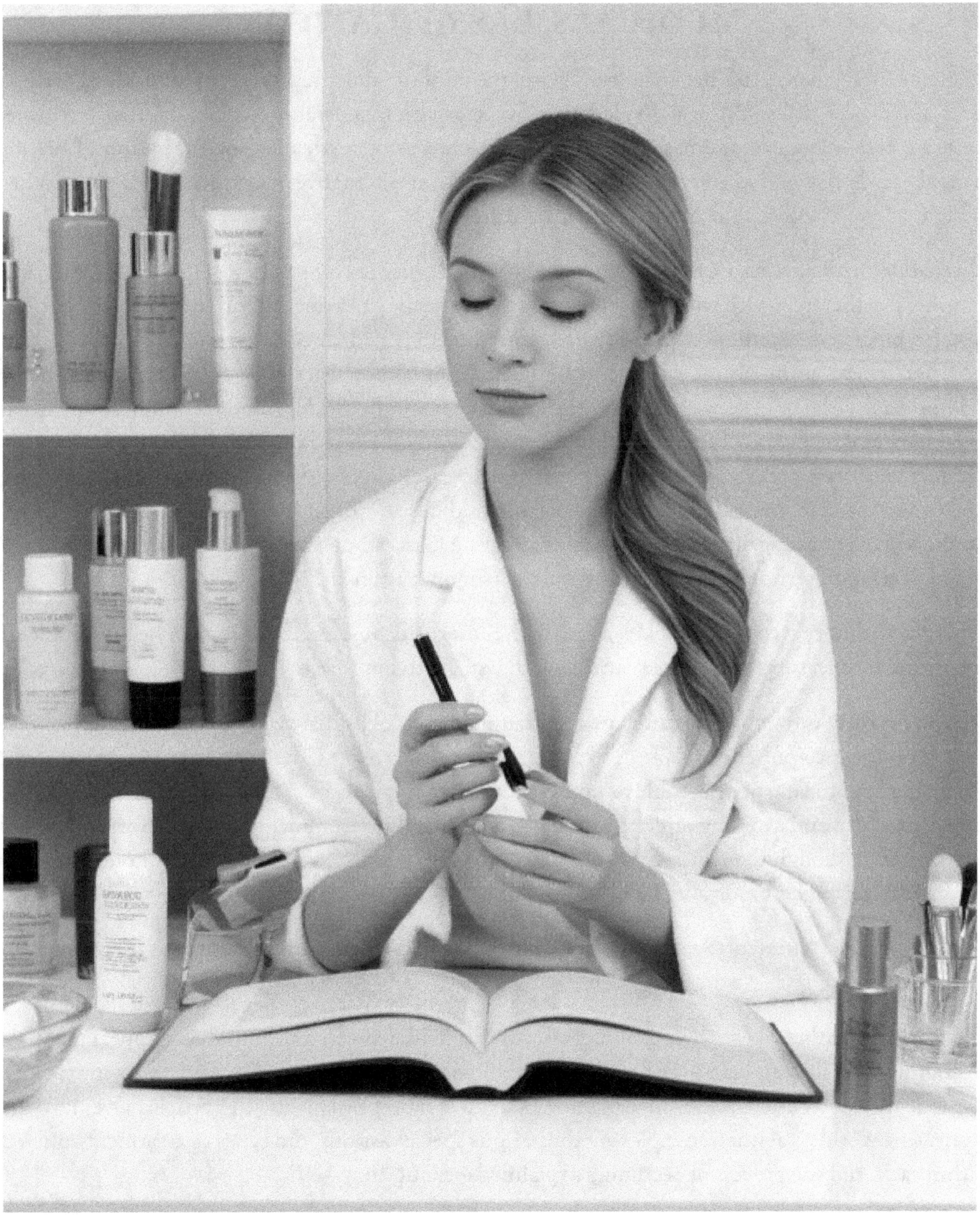

MEDICAL CLASSIFICATION

Medicine is a science and art that deals with the healing and prevention of disease, as well as the maintenance of health. It is divided into five specialties: general medicine, internal medicine, intensive care medicine, alternative medicine, and preventive medicine. For the purposes of this manual, aesthetics and cosmetology are grouped within alternative medicine, along with other therapies that we will explore in the following chapters.

Alternative medicine, also called complementary medicine, encompasses a set of exogenous and non-invasive therapies with widely accepted health and healing treatments. It is influenced by ancient Eastern medicine techniques, homeopathy, and holistic medicine. Thus, we see how Eastern medicine focuses primarily on massage techniques, acupuncture, macrobiotics, and medicinal herbs to improve health conditions or defects. Homeopathy is another widely used technique, established by Samuel Hahnemann, who proposed that healing should be rapid, safe, and permanent. In acute treatments, homeopaths have knowledge of the disease, its etiology, and pathology, and have established the cure in small portions, such as pills and doses. Holistic medicine, on the other hand, is defined as the healing of the body and mind, treating it as a whole, which may include one or more mental relaxation techniques and stress or muscle pain management.

Similarly, within preventive medicine, along with biosecurity, researchers of human health problems also introduce measures that people can take individually to improve their health.

Among the main preventive measures are maintaining personal hygiene with constant hand washing, the use of masks to prevent the spread of viruses such as the recent Covid-19 virus, practicing social distancing, and the use of disposable or homemade gloves to protect the lungs from free radicals. The use of sunscreen and avoiding prolonged sun exposure are also recommended in an effort to prevent skin cancers, although these measures have been shown to be ineffective against melanoma, the skin cancer with the highest mortality rate.

**Unveiling the World of Aesthetics: Specialties, Applications, and the Path to Becoming an Esthetician

The world of aesthetics is a diverse and ever-evolving field dedicated to improving appearance and promoting overall well-being. From non-surgical skin resurfacing to advanced laser treatments, aesthetic specialists offer a wide range of services to meet individual needs. This article delves into the captivating world of aesthetics, exploring the various specializations, the types of treatments offered within each, and the process of becoming a qualified esthetician.

Classifications of Aesthetic Specialties: The broad field of aesthetics encompasses a range of specializations, each focusing on specific areas of treatment. Here's a breakdown of some key classifications:

* **Skin Care Specialists:** These professionals excel in the art of healthy skin. They provide treatments such as facials, microdermabrasion, chemical peels, and acne management. Their expertise lies in understanding skin types and recommending personalized skin care routines for a radiant complexion.

* **Laser Specialists:** This specialization revolves around the use of medical-grade lasers for various purposes, such as hair removal, tattoo removal, wrinkle reduction, and the treatment of vascular lesions. Laser specialists possess in-depth knowledge of laser technology, ensuring safe and effective treatment results.

* **Body Contouring Specialists:** This area focuses on non-surgical body sculpting techniques, such as radiofrequency (RF) treatments, ultrasound cavitation, and cryotherapy. These treatments aim to refine the body's shape, reduce cellulite, and tighten loose skin. ***Injection Specialists:** This specialization involves the use of injectable materials such as Botox, fillers, and Kybella to achieve aesthetic alterations. Injection specialists have a keen eye for facial anatomy and artistry to create natural-looking results, addressing wrinkles, lines, and facial volume loss.

* **Permanent Makeup Artists:** These professionals offer services such as eyebrow microblading, permanent eyeliner, and lip blush. They use specialized techniques to create semi-permanent makeup solutions that enhance facial features and reduce daily makeup routines.

* **Consultants

Aesthetic Consultants: Often found in medical spas and cosmetic surgery clinics, aesthetic consultants provide comprehensive consultations to clients, assessing their needs and recommending appropriate treatments or procedures. They possess extensive knowledge of aesthetic options and can guide clients toward achieving their desired results.

HISTORICAL EVOLUTION

Amarna in Egypt, built around 1350 BC. Small versions of these same facilities existed for women.

In Rome, Italy the Bath of Dioclesano was preserved, which today became the Church of Santa María de los Ángeles, it was the place where water was brought from distant sources through aqueducts.

To heat the interior of all the rooms, a series of hot water pipes were used, located under the floors, which were covered with decorative mosaics. The architectural layout of the Bath of Dioclesano is similar to that of the rest of those that are preserved throughout the Roman Empire. Around a central courtyard called the palestra, where you can practice exercise, is the apodyterium or changing room; the caldarium or alveus room or hot water pool, followed by the laconicum or steam bath, and the frigidarium or cold pool.

In ancient Greece, three different gymnastic exercise programs were developed: one for fitness maintenance, another for military training, and a third as part of the training regimen for athletes.

Each Greek City had a gymnasium, where the exercises were The first Greek fitness teachers (paidotribes) were the pioneers in designing physical activity systems, both for athletes and for all citizens.

These programs, including gymnastic exercises, were considered essential in the education of children. The Greeks believed that the unity of mind and body could be achieved only through participation in physical exercises. Gymnastic systems designed to prepare the military were widely used by the Romans. Today the healthy practice of doing "detox" or detoxification continues to be fashionable. Make a diet that removes excesses from the body, cleanses us of impurities and thus restores us to health. It is achieved through various techniques such as vegetable soup, with natural juices and semi-thick shakes, pills from manufacturing industries, in tea and for the most intense detox with long stay trips where they are secluded in clinics or spas away from the City in the midst of a tuxedo free climate that promises to restore you to your lost health.

Sometimes their result does not stand out to the naked eye, but it takes many sessions for a type of months to recognize them. Seeking well-being with exotic techniques turns each treatment into a relaxation ceremony, for one or as a couple it is a delight. Today we can find the My Blend by Clarins sap, housed at the Ritz Carlton hotel in Toronto, offering the best way to connect with the Float in the Clouds treatment, designed to tempt the senses. The romantic escape from the Hela Spa in Mexico City includes champagne body wraps and Milan's Amala Bulgari provides a unique experience. Classification of aesthetic subspecialties Medicine is a science and art that deals with the cure and prevention of disease, as well as the maintenance of health. It is divided into five specialties which are: General Medicine, Internal Medicine, Intensive Medicine, Alternative Medicine and Preventive Medicine. For the purposes of this manual, aesthetics and cosmetology are grouped within alternative medicine along with other therapies that we Will learn about in the following chapters.

Alternative medicine, also called complementary medicine, encompasses a set of exogenous and non-invasive therapies with widely accepted health and healing treatments. The influence of ancient techniques of oriental medicine, homeopathy and holistics. Thus we see how oriental medicine focuses more on massage techniques, acupuncture, macrobiotics and medicinal herbs to influence an improvement in the conditions or defects of health. Homeopathy is another widely used technique which was established by Samuel Hahnemann and proposed that healing should be fast, safe and permanent.

The homeopath has in acute cures the knowledge of the disease, etiology, pathology and established the cure by small portions such as pills and doses. Holistics, on the other hand, is defined as the healing of the body and mind taking care of it as a whole, for which it can include one or more techniques of mental relaxation and management of stress or muscle pain.

Similarly, within preventive medicine alongside biosafety, researchers of human health problems also introduce measures that people can take individually to improve their health. Among the main prevention measures are maintaining personal hygiene with constant hand washing, the use of masks or face masks to prevent the proliferation of viruses such as the recent Covid 19, practicing social distancing and the use of disposable or homemade gloves, to protect the lungs from free radicals. Using sunscreen and avoiding prolonged sun exposure is also advised in an effort to prevent skin cancers, although these measures have been shown to be ineffective against melanoma, the skin cancer with the highest mortality rate.

DERMATOLOGY

Among the scientific specialties, dermatology is the one that most closely approximates the precepts and techniques of cosmetology aesthetics. This is responsible for the study of the structure and protective and purifying functions of the skin, in addition to treating diseases pharmacologically. Dermatologists are doctors who, after completing a degree that has an average duration of 4 years, specialize in dermatology and become qualified in diagnosing, preventing and indicating the most appropriate treatment.

Skin diseases sometimes appear isolated as vitiligo, however on Other occasions they are externalizations of internal ailments as occurs in skin cancer and Other conditions. In addition to knowledge of infectious diseases, they must have knowledge of immunology, neurology, rheumatology, and endocrinology.

COSMETIC DERMATOLOGY: It is a sub-specialty of this branch of health that uses various cosmetic and appliance techniques to treat scars left by acne using lasers, application of botox for lips and wrinkles, among Other injectable treatments with proven effects. Dermatological pathologies are grouped into infectious, specific disorders, carcinogenic, congenital and Others, as detailed in the following graph.

The field of aesthetics has seen a dramatic increase in popularity in recent years. People are increasingly seeking non-surgical and minimally invasive procedures to improve their appearance and boost their confidence. But what exactly is aesthetics, and what does it take to establish a successful clinic? This article delves into these questions, unpacking the various aspects of aesthetics and providing a roadmap for aspiring clinic owners. **Defining Aesthetics: Beyond Physical Beauty** Aesthetics, in the context of this article, refers to the practice of enhancing a person's appearance through non-surgical or minimally invasive procedures. While some may view aesthetics as focused solely on physical beauty, it encompasses a broader scope. It can address concerns such as: * **Skin health: Addressing wrinkles, acne, sun damage, and uneven skin tone. * **Body contouring:** Non-surgical procedures such as fat reduction and cellulite treatment. * **Hair Removal:** Laser hair removal and electrolysis.

* **Facial Rejuvenation:** Botox injections, fillers, and laser treatments.

* **Anti-Aging Concerns:** Procedures that address wrinkles, fine lines, and loss of facial volume.

Types of Aesthetic Treatments: A Diverse Landscape

The world of aesthetics offers a variety of treatments to address individual needs and preferences. Here's a breakdown of some popular categories:

* **Skin Rejuvenation:** This encompasses procedures such as chemical peels, microdermabrasion, microneedling, laser skin resurfacing, and injectable fillers. These treatments aim to improve skin texture, tone, and elasticity.

* **Neuromodulators (Botox):** Botox injections relax targeted facial muscles, reducing the appearance of wrinkles and fine lines.

* ** Dermal Fillers:** Fillers are injected into the skin to fill wrinkles, restore lost volume, and enhance facial features like the lips and cheeks.

* ** Body Contouring:** This category includes non-surgical fat reduction treatments like CoolSculpting and Laser Lipolysis. These procedures target stubborn fat deposits for a more sculpted physique.

* ** Laser Treatments:** Lasers can be used for hair removal, skin resurfacing, and the treatment of vascular lesions.

* ** Microneedling:** Tiny needles create controlled injuries in the skin, triggering collagen production to improve skin texture and reduce scarring.

* ** Chemical Peels:** Chemical solutions are applied to the skin to remove the outer layer, revealing a smoother, brighter complexion. ** Organizational Structures in Aesthetics: Finding Your Niche** Before setting up your clinic, consider the different organizational structures within the aesthetics field. Here are some common models:

* **Dermatologist-Owned Clinics:** Dermatologists are physicians who specialize in skin conditions. They can offer a wide range of aesthetic treatments, often in conjunction with medical dermatology services.

* **Plastic Surgeon-Owned Clinics:** Plastic surgeons can perform surgical and nonsurgical aesthetic procedures. This model offers a broader spectrum of services, including more invasive options.

* **Medspa Model:** Medspas are typically owned by a physician but are staffed by various professionals such as nurses, estheticians, and laser technicians. They offer a range of nonsurgical aesthetic treatments in a spa-like setting.

* **Nurse-Owned Clinics:** Registered nurses with additional training and certifications can provide some nonsurgical aesthetic treatments under the supervision of a physician. * **ESPLAYERS OWNED BY AESTHETICIANS:** Estheticians are licensed professionals who can offer skin care treatments but are not authorized to perform certain medical procedures such as Botox injections.

The Essential Guide to Establishing Your Aesthetic Clinic Now that we've explored the different aspects of aesthetics, let's navigate the steps involved in establishing your own clinic:

1. **Develop a Business Plan:** This plan outlines your clinic's concept, target market, services offered, financial projections, and marketing strategy. 2. **Licenses and Regulations:** Research and obtain all necessary licenses and permits to operate an aesthetic clinic in your area. This could involve permits for specific procedures or equipment.

3. **Location and Environment:** Strategically choose a location with good accessibility and visibility. Design a welcoming and professional space that reflects your brand and creates a relaxing environment for clients.

4. **Equipment and Technology:** Invest in high-quality equipment that aligns with the procedures you plan to offer. Ensure proper maintenance and staff training on how to use the equipment safely and effectively.

5. **Assemble Your Team:** Recruit qualified and experienced professionals such as doctors, nurses, aestheticians, and support staff. Ensure ongoing training to stay up-to-date on the latest advancements.

6. **Marketing and Client Acquisition:** Develop a comprehensive marketing strategy to reach your target audience. Use online advertising, social media marketing, and community outreach to build brand awareness.

7. **Compliance and Patient Safety:** Prioritize patient safety by complying with all hygiene protocols, being clear.

AESTHETIC ORGANIZATION AND FURNITURE

The world of aesthetic medicine is booming, offering a variety of treatments to enhance natural beauty and boost confidence. But beyond advanced technology and skilled practitioners, the success of an aesthetic clinic depends on its organization and environment. This article delves into the essential aspects of setting up your aesthetic clinic, from organizational structures to furniture selection. We'll explore different clinic models, navigate the application process, and provide tips on how to create a space that is both functional and appealing to patients.

Understanding Clinic Organizational Structures

Choosing the right organizational structure lays the foundation for your clinic's operations. Here are the main models:

* **Solo Practitioner:** Smaller clinics are often run by a single qualified practitioner, usually a dermatologist, plastic surgeon, or registered nurse. This model offers flexibility and control for the practitioner, but may limit the services offered due to individual expertise.

* **Partnership:** Two or more qualified professionals may join forces to create a partnership. This structure allows for a broader range of services and expertise, which could attract a larger clientele. Sharing resources can also reduce overhead.

* **Medical Spa:** These clinics offer a wide range of non-surgical aesthetic treatments, often combining medical expertise with spa services such as massages and facials. Medical spas may be owned and operated by a physician who oversees a team of nurses and aestheticians.

* **Independent Clinic:** This model is typically a larger clinic with multiple staff members, including physicians, nurses, aestheticians, and administrative staff. Independent clinics often offer a broader menu of services, incorporating surgical and non-surgical procedures. The ideal structure depends on your budget, experience, and long-term vision. Consider your desired range of services, financial resources, and the number of qualified professionals involved before making your choice.

The Application Process: Turning Vision into Reality

Once you've chosen your organizational framework, it's crucial to obtain the necessary licenses and permits. This process involves multiple steps, which may vary depending on your location. A general overview includes:

1. **Business Registration:** Register your clinic as a business entity, such as a sole proprietorship, partnership, or limited liability company (LLC).

2. **Licensing:** Obtain the necessary licenses to operate in your area. This could involve a business license, a medical license for practitioners, and specific licenses for specific equipment or procedures.

3. **Permitting:** Acquire permits for renovations, waste disposal, and other activities specific to your location.

4. **Compliance with Health Regulations:** Ensure your clinic adheres to all relevant health regulations, including those related to patient privacy, hygiene protocols, and waste disposal. Contact your local health department for detailed information.

5. Insurance: Obtain the appropriate malpractice, property, and business interruption insurance coverage. Navigating the application process can be complex. Consider consulting with a business attorney or healthcare consultant to ensure you comply with all regulations and avoid delays.

Crafting Your Clinic's Identity: Furnishing for Functionality and Appeal Now comes the exciting part: shaping the physical space! The furniture you choose plays a vital role in creating a welcoming and functional environment for both patients and staff. Here's a breakdown of the key areas and furniture essentials:

Reception Area:

Reception Desk: A stylish and functional reception desk serves as the first point of contact for patients. Choose a design that reflects your clinic's brand and offers ample space for paperwork and patient interaction.

Comfortable Seating: Comfortable chairs with side tables provide a welcoming waiting area for patients. Consider incorporating a mix of chairs and a small sofa to meet different needs.

* **Coffee Table and Magazines:** A low table with current magazines or brochures breaks the ice and allows patients to relax and learn about your services.

* **Information Screen:** A digital signage screen displays clinic information and before-and-after photos (with consent)

SPA: DEFINITION AND BENEFITS

It is health through water, currently the use of the word «spa" is related to leisure and health establishments, where therapies are used mainly with water, through swimming pools, Jacuzzi, whirlpools and saunas, medicinally they are called spas, also Massages and treatments of tradition or cultural heritage are offered according to each region of the planet. Among the benefits of the spa are:

Physical improvement: Physical improvement of muscle pain and certain bone problems such as arthritis is achieved.

Psychic improvement: Stress reduction, based on the relaxation that is obtained.

Aesthetic improvement: Relaxation and a feeling of well being and tranquility is reflected in our appearance, through the different beauty treatments that can be performed.

Types of Spa

Five types of spa are known that are classified according to the types of treatments they offer.

Urban Spa or Day Spa: These are those that are usually used as a quick relaxation and anti-stress treatment.

Spa Hotel: It is the main service of a hotel for the stay of its guests and offers long-term treatments.

Wellness Center. These are spas aimed at improving the health of customers through eating habits and exercise routines in the gym.

Holistic Spa: offers treatments for the body and mind to find inner peace.

Medical Spa: These are Spas specialized in medical treatments for their patients in order to complement the health and wellness offer, to which Other techniques have been added. In hydro massage bathtubs they usually have a lighting system called chromotherapy and some incorporate a fragrance induction system to provide aromatherapy in the water.

ESTHETIC CLINICS

This postmodern concept of "clinicn has its origins in antiquity, linked to the science and art of medicine, when Greek doctors like Hippocrates in the 5th century BC invented it, continuing into the Middle Ages. Its etymological meaning comes from the Greek term "kliní", which means bed or bed. This place was destined to the investigatory process, or anamnesis, and oriented to the diagnosis of the pathological situation that the inhabitants of the villages, towns and cities presented since those centuries. These symptoms were appearing more and more frequently and were thus forming the pictures that determined the signs for doctors to recognize each given disease, according to their specialty, as we know them today.

The physical examination, which can be from the office or at the foot of a bed is where we recounts or describes their condition and his impressions of the appearance of pain. This is in conjunction with complementary laboratory scans and imaging tests for tumors and fractures. After this review of the patient, a treatment more appropriate to the budget, predisposition or type of the skin is determined, which in the case of aesthetic clinics are mainly external and if they are serious diseases, they are immediately referred to a specialist in dermatology, general medicine or in the worst case to oncology, where Other cure options are determined.

Beyond the primitive methods, the patient is treated by a healer or shaman who, through dances, concoctions and even trepanations similar to surgical interventions, was intended to expel the spirit or demon that brought the disease out of the body, today the medicines Modern are manufactured and processed with meticulous techniques. The greatest achievement of the time was the use of plant extracts, whose narcotic and stimulating properties were gradually being discovered.

They have proven so effective that they are Still used today.

In primitive societies surgical techniques such as cleaning and treating wounds by cauterization, poultices and sutures, reduction of dislocations and fractures, with the use of splints (or splints), were practiced. Other additional therapies included purges, diuretics, laxatives, emetics, and enemas.

BEAUTY SALON

It is a commercial establishment dedicated to offering various cosmetic treatments for women mainly and Other similar ones for men. Among these are:

- Cut off
- Dye
- Hairstyle
- Make-up and waxing of the face
- Hair extensions, eyebrows, wigs and product sales.

The oldest reference we have on the existence of cosmetic hair care takes us back to Egypt, where they began to make the most significant changes in terms of hair cosmetics. In that culturally large nation, the City as happened in many others were taking off, although not so much the priests and members of the ruling elite, who were dedicated to taking care of their hair playing with different hairstyles and shades. The wigs also had their peak, and traditional straight hair predominated, with bangs, very even in a length that reached the shoulders. But another great contribution of the Egyptians was in terms of color, since they discovered the usefulness of henna, which allowed them to obtain reddish and mahogany colors.

There are also Other variations of the type of business where a beauty salon is combined with a spa that includes only some of the extended, non-invasive aesthetic services for facial health such as:

- Eyebrow wax
- Facial
- Artificial tan

• Manicure

• Pedicure

• Oxygen therapy

• Mud baths

• Aromatherapy

Beauty salons have proven to be an industrial executor of economic recession in developed nations spreading to underdeveloped countries at all times. Although sales have declined since 2008 due to the Great Recession, they are Still strong on a long term projection. It is even believed that during recessions consumers tend to be more price conscious, and these costs are continually increasing. with the increase in per capita income in the United States since 2015, beauty salons are emerging with the industry generating $ 56.2 billion, proof of this is when we see many entertainment stars or singers who invest their fortunes in perfume lines and makeup. Haircare is the largest segment with 86,000 locations. They expect the skincare industry to generate $ 11 billion in revenue by 2018. This increase is due to the numerous campaigns on skin cancer and the aging possibilities of anti-cancer discoveries being offered to women, and especially to men. Start-ups or entrepreneurs also compete with large chains that are financed on average through online sales and marketing on the Web. The labor office estimates that 20% of the jobs created between 2008 and 2014 are represented by the skin care specialist industry.

Hairdressing tools can be classified into five essential groups for the facilitation of their study:

• Main tools: are those instruments with which hairdressing tasks are carried out: combs, brushes, scissors, tweezers, etc.

• Auxiliaries: are those objects that are used to facilitate the work with the first and also as protection material: rollers, hair nets, gloves, caps, towels, cutting capes, etc.

• Laboratory tools: are those materials that are used to make chemical mixtures (dyes, hydrogen Froxide, etc.): glass containers, litmus paper, etc.

• Device: set of devices designed for the performance of hairdressing techniques, as well as for the detection and treatment of hair problems that occur most frequently in the salon.

• Hairdressing: hairdryers, vaporizers, sterilizers, micro-viewer, infrared lamp for baldness, etc.

• Decoration material: these are those elements of the furniture that participate in the execution of the hairdressing and customer service tasks: washbasins (previously called barber's bowl), auxiliary tables, mirrors, armchairs, etc.

BARBERSHOP

They are places dedicated to the exclusive haircut and beard service for men and short Styles for women, which are Still preserved in some Mediterranean and Latin American countries where they have not yet been replaced by unisex beauty salons. The name of barber comes from the treatment for the growth of the beard that was done since ancient times, and the barber is the person in charge of shaving, cutting and conditioning the hair of the clients. A barber of today must have a lot of manual precision and have the artistic qualities to reproduce the various levels of styles in order to obtain an excellent result and the expectations of his clientele, which generally becomes frequent.

Among the functions performed by a barber or hairdresser are:

• Carry out daily maintenance to keep razors in good condition, this means that they Will always be hair-free and oiled.

• Avoid reusing disposable razors of those that are reusable such as those of European import.

• You should have several combs and scissors to permanently sterilize them in primary grade alcohol, with minimal dissolution, and antiseptic such as isopropanol.

• You must stock up on swabs, cottons, antiseptic towels for customer care.

• Stock up on shaving creams, ointments, shampoo, and Other hair care products.

• Keep mirrors visible and clean, as well as collect hair from the floor to dispose of debris in plastic bags daily.

Dyes for gray coverage and gray hair removal are also a specialty when grooming the heads of young people and adults. A barber must first know the client's Style tastes in order to follow established fashions or invent new ones. In the treatment of the beard, we proceed to place a cloth napkin under the client's chin and prepare the knives, placing the razor that is placed with the edge of the razor flush. Finally, it is applied to the shave with menthol red alcohol, aromatic talcum powder or another type of after product to relieve the itching sensation and tone the skin.

In ancient times, hairdressers, later called shearers, were brought from Sicily to Rome by a certain Fr. Ticinio Menas, in the year 451 after the founding of the city. The long-standing fashion in Greece for short hair and a clean beard spread quickly thanks to Scipio, the second African, who shaved every day. The shearers began exercising their industry in the open air, but later this use subsisted only for the common people and the slaves and the tents of the barbers announced by a presentation of knives, razors and mirrors became meeting points for the idle and for journalists.

Because it is a public health service, the diseases that must be avoided with the application of strict hygienic measures are lice and conjunctivitis. True lice or suckers have a type of mouth sucking apparatus and lack wings. There are three types of sucking lice that infect humans. Crabs are broad, greyish-white, about 3 mm in length, and are generally found in the hair of the pubic region. In addition, there are two Other types of lice that are narrower, gray and also about 3mm in length: the body louse, which is usually found on clothing, and the head louse, which is found on the hair. Another is inflammation of the conjunctiva. This is a mucous membrane that covers the inner surface of the eyelids and the outer surface of the eyeball on its anterior face (except in its anterior ple, where the cornea is located). The cause of conjunctivitis can be an infection, an allergy, or a trauma. It is characterized by redness, inflammation, a foreign body sensation when blinking, and excessive sensitivity of the eye to light (photophobia). In severe cases, a thick mucus exudation occurs. If the cause is an infection, there is a discharge of pus. Acute infectious conjunctivitis is caused by various bacteria and viruses and is generally epidemic. Most bacterial conjunctivitis is successfully treated with antibiotics or sulfonamides. Viral conjunctivitis usually heals within two weeks, although treatment may be necessary when are some complications.

TATTOOS AND CARE

The skin is an external and delicate organ of our body, so we have not been able to leave out this book this skin decoration technique which, far from disappearing due to its possible adverse effects, continues to be perfected and continues to be accepted by a significant group of people, such as a modern cultural and ethnic expression. The tattooed motifs or designs are inserted by means of coloring substances under the epidermis in a somewhat painful process, depending on the area of the body and the sensitivity of the persons skin, piercing with a sharp object that is often an electric needle.

Due to warnings from health authorities that tattoo needles can be a means of spreading infectious diseases, especially hepatitis, in recent times this custom has fallen into the spotlight. Easily removable body paints and adhesive decorations are being used more and more. Tattoos made with a needle can be removed with a laser.

Traditional tattoos leave a fixed mark on the skin. The tattoo artist injects ink underneath with a special needle. Healthy skin and remains the etched design forever. Does it scare you what "forever" sounds like? The alternative is to opt for a temporary tattoo. Like those made with an ink called henna, of Hindu origin. Permanent tattoos can only be removed by laser or other means that cost money (sometimes a lot). The henna ones disappear after a short time of three to five days.

This process temporarily weakens the surface of the skin making it susceptible to bacteria and infections, so it is essential to take some measures after getting a tattoo, since a tattoo is really a wound on the skin and special care must be followed. Help a tattoo become a good experience, far from being an ugly scar or incurable wound in cases of diabetics ones.

• Cover the tattoo with a bandage: during the first hours, the tattoo artist places a bandage and adhesive tape that must remain so to protect from dust, sunlight and bacteria. It should not be removed until after 2 to 4 hours. You should not use plastic as it increases the temperature and helps to collect fluids in the area. You should not be tempted to show it to someone.

• Cleaning the tattoo: during the first month the tattoo area should be cleaned with mild soap, avoiding perfumed and alcoholic products as they can irritate. They can be cleaned up to three times a day with a sponge or towel to dry it well, avoiding scratches.

• Use of antiseptic creams: This prevents MRSA which stands for methicillin, resistant Staphylococcus aureus infection and occurs as a result of people who share razors, people who have tattooed and work in public, people who are operated and those who take drugs or antibiotics that do not work.

Therefore, it is preferable to use topical creams with antibiotic effects. They are signs of kidney failure and a weak immune system so you should consult a dermatologist.

• Hydration of the wound: moisturizers enriched with vitamins A and D are recommended, although there are products without oils and lanolin or waxes that are more expensive and effective.

• Avoid soaking baths: this could erase part of the tattoo, and it should not be exfoliated for at least 3 weeks. It also applies to swimming pools or the sea, since the dirt contained in these waters could trigger infections.

• Use of sunscreen: if you go to the beach or in summer, the tattoo is recommended to apply the cream blocking factor 30 or higher and not to expose a lot of time to the sun.

• Ventilation and bandaging: it should never be kept bandaged after 4 hours of tattooing, so that the wounds are better oxygenated in the open air.

• Monitoring for any discomfort: You should never scratch excessively, and you should be careful during the healing period.

• Complete healing: if after a month you have not noticed discomfort or signs of burning, itching or scabs, you can consider that it has healed, there is less chance of infection and that you only need to take care of excessive sun exposure.

As for piercing, we can say that it is the practice of piercing or cutting a part of the human body, generally to insert earrings. These piercings are a form of cultural modification and reflect cultural, religious and spiritual values, and are also part of fashion, eroticism, nonconformity or identification with a subculture. In Western history, traditionally only women had a single hole in their ears from childhood throughout their lives; however, in other cultures around the world and in western culture today and in ancient times, various parts of the body are also pierced in both sexes.

Usually, they are small hoops covered with a sphere, metallic or plastic.

However, the larger ones vary in shape and material. Whoever decides to wear an earring should pay attention, since it is like placing an element that Will be foreign to the body and that can react negatively, so it must always be cleaned very well and correctly, not mistreated, or exceed the healing of the piercing. And of course, do not try to exchange the piece with another person as a sanitary measure to avoid infection and even the transmission of diseases.

PLASTIC SURGERIES

Plastic surgery is the branch of surgery that deals with reshaping any part of the human body affected by an injury or deformity. The malformation can be congenital, that is, be present from birth, as in the case of children born with a cleft palate or lip or Other congenital anomaly. The disfigurement can also be the consequence of an injury or surgical deformity necessary for the treatment of diseases such as cancer. The main goals of plastic surgery are correcting abnormalities, restoring lost functions, and improving the appearance of disfigured parts.

Plastic surgery is one of the oldest surgical practices. Nose reconstruction operations were likely performed in ancient India as early as 2000 BC, when nose amputations were a form of punishment; over time, the potter caste devised a method to rebuild the nose using part of the forehead, a technique that is Still used today. Some allusions to this type of surgery also appear in ancient Greece and Rome. However, the most significant development of surgical techniques did not take place almost until the 16th century, particularly in the work of the Italian physician Gasparo Tagliacozzi.

During the 20th century, the psychotherapeutic importance of plastic surgery was demonstrated after World War II; victims of war wounds and burns recovered the function of their injured body parts and the external disfigurement, which usually leads to depressive states, was repaired.

The world of plastic surgery is vast and constantly evolving. From reconstructive procedures that restore form and function to cosmetic surgeries that enhance appearance, this field offers a spectrum of options for people seeking physical transformation. This article delves into the different types of plastic surgery, their applications, and crucial factors to consider before undergoing any procedure.

Understanding Plastic Surgery: Plastic surgery is a surgical specialty dedicated to the restoration, reconstruction, or alteration of the human body. It encompasses two main categories: *

Reconstructive Surgery: aims to correct abnormalities caused by birth defects, accidents, burns, disease, or trauma. It focuses on restoring function, improving appearance, and enhancing a patient's quality of life.

* **Cosmetic Surgery:** Focuses on improving appearance to achieve desired aesthetic goals. These procedures are elective and not medically necessary.

Reconstructive Surgery: Reconstructive surgery plays a vital role in restoring normalcy to people who have suffered physical alterations. Here are some common areas of focus:

* **Craniofacial Surgery:** Addresses facial deformities due to birth defects, trauma, or tumors. Procedures may involve cleft lip and palate repair, jaw reconstruction, and facial bone reconstruction after accidents.

* **Hand Surgery:** Specializes in restoring the function and appearance of hands after injuries, burns, or arthritis. Reconstructive techniques can improve dexterity, grip strength, and overall hand functionality.

* **Microsurgery:** Uses specialized techniques and instruments to perform delicate surgeries involving tiny structures such as nerves and blood vessels. This allows for intricate procedures such as tissue transfer and flap reconstruction.

* **Burn Surgery:** Focuses on the treatment of burns and their aftereffects. Techniques include skin grafting, scar revision, and restoring function to burned areas.

* **Breast Reconstruction:** Helps women who have undergone a mastectomy (breast removal) due to cancer or other reasons regain a sense of normalcy. Reconstructive procedures can recreate the breast mound and restore symmetry.

Cosmetic Surgery: Cosmetic surgery offers a wide range of procedures to enhance appearance. While these procedures are not medically necessary, they can boost self-confidence and address aesthetic concerns. Here are some popular options:

* **Facelift:** Aims to address signs of facial aging by tightening sagging skin and reducing wrinkles.

* **Rhinoplasty (Nose Job):** Reshapes the nose to improve its size, bridge, or tip.

* **Blepharoplasty (Eyelid Lift):** Corrects drooping eyelids or removes puffiness for a more youthful appearance.

* **Liposuction:** Removes unwanted fat deposits from specific areas of the body for body contouring.

* **Breast Augmentation:** Increases breast size through implants or fat transfer.

* **Breast Reduction:* Reduces breast size and weight to relieve discomfort and improve posture.

* **Tummy Tuck:** Removes excess skin and tightens abdominal wall muscles for a flatter stomach.

* **Body Lift:** Tightens loose skin and improves body contours after significant weight loss or pregnancy.

Important Considerations Before Plastic Surgery: Consider that plastic surgery is a major decision. Here are some crucial factors to weigh before proceeding:

* **Realistic Expectations:** It is essential to have realistic expectations about the outcome of any procedure. Thoroughly discuss your desired results with your surgeon and understand the limitations of the surgery. * **Board Certification:** Always choose a board-certified plastic surgeon with

extensive experience and a proven track record. Research their qualifications, credentials, and patient reviews.

* **Consultation:** During your consultation, discuss your medical history, desired outcome, and any concerns you may have. The surgeon will assess your suitability for the procedure and explain the risks, potential complications, and recovery process.

* **Cost and Insurance:** Plastic surgery can be expensive. Understand the associated costs, including the surgeon's fee, facility fees, anesthesia, and postoperative care.

Surgical. Some insurance plans may offer partial coverage for reconstructive procedures, but typically not for cosmetic surgery.

* **Health Considerations:** You must be in good health to undergo surgery. Inform your surgeon of any medical conditions or medications you are taking.

* **Recovery Time:** Each procedure has a specific recovery timeline. Understand the time commitment involved, including postoperative limitations and potential discomfort.

* **Psychological Factors:** Consider the psychological impact of surgery. Make sure you are undergoing the procedure for the right reasons and not because of pressure from others.

Additional Considerations About Your Non-Surgical Alternatives: Explore non-surgical options such as injectables, fillers, or laser treatments that can achieve the desired results without surgery.

* **Maintenance:** The results of some procedures may not be permanent. Discuss with your surgeon the need for follow-up procedures or maintenance strategies.

* **Ethical Considerations:** Consider the ethical implications of cosmetic surgery, especially as they relate to societal beauty standards.

PLASMATHERAPY AND AUTOHEMOTHERAPY

In the dynamic world of aesthetics, the quest for timeless beauty and youth has driven the development of innovative techniques that promise effective and long-lasting results. Among these techniques, plasma therapy has emerged as a promising option, captivating the attention of professionals and patients alike.

What is plasma therapy?

Plasma therapy, also known as platelet-rich plasma (PRP), is an aesthetic procedure that harnesses the body's own regenerative potential to improve the appearance of the skin. This technique is based on the extraction of a small amount of the patient's blood, which is centrifuged to separate the plasma, a portion rich in platelets and growth factors.

What are the benefits of plasma therapy in aesthetics?

The benefits of plasma therapy in the field of aesthetics are diverse and cover a wide range of applications:

1. Facial Rejuvenation:

* **Wrinkle and Fine Line Reduction:** PRP stimulates the production of collagen and elastin, essential components for smooth, firm skin.

* **Improves Skin Texture:** Plasma helps reduce the appearance of enlarged pores, scars, and stretch marks.

* **Brightening:** PRP revitalizes the skin, giving it a more radiant and healthy appearance.

2. Hair Treatment:

* **Hair Strengthening:** PRP stimulates hair growth, combating hair loss and brittleness.

* **Baldness Prevention:** Plasma can help prevent androgenetic alopecia in men and women.

* **Hair Volume Increase:** PRP promotes hair thickening, providing greater density.

3. Body Rejuvenation:

* **Stretch Mark Reduction:** Plasma stimulates collagen production, improving the appearance of stretch marks.

* **Skin Toning:** PRP helps firm loose skin in areas such as the abdomen, thighs, and arms.

* **Cellulite Improvement:** Plasma can help reduce the appearance of orange-peel skin.

How is the plasma therapy procedure performed?

The plasma therapy procedure is relatively simple and performed on an outpatient basis:

1. **Blood Collection:** A small amount of blood is drawn from the patient, usually from the arm.

2. **Centrifugation:** The blood is centrifuged to separate the plasma from other blood cells.

3. **Plasma Application:** Platelet-rich plasma is injected into the treatment areas using a fine needle.

What are the side effects of plasma therapy?

The side effects of plasma therapy are usually mild and temporary, and include:

* **Redness**

* **Swelling**

* **Mild discomfort at the injection site**

In what cases is plasma therapy contraindicated?

Plasma therapy is not suitable for all patients. Some contraindications include:

* **Pregnancy or breastfeeding**

* **Autoimmune diseases**

* **Infections at the treatment area**

* **Blood clotting disorders**

Is plasma therapy an option for you?

If you are considering plasma therapy as a cosmetic treatment, it is important to consult with a **qualified medical professional** to evaluate your case and determine if this procedure is right for you. The doctor can provide you with personalized information about the benefits, risks, and expectations of the treatment. **In conclusion,** plasma therapy presents itself as a promising alternative in the field of aesthetics, offering a natural and effective approach to improving the appearance of skin and hair. However, it is crucial to consult with a medical professional to determine if this treatment is right for your individual needs and expectations.

BIOPOLYMERS RISKS

Surgery techniques have obtained some successes in recent decades but also misleading in relation to the substances used to supposedly increase the volume of different areas of the body or face of patients desperate to improve their aesthetic appearance. For this reason, it was believed at first that these invasive substances would not have adverse effects, but as time passed, the warning voices of patients affected many times by surgeons without suitability or scruples to apply such aesthetic procedures began to emerge.

Biopolymers are synthetic substances that range from paraffin, liquid silicone, bone cement, and even oils for industrial use. The risk to the health of patients arises when they begin to experience discomfort in the operated area with Iatrogenic allogenosis with degeneration of the skin tissue, in addition to the symptoms of the syndrome known as Asia, with ailments such as joint and muscle pain, physical exhaustion, depression, memory loss, dry eyes and mouth, among others.

The solution to this reaction is the partial removal of biopolymers and it is a surgical procedure performed by plastic surgeons and comprises a set of surgical techniques that seek to eliminate deposits of the injected material including buttocks, lumbar region (lower back), thighs, legs, among other area.

This surgery can be done for a number of reasons:

• To decrease the inflammatory response.

• To try to stop the degenerative process of healthy tissues. To improve the appearance of symptoms compatible with autoimmune diseases. To treat the facial, body or breast contour, which presents deformities due to the substance that has been injected.

• To treat pain.

• As a reconstructive technique in certain situations. In most cases, the best option is to remove the substance, even if no symptoms have occurred, in fact, it is better to remove the biopolymers as soon as possible, preventing the substance from causing serious damage to the body that prevents surgery due to the high risk of the procedure for the health and life of the patient, points out the Internet site "Colombia.com".

AUTOLOGOUS MATERIALS

Autologous materials are those obtained from the individual's own tissues, that is, they are **autogenous** biomaterials. They are characterized by being:

* **Biocompatible:** they do not generate rejection in the body.

* **They reduce the risk of infections:** as they do not come from external sources.

* **They decrease the need for grafts:** by using the individual's own tissues.

* **They promote tissue regeneration:** by containing viable cells and growth factors.

* **Wide range of applications:** in reconstructive, orthopedic, maxillofacial, and other surgeries.

Examples of autologous materials:

* **Autologous bone:** obtained from the individual for bone grafts.

* **Autologous cartilage:** used to repair joint injuries.

* **Cultured skin:** to cover wounds and burns.

* **Autologous fats:** for aesthetic and reconstructive grafts.

* **Stem cells:** with the potential to regenerate various tissues.

Autologous materials offer a promising alternative in the field of regenerative medicine, with great potential to improve patients' quality of life.

TYPES AND TECHNIQUES OF EPIDERMAL GRAFTS

One of the main techniques of plastic surgery is the graft, transplantation or implantation of living tissue from one part of the to another, or from one person to another, with the aim that the tissue takes hold and grows to replace a lost part. Different skin grafting techniques are generally used. One is the transfer of tissue from an adjacent area to the defect by transport or rotation of detached skin fragments. Another frequently used technique, especially in minor facial anomalies, is the full-thickness graft, in which complete skin fragments, that is, with all the layers that compose it, are extracted and transferred as a free transplant to the area in question.

A third technique, called a partial thickness graft, is used in severely burned patients who have deep burns over large areas of the body. Using an instrument called a "dermatome", a piece of skin of a specified thickness can be obtained from the donor area that contains enough live dermal cells to cover the burned area, leaving enough cells in the donor area for the skin to grow back. Sometimes the life of a burn patient can be saved by temporarily covering the surviving skin cells in the burned area with skin grafts from genetically incompatible donors. These grafts do not survive permanently and can be rejected by the immune system.

More complicated cases require other types of skin coverings, such as loss of full thickness of the cheek or loss of the entire nose. The transplant must be irrigated by the blood vessels in its original area until it has taken hold in its new location. In these cases, a tube or skin flap with underlying tissue is left to connect the transplant with its original blood supply. The requires a two-stage operation; the second stage involves excision of the connecting pedicle after the transplanted part has acquired a new blood supply from the recipient area.

Other types of grafts are also used in plastic surgery. For example, cartilage obtained from a patient's rib is modeled to reproduce the shape of a missing ear. the cartilage is transplanted to the area of the new ear. Bone grafts obtained from the pelvis or ribs are used to reconstruct different types of abnormalities, such as to replace the jaw. Nerve grafts are also used in the treatment of facial paralysis if the facial nerve has been injured as a result of trauma.

CHAPTER 3 COSMETOLOGY & PRODUCTS

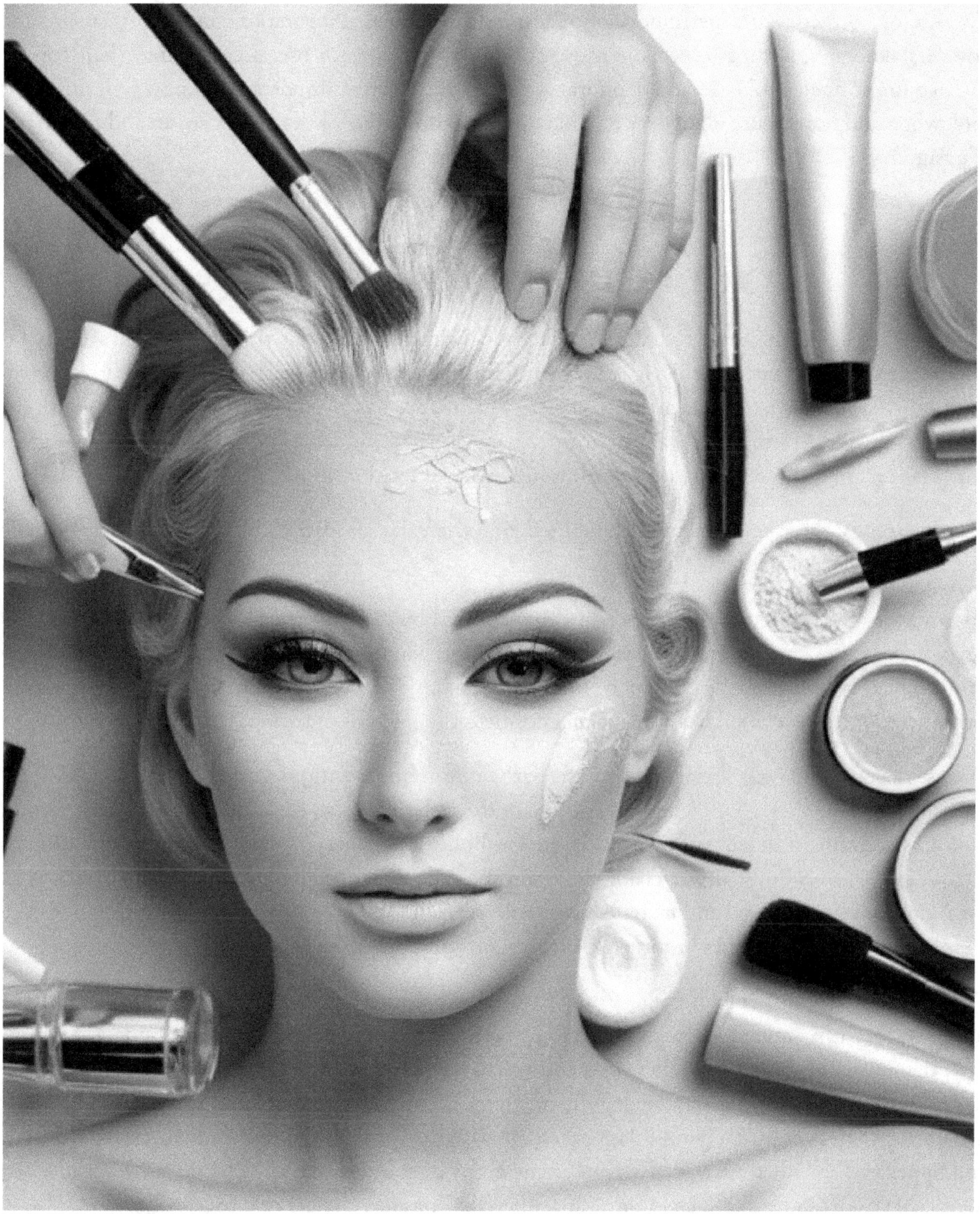

The use of cosmetics and perfumes is not limited to women. Preparations used by men include powders, colognes, lotions (especially those containing alcohol for use after shaving), hair toners, with a quinine or alcohol base, and deodorants. Therefore, it is very important to know well this work tool, when and how to use it and to do so have a basic knowledge of the composition and properties of cosmetics.

INTRODUCTION TO COSMETOLOGY

The annual sales of beauty products for men and women mean that this industry has today an important development and that it is very profitable. Cosmetology arises to meet a person's own needs, such as improving the anti-aging qualities that nature has given us and maintaining youth for as long as possible. Both aspects aimed at improving appearance, something that currently has great importance, not only on a personal level, but in our social relationships.

In cosmetology, three key aspects are combined, one scientific, another technical and another artistic in relation to the color line.

To introduce the beautician in the broad field of cosmetology, we first need to know what cosmetics are, which is the general term that is applied to all preparations and elements for external use to condition and beautify the body, which clean, color, soften or protect the skin, hair, nails, lips or eyes. Perfumery is often excluded from the field of cosmetics.

The use of cosmetics is universal and dates from the most remote antiquity. Despite the general belief that cosmetics, as they are now known, originate from the Far East, the study of primitive cultures indicates their use in all parts of the world. The symbolic or magical paintings of indigenous cultures, tattoos and scarifications (superficial incisions in the skin) practiced by many peoples (for example, the Maori of New Zealand and many African cultures), and the use of dyes to decorate the body are all forms of cosmetics used both for psychological intimidation of the enemy and for decoration.

The earliest known cosmetics come from the First Dynasty of Egypt (c. 3100-2907 BC). In the tombs, vases with ointments that appeared to be perfumed have been found, as later finds show. Both Egyptian men and women used these preparations as well as scented oils with great profusion to keep their skin supple and smooth in the dry climate of their country. Likewise, they discovered the art of decorating their eyes by applying a dark green color to the lower eyelid and darkening the eyelashes and upper eyelid with kohl, a preparation of antimony or soot. It seems likely that the Jews adopted the use of cosmetics from the Egyptians, since the Old Testament refers to face paints.

In the middle of the Ist century BC. the Romans used some cosmetics such as kohl to darken the eyelashes and eyelids, chalk (or chalk) to whiten the face, blush, depilatories (hair removal compounds) and pumice stone to clean the teeth. During the Middle Ages the Crusaders observed the use of cosmetics in the Middle East, and it was they who spread it throughout Europe.

The almost universal use of cosmetics in modern times has grown along with the scientific study of the ingredients used. This research, which was stafted in the 19th century by the French, led to the development of more and better products at a lower price.

TYPOLOGY AND SKIN CARE

To establish the client's skin type, these guidelines must be followed, such as observing the skin, establishing a dialogue in order to obtain useful information on our purpose and finally drawing the final conclusion. There are several ways to classify skin types such as their thickness, temperament and morphological variations, etc.

However, the most widely used classification is based on the secretory nature of the skin.

By virtue of the epicutaneous emulsion, as well as data collected during the skin study, the client's skin typology can be determined. two groups of epicutaneous emulsion are established:

• Matte skin type: They do not have shine and their appearance is normal or dry. (from epicutaneous O / A emulsion) Dull skins can be normal or eudermic where the hydrolipidic emulsion is adequately formed. Dry skin can be atypical dry skin, when sebaceous secretion is insufficient, and dehydrated skin when there is excessive dehydration of the horny layer.

• Shiny skin: It has a certain shine because the oily phase predominates. (A / O epicutaneous emulsion) They can be classified according to their behavior, degree of sebaceous secretion and external manifestations in: normal oily skin, where there is a variation in the amount of components and emulsifiers determining the external phase. Dehydrated oily skin where the external oily phase is usually formed in a defective way because the sebum is altered in its composition. Oily occluded skin where the sebaceous secretion is modified and does not come out, causing a tendency to acne.

• Mixed skin: In cases of combination skin, there are areas on the face where the fat or midface region is located, and also areas that have a dry or normal appearance, such as the cheeks. The condition of the skin is influenced by multiple external factors such as mechanical, environmental, or biological aggression, as well as internal ones related to nutrition and aging.

MAKEUP

Some of us might consider that the origin of makeup belonged to the ancient civilizations of the Middle East, but it is known that tribes around the world used makeup with pigments taken from nature to indicate a certain degree of hierarchy between members. It even emerged jointly with the characterization of characters from Greek, Roman, Japanese and Other theater. It is used to conceal, cover defects of the face of people, and accentuate a natural and clean appearance in the contour of the face.

CHEMICAL COMPOSITION. The basic components of makeup are talc and starch. Talc is a soft, fatty mineral substance with a granular or fibrous texture composed of magnesium acid metasilicate. Its color can range from White, Silver or gray to apple green and shines with a pearly luster.

It is mined from metamorphic rock beds and is heat resistant. In addition to being used as the base powder for cosmetics due to its pigment tones, it is an ingredient in soaps, lubricants and tailor's chalk. On the Other hand, starch is a tasteless and colorless carbohydrate in the form of powder or grains, abundant in the seeds of cereals and tuber bulbs. Starch is hardly soluble in cold water and in alcohol, but in boiling water it causes a colloidal suspension that turns gelatinous when cooled. The hot water acts slowly on the starch, creating smaller molecules called dextrins. This reaction is an example of hydrolysis catalyzed by acids and some enzymes.

Dextrins, like starch, react with water to form even simpler molecules, to finally obtain maltose.

Other ingredients that are also added to cosmetics are magnesium carbonate to fix perfumes and achieve lightness with its powdery texture. Zinc stearate, antioxidants to stabilize and preserve. The application protocol for makeup products is simple:

Make-up artists recommend preparing the facial skin by first applying a moisturizer (moisturizing) with a cotton ball, removing the fat from the client's face.

The second step is to apply the primer that helps to set the makeup to the skin for the rest of the day.

The concealer is applied under the eyes, covering from the outside towards the nose any marks of dark circles.

The powder or liquid foundation is applied to the forehead, nose and chin.

The pencil is used and the eyebrows are outlined according to the client's hair tones

The shadow is applied to the eyelid using a thin sponge in two to three shades to create contrast.

The contour of the eye is delineated.

Apply the eyelash curler.

Apply lipstick, and glitter unnecessary.

Finally, using the Wide brush, apply the blush to the cheeks in a shade lighter or darker than the client's skin tone.

MAKE-UP TECHNIQUES.

Currently, makeup artists and beauty professionals advise wearing one of these three basic makeup techniques that are applied depending on the physical characteristics of the face of the model or client, and they are:

- Contouring:

After applying the base, contouring is carried out using concealers and bronzers, in powder or cream presentations. This technique is used to define or highlight cheekbones, chin, nose, reduce forehead or chin, or lighten the jaw.

- Baking:

Using translucent powders and this technique serves to show off a dull or matte effect and a long-lasting effect on the area to be highlighted. It is usually used in the area of the dark circles and jaw, to prolong the makeup in that area and help not to mark the wrinkles of the same.

- Strobing: The technique is done to obtain a natural appearance to give light to the face, no bronzers are applied, accentuating the points of light such as the cupid's bow, chin, nose and cheekbones and the arch of the eyebrows, using powder highlighter, liquid or sticks. We can also illuminate with corrector in a matte finish of shades lighter than the skin to be worked on.

COSMETICS PRODUCTS

The companies that produce the different types of cosmetic offer us a wide variety of options from creams, balms, oils, soaps, perfumes and detoxifying drinks. For this reason, we must clearly understand what its atomic measurements, effects and its usefulness are when choosing which cosmetic products are indicated for each case of the patients of a spa or aesthetic clinic. In the field of cosmetics the measure used is the kilodalton.

In 1808 the work "New system of chemical philosophy" was published, which included the atomic masses of various known elements in relation to the mass of hydrogen. Their masses were not entirely precise but they form the basis of the modern periodic classification of the elements. Dalton arrived at his atomic theory through the study of the physical properties of atmospheric air and Other gases.

In the course of his research, he discovered the law known as 'Dalton's law of partial pressures', according to which the pressure exerted by a mixture of gases is equal to the sum of the partial pressures that each of the gases would exert if he Will only occupy the total volume of the mix.

The basic products are three:

- Cleanser: removes oil, lymphatic debris from the upper layer of the skin and removes dead cells. Examples of cleaning substances are red wine, oatmeal, cucumber, and sugar.

- Astringent: It is any substance, such as alum, that is used for medical or industrial purposes to contract tissues and reduce mucus and Other secretions. Mineral salt solutions are generally astringent; vegetable astringents contain tannins.

- Moisturizer: Exposed skin suffers dryness from the environment, heat and polluted air, so moisturizing cream is applied to keep the skin soft. Humectants are surface active substances that work by dissolving in water causing a lower contact angle between a substance and a hydrophobic surface. The surfactant absorbs the fat and the solid surface, favoring the migration of particles. Some examples of moisturizing products are Wakame's Shea and seaweed creams that create a layer resistant to sudden changes in temperature, preventing wrinkles and stretch marks on the hips.

Some of the most common ingredients at the moment for body and facial treatments are the following:

Hyaluronic Acid:

It was discovered in Columbia, New York in 1934 by a couple of German-born research pharmacists. It has several sources of natural extraction such as the poultry comb for its high content of this acid. In the 1970s it was used as an anti-inflammatory by veterinarians at racetracks and thanks to many subsequent studies it was approved as a medicine in humans and today it is used in medicine since 1996. In simple terms, hyaluronic acid maintains collagen and stimulates its production that is part of the original structure of the skin, providing a filling effect between the pores. This substance is marketed in moisturizing and anti-aging creams, in skin injections and others. The results prolong the rejuvenating appearance of the treated skin area, contouring the lips and cheekbones, as well as to smooth the forehead and reduce scars from severe acne and Other skin problems that cause loss of the skin's protective layer. This product comes in three presentations according to its measurement of kilodaltons, KDa (kilodalton). The molecular weight of hyaluronic that we find in cosmetics is very diverse, and that makes some products better than others and more suitable for each skin. The hyaluronic of 320 KDa or more does not guarantee the filling effect, but it does guarantee the hydration. Hyaluronic 20 kDa or less has such a penetrating ability that it can be irritating to some people. For this reason, there are products that combine high weight hyaluronic with low weight. To avoid possible irritations, low-weight 50 kDa hyaluronic is used in products formulated for sensitive skin. In addition to cosmetics, they are used in dentistry and plastic surgery.

• Boric Acid:

White crystalline powder, with the formula H3B03. Although boric acid is barely soluble in water at room temperature (I g dissolves in 18 g of water), it dissolves more easily in hot water (l g dissolves in less than 4 g of water) as well as in alcohol and glycerin. It is slightly volatile. Significant amounts of boric acid are found in hydrothermal crevices in Tuscany, Italy, but it is not otherwise naturally found. Boric acid can be easily obtained by treating borax with sulfuric acid. Boric acid in solution is slightly acidic and acts as a mild, non-irritating astringent antiseptic, suitable for use in eye hygiene.

• Glycerol: In 1779 the Swedish chemist Carl Scheele formalized the discovery that natural fats and oils contain glycerin. It is one of the main products of the digestive degradation of lipids, an intermediate of alcoholic fermentation. It comes in the form of a colorless, viscous liquid with a sweet taste. It is believed that its continued use helps to firm the outer surface of the skin avoiding and expression lines on the face.

• Allantoin: It is a nitrogenous substance of a complex series that contains two molecules of urea or their radicals, such as uric acid or allantoin. Many nitrogenous organic compounds are found in some plants and in the urine of some mammals. Allantoin is a natural healing agent. It is characterized by accelerating the process that the skin does to shed dead or aging cells and replace them with new and healthy ones.

It promotes and accelerates natural healing «that is, it helps the skin to help itself. It has also been mentioned that it is a cell proliferator and stimulant of epithelialization and a debrider, this means that it helps to clean and get rid of necrotic tissue, accelerating the growth ofhealthy new tissue " Allantoin has shown to stimulate skin epithelialization by stimulating cell proliferation. It helps to eliminate necrotic, unreliable tissues, replacing them with new tissues. Another of its actions is to act as an anti-irritant, protecting the skin from the action of acidic or alkaline substances, soaps or oils. The and Drug Administration, the American Drug Testing Agency, approves the use of allantoin in various indications for maintaining skin condition.

BASIC PROPERTIES OF COSMETICS

** Botanical Properties of Cosmetic Ingredients on the Skin

The world of cosmetics has experienced a boom in the use of botanical ingredients derived from plants, flowers, fruits, and other natural components. These ingredients offer a wide range of beneficial properties for the skin, from cell regeneration to sun protection. The most common botanical properties used in cosmetics are described in detail below:

1. Regenerative Properties:

Botanical ingredients with regenerative properties stimulate cell renewal and the production of collagen, elastin, and other essential skin components. Some examples include:

* **Aloe vera:** rich in vitamins, minerals, and enzymes that promote healing and skin regeneration.

* **Centella asiatica:** stimulates the synthesis of collagen and elastin, improving skin firmness and elasticity.

* **Rosehip:** rich in essential fatty acids and antioxidants that help repair damaged skin and reduce wrinkles.

2. Astringent Properties:

Astringent ingredients help tone the skin, tighten pores, and control oil production. Some examples include:

* **Witch Hazel:** a natural astringent that helps clear pores and reduce inflammation.

* **Green Tea:** rich in antioxidants that fight free radicals and tone the skin.

* **Cucumber:** has cooling and soothing properties that help reduce swelling and redness.

3. Antiseptic and Antimicrobial Properties:

Antiseptic and antimicrobial ingredients fight bacteria and fungi that can cause skin infections. Some examples include:

* **Tea Tree Oil:** a powerful natural antiseptic that helps fight acne and other skin infections.

* **Lavender:** has anti-inflammatory and antiseptic properties that help soothe irritated skin.

* **Rosemary:** a natural antioxidant that helps fight free radicals and prevent cell damage.

4. Soothing Properties:

Soothing ingredients help soothe irritated skin and reduce stress. Some examples include:

* **Chamomile:** has soothing and anti-inflammatory properties that help relieve itching and redness.

* **Lavender:** known for its relaxing aroma that helps calm the mind and body.

* **Calendula:** has anti-inflammatory and healing properties that help soothe irritated skin.

5. Tonic Properties:

Tonic ingredients help stimulate blood circulation and tone the skin. Some examples include:

* **Rosewater:** a natural toner that helps hydrate and refresh the skin.

* **Apple Cider Vinegar:** helps balance the skin's pH and remove dead skin cells.

* **Witch Hazel:** has astringent and tonic properties that help tighten pores and tone the skin.

6. Emollient Properties:

Emollient ingredients help moisturize the skin and prevent dryness. Some examples include:

* **Coconut Oil:** rich in fatty acids that help hydrate and nourish the skin.

* **Shea Butter:** a natural emollient that helps protect the skin from dryness and environmental factors.

* **Jojoba Oil:** similar to the skin's natural sebum, it helps hydrate and balance the skin.

7. Exfoliating Properties:

Exfoliating ingredients help remove dead skin cells, improving its texture and radiance. Some examples include:

* **Sugar:** a natural exfoliant that helps remove dead skin cells without irritating the skin.

* **Ground coffee:** a natural exfoliant that helps stimulate blood circulation and reduce cellulite.

* **Sea salt:** a natural exfoliant that helps remove impurities and tone the skin.

8. Healing properties:

Wound-healing ingredients help accelerate wound healing and reduce the appearance of scars. Some examples include:

* **Aloe vera:** rich in vitamins, minerals, and enzymes that promote healing and skin regeneration.

* **Rosehip oil:** rich in essential fatty acids and antioxidants that help repair damaged skin and reduce wrinkles.

* **Centella asiatica:** stimulates the synthesis of collagen and elastin, improving wound healing.

FREQUENTLY USED COSMETIC INGREDIENTS

In the vast world of beauty, soap is positioned as a fundamental element, an indispensable ally for skin and body care. Its simplicity and versatility make it a basic tool both in the professional and home settings.

** Key Ingredients in Soap: A Blend of Cleansing and Care

The composition of soap varies depending on its purpose and type, but some basic ingredients are essential for its cleansing function:

1. Surfactants: These are the backbone of soap, responsible for lathering and removing dirt, oil, and sweat. The most common are **alkyl sulfates**.

2. Foaming Agents: These help generate a rich lather, improving the user experience and facilitating cleansing. Some examples are **cocamide DEA** and **betaine**.

3. Emollient Agents: These counteract the drying effect of surfactants, keeping skin hydrated and soft. Among them are **glycerin**, **coconut oil**, and **shea butter**.

*4. pH Regulators:** They help maintain the skin's acid-base balance, preventing irritation and dryness. **Citric acid** and **triethanolamine** are common examples.

5. Fragrances and Dyes: These are added to provide a pleasant aroma and an attractive aesthetic. However, it is important to choose soaps with natural fragrances and mild dyes to avoid irritation to sensitive skin.

**Types of Soap: Adapting to Every Need

The variety of soaps available allows you to find options for every skin type and need:

1. Neutral Soap: Ideal for sensitive skin, as it is gentle and contains no fragrances or dyes.

2. Antibacterial Soap: Fights bacteria and germs, being useful for oily or acne-prone areas.

3. Moisturizing Soap: Contains moisturizing agents that help keep skin hydrated and protected.

4. Exfoliating Soap: With fine abrasive particles that remove dead skin cells, promoting cell renewal.

5. Body Soap: Designed for deep cleansing of the body, removing impurities and leaving a feeling of freshness.

** Uses of Soap: Beyond Basic Cleansing

Soap not only cleanses the skin, but can also be used for various aesthetic purposes:

1. Facial Cleansing: The first step in any facial care routine is cleansing with soap. It is important to choose a soap appropriate for your skin type and avoid harsh products that can dry it out.

2. Makeup Removal: Some specific facial soaps are formulated to remove makeup effectively and gently.

3. Body Cleansing: Body soap cleanses the skin, removing impurities and leaving a feeling of freshness.

4. Moisturized Hands: Frequent handwashing with soap not only eliminates germs, but can also keep your hands moisturized if you choose a soap with moisturizing ingredients.

5. Foot Soak: A foot bath with warm soap and water helps soften the skin and remove calluses.

** Soap Procedures: Correct Techniques to Maximize Benefits

To take full advantage of soap's properties, it is important to follow proper technique:

1. Moisture: Moistening the skin before applying soap facilitates its cleansing action and prevents irritation.

2. Lather: Gently rub the soap into your skin until a rich lather forms.

3. Rinse: Rinse thoroughly with warm water to remove any soap residue.

4. Dry: Dry your skin with a soft towel, avoiding rubbing.

5. Moisturize: Apply a moisturizer or lotion after washing to keep your skin moisturized and protected.

6. Frequency: Washing with soap should be appropriate for your skin type and physical activity. In general, twice a day is usually sufficient.

*** Additional Considerations: Choosing the Right Soap

When selecting a soap, it is important to consider:

1. Skin Type: Oily, dry, sensitive, or combination skin determines the ideal soap formulation.

2. Ingredients: Avoid soaps with parabens, harsh sulfates, or artificial fragrances that irritate the outer layer.

** The Fascinating World of Serums: A Complete Guide to Skin Care

In the vast universe of facial care, serums have emerged as undisputed protagonists, winning the hearts of beauty lovers for their effectiveness and versatility. These concentrates of cosmetic active ingredients offer a precise dose of nutrients and active ingredients that penetrate deep into the skin's layers, combating various problems and delivering visible results.

** What is a serum?

A serum is a cosmetic product with a light texture and rapid absorption that is characterized by its high concentration of active ingredients.

MICRODERMABRASION

What is microdermabrasion?

Microdermabrasion is a dermatological procedure that uses a device with a diamond tip or aluminum crystals to gently exfoliate the surface layer of the skin. This process removes dead skin cells, dirt, and debris that clog pores, revealing smoother, brighter, and more even-toned skin.

The benefits of microdermabrasion are numerous and cover a wide range of aesthetic needs:

* **Fine Line and Wrinkle Reduction:** Stimulates collagen and elastin production, softening the appearance of fine lines and wrinkles.

In the dynamic world of aesthetics, the quest for radiant, healthy skin is a constant.

Among the various treatments available, microdermabrasion has established itself as an effective and minimally invasive technique for revitalizing the skin and combating the signs of aging.

What are the benefits of microdermabrasion?

An Ally for Renewed Skin

Microdermabrasion

* **Scar and stretch mark reduction:** Reduces the appearance of scars caused by acne or surgical procedures, as well as stretch marks.

* **Improves the appearance of enlarged pores:** Reduces the size of enlarged pores, giving the skin a more uniform appearance.

* **Spot Lightening:** Reduces uneven pigmentation and spots caused by sun exposure or aging.

* **Improves product absorption:** Prepares the skin for better absorption of subsequent topical treatments.

In which areas of the face can microdermabrasion be applied?

* **Deep Exfoliation:** Removes dead skin cells, improving overall texture and tone.

1. **Facial cleansing:** A deep cleansing of the face is performed to remove any residue or impurities.

5. **Sun Protection:** It is essential to apply broad-spectrum sunscreen after the procedure to protect your skin from UV rays.

Microdermabrasion is a versatile treatment that can be applied to various areas of the face, including:

2. **Application of topical anesthetic:** In some cases, a topical anesthetic may be applied to minimize discomfort during the procedure.

* Forehead

3. **Microdermabrasion:** The device with a diamond tip or aluminum crystals is used to exfoliate the skin in a controlled manner, making gentle passes over the selected areas.

How is the microdermabrasion procedure performed?

The microdermabrasion procedure is simple and quick, taking approximately 30 to 45 minutes. The general steps are detailed below:

* Upper lip

How many microdermabrasion sessions are recommended?

* Neck

The number of recommended microdermabrasion sessions will depend on each patient's specific needs and treatment goals. Generally, 3 to 6 sessions are recommended, with an interval of 1 to 2 weeks between each session.

* Cheeks

4. **Application of a soothing mask:** Once the exfoliation is complete, a soothing mask is applied to hydrate and refresh the skin.

* Nose

In most cases, these side effects disappear within hours or days.

* **Active acne**

It's important to remember that it's always a good idea to consult with a dermatologist or aesthetician to determine if microdermabrasion is the right treatment for you.

What are the side effects of microdermabrasion?

Who are the ideal candidates for microdermabrasion?

MICRONEEDLING

Microdermabrasion is a safe and effective procedure for most people, however, it is not recommended in the following cases:

Side effects of microdermabrasion are generally mild and temporary, and may include:

Slight sensitivity

* **Very sensitive skin**

A journey to radiant skin

* Itching

In conclusion, microdermabrasion has become a valuable tool in the field of aesthetics, offering a noninvasive and effective alternative for improving skin's appearance. If you're looking for a treatment to revitalize your face, combat the signs of aging, and achieve brighter, more even skin, microdermabrasion may be an excellent option.

* Swelling

* **Skin wounds or infections**

* **Skin diseases such as herpes or eczema**

* **Pregnancy or breastfeeding**

Redness

* People with **mature skin** looking to combat the signs of aging.

* **Alopecia:** Stimulates hair growth in areas with baldness or thinning.

In the dynamic world of aesthetics, the quest for perfect skin is a constant. Among the most innovative and promising techniques is microneedling, a non-surgical procedure that has gained popularity for its effectiveness in facial revitalization.

* **Enlarged pores:** Reduces the size of enlarged pores, improving the overall appearance of the skin.

What is microneedling?

Who is microneedling suitable for?

* **Stretch marks:** Helps improve the appearance of stretch marks on the abdomen, thighs and buttocks.

* **Scars:** Promotes the reduction of surgical and burn scars.

* **Facial Rejuvenation:** Significantly reduces fine lines, wrinkles and acne scars, improving the overall texture and tone of the skin.

* People with **acne** or **acne scars**.

* **Spot and pigmentation treatment:** Reduces the appearance of dark spots, hyperpigmentation and melasma.

* People with **spots** or **hyperpigmentation**.

Microneedling, also known as collagen induction therapy, involves applying a device with sterile microneedles that create tiny, controlled perforations in the epidermis and dermis of the skin.

These microinjuries activate a natural repair and regeneration process, stimulating the production of collagen and elastin, essential proteins for keeping skin firm, smooth, and radiant.

Microneedling is a versatile procedure that can be beneficial for a wide range of people, including:

Benefits of microneedling:

4. Serum application: A specific serum is applied to stimulate the production of collagen and elastin.

What are the side effects of microneedling?

* **Sensitivity**

* People with **stretch marks**.

5. Sun protection: It is important to apply a broad-spectrum sunscreen after the procedure.

How many microneedling treatments are needed?

* People with **hair loss**.

2. Anesthesia: A topical anesthetic cream may be applied to minimize discomfort.

* **Swelling**

3. Microneedling: The microneedling device is applied to the skin using precise movements. The

depth of the needles is adjusted according to the area being treated and the specific needs of the skin.

* **Itching**

The microneedling procedure typically takes between 30 and 60 minutes and can vary depending on the area being treated and the depth of the needles used. The general steps are detailed below:

Side effects of microneedling are usually mild and temporary, and include:

1. Cleansing: The skin is thoroughly cleansed to remove any impurities or makeup.

* **Redness**

* People with **enlarged pores**.

Microneedling results are **gradual and progressive**. A minimum of **3 sessions** is recommended, with an interval of **4 to 6 weeks** between each session for optimal results.

What does the microneedling procedure consist of?

Unlike traditional tattooing, this procedure uses biocompatible pigments that are deposited in the superficial layers of the skin, creating subtle and long-lasting aesthetic effects.

In conclusion, microneedling has become a powerful tool in the field of aesthetics, offering a safe and effective alternative for rejuvenating the skin, treating various conditions, and improving its overall appearance. If you're looking for a procedure to help restore the radiance and vitality of your skin, microneedling may be the perfect option for you. Always consult with a qualified professional for a personalized evaluation to determine if this procedure is right for you.

It is important to note that microneedling must be performed by a qualified professional to ensure the safety and effectiveness of the procedure.

MICROPIGMENTATION

Contraindications of microneedling:

Art and beauty in today's face

* People with metal allergies.

Uses and applications of micropigmentation:

* People with active skin diseases such as herpes or psoriasis.

An ancient art with modern applications

* People with blood clotting disorders.

The roots of micropigmentation date back to ancient civilizations, where similar techniques were used to adorn the body. However, today, this technique has evolved considerably, incorporating technological advances and adapting to modern aesthetic demands.

Microneedling is not indicated for:

In the dynamic world of aesthetics, **micropigmentation** has emerged as a revolutionary technique that redefines facial beauty.

Pregnant or breastfeeding women.

4. Hair pigmentation: In cases of alopecia or fine hair, hair micropigmentation can help create the illusion of greater hair density. Pigments are implanted into the scalp to simulate hair follicles, which adds volume and texture to the hair.

5. Breast Areolas: Micropigmentation is a technique used to reconstruct or correct the breast areola, especially in women who have undergone mastectomies or breast reconstruction.

Realistic areolas can be created with appropriate color and symmetry, providing greater patient confidence and satisfaction.

Micropigmentation procedures and techniques:

3. Lips: Micropigmentation offers solutions for pale, thin, or asymmetrical lips. It can be used to define the lip contour, increase volume, correct imperfections, and add color to the lips, creating a healthier and more attractive appearance.

6. Scar camouflage: Micropigmentation offers an effective alternative for camouflaging facial and body scars. By depositing pigments that resemble the skin tone, it helps blur the scar, making it less visible and improving its aesthetic appearance.

2. Eyeliner: Permanent eyeliner, also known as "permanent makeup," is one of the most popular applications of micropigmentation. It allows for subtle yet long-lasting definition of the eye contour, enhancing the look and eliminating the need for daily makeup.

1. Eyebrow Design: Micropigmentation has become an invaluable tool for restoring or enhancing the shape and volume of eyebrows. It allows you to create full, symmetrical, and natural-looking eyebrows, correcting asymmetries, filling in sparse areas, or even designing completely new eyebrows.

1. Evaluation and Design: The specialist performs a thorough evaluation of the client, considering their skin type, hair color, facial features, and aesthetic goals. From this, the procedure is designed, selecting the appropriate color and shape for each patient case.

The micropigmentation process generally involves the following steps:

* Periodic touch-ups are recommended to maintain the desired effect over the long term.

Ultimately, micropigmentation represents an art that transforms, bringing beauty and naturalness to the face, and contributing to emotional well-being and personal satisfaction.

2. Anesthesia: A topical anesthetic cream is applied to minimize discomfort during the procedure.

Micropigmentation, an art that transforms:

More than just a cosmetic technique, micropigmentation has become a tool for improving self-esteem and self-confidence. It allows people to feel more beautiful and confident in their physical appearance, correcting imperfections and enhancing their natural features.

3. Pigment Implantation: Using a device similar to a dermograph, the specialist introduces the pigments into the superficial layers of the skin with precision and delicacy.

* It is essential to avoid direct sun exposure during the first weeks.

* It is important to choose a certified and experienced micropigmentation professional.

MICROBLADING

* The specialist's instructions regarding hygiene and post-procedure care should be followed.

The art of microblading: A touch of natural beauty for your eyebrows

4. Healing and Touch-Ups: The healing process typically takes a few days. A touch-up is then performed to perfect the final result and ensure the desired symmetry and color.

With its multiple applications, micropigmentation has revolutionized the world of aesthetics, offering long-lasting and aesthetic solutions for a wide range of needs.

Recommendations and aftercare:

* **Fill in sparse eyebrows:** It is ideal for people with thin, sparse or bald eyebrows.

* **Time Saver:** Forget about doing your eyebrow makeup every day.

In the world of aesthetics, eyebrows have taken on an undeniable role. Their shape, thickness, and definition frame the face, adding character and expressiveness. For those who desire full, defined, and natural-looking eyebrows, microblading has become a revolutionary technique that has taken the beauty world by storm.

Microblading gives you a permanently groomed look.

What is microblading?

* **Boost Self-Esteem:** Beautiful, well-groomed eyebrows can boost self-confidence.

* **Natural look:** The hair-by-hair technique simulates natural eyebrow hair, providing a realistic and harmonious result.

* **Improves symmetry:** Microblading allows you to correct asymmetries in the eyebrows, creating facial balance.

Benefits of microblading:

* **Define the contour of the eyebrows:** Helps shape the eyebrows and correct asymmetries.

* **Full, defined brows:** Microblading fills in gaps and defines the contour of your brows, creating a thicker, more even appearance.

* **Camouflage scars:** It can be used to camouflage scars or sparse areas on the eyebrows.

Microblading, also known as eyebrow micropigmentation, is a semi-permanent makeup technique that uses a handheld tool called a "tebori" or "blade" to implant pigment into the superficial layers of the skin, mimicking natural eyebrow hair.

Uses of microblading:

Unlike traditional tattooing, microblading is performed with finer, more delicate needles, allowing for precise, hair-by-hair strokes, achieving a natural and long-lasting effect.

Microblading durability:

* Avoid touching or manipulating your eyebrows.

* Presence of cold sores or folliculitis in the area to be treated.

* **Recreate missing eyebrows:** In cases of alopecia or total loss of eyebrows, microblading allows them to be reconstructed naturally.

* Do not expose yourself to direct sunlight or swimming pools during the first week.

* Allergies to the pigments used.

Microblading procedure:

*

Aftercare:

Pregnant or breastfeeding women.

* Keep the area clean and dry for the first few days.

* People with diabetes or autoimmune diseases.

3. **Pigment implantation:** With Tebori, precise strokes are made imitating natural hair, depositing the pigment in the superficial layers of the skin.

Microblading is a semi-permanent treatment that can last between 1 and 2 years. The duration depends on various factors such as skin type, aftercare, and use of cosmetic products. Touch-ups are recommended every 6-12 months to maintain eyebrow color and definition.

4. **Touch-up:** A touch-up is recommended every 4-6 weeks to perfect the result and ensure durability.

Contraindications:

1. **Evaluation and Design:** The specialist evaluates the face, natural eyebrow shape, and hair color to determine the ideal design.

Follow the specialist's recommendations.

Important considerations:

2. **Topical anesthesia:** An anesthetic cream is applied to minimize discomfort during the procedure.

Types of Peeling: Adapting to Every Need

Microblading has become an invaluable tool for those looking to improve the aesthetics of their eyebrows and boost their self-esteem. With the proper procedure and the necessary aftercare, you can achieve perfect, natural, and long-lasting eyebrows that enhance your natural beauty.

* It is essential to choose a certified and experienced microblading professional.

PEELINGS TYPES AND INDICATIONS

Discovering the Art of Peeling: A Journey to Radiant Skin

Follow the specialist's instructions to obtain a result * **Microdermabrasion:** Uses fine crystals to exfoliate the surface layers of the skin, removing impurities and improving texture, optimal and avoid complications.

* **Dermabrasion:** A more invasive technique that uses a rotating abrasive device to remove deeper layers of the skin, indicated for treating scars and deep wrinkles.

* Perform an allergy test prior to the procedure.

To better understand peeling techniques, it is essential to know their different types, each with its own specific characteristics and applications:

1. Physical Peeling:

Ensure that quality materials and pigments are used

In the fascinating world of aesthetics, peeling has become a fundamental technique for revealing renewed and radiant skin. This procedure, which involves the controlled exfoliation of the skin's superficial layers, offers a wide range of benefits, from removing dead cells to stimulating collagen and elastin production biocompatible.

* **Retinoic Acid:** A derivative of vitamin A that promotes cell renewal and improves skin texture, indicated to treat photoaging and pigmented spots.

3. Enzyme Peeling:

* **Bromelain Enzymes:** Ideal for sensitive skin, as they are less irritating than other types of peels.

Key Ingredients for Effective Exfoliation

* **Salicylic Acid:** A beta hydroxy acid (BHA) effective for oily and acne-prone skin, as it clears pores and reduces inflammation.

* **Papaya Enzymes:** Gentle and effective for all skin types, removes dead cells and provides luminosity.

* **Glycolic Acid:** An alpha hydroxy acid (AHA) ideal for dry and mature skin, as it stimulates collagen production and reduces the appearance of fine lines and wrinkles.

2. Chemical Peeling:

* **Enzymes:** Papain, bromelain. They gently exfoliate and are ideal for sensitive skin.

* **Retinoids:** Vitamin A and its derivatives. They stimulate cell renewal, reduce fine lines and wrinkles, and improve skin texture.

* **Betahydroxy Acids (BHA):** Salicylic Acid. They clear pores, fight acne, and reduce inflammation.

Procedure: A Beauty Ritual

Beyond the type of peel chosen, the ingredients used play a crucial role in its effectiveness:

* **Alpha Hydroxy Acids (AHAs):** Glycolic acid, lactic acid, citric acid. They help remove dead cells, stimulate collagen production, and reduce the appearance of fine lines and wrinkles.

Contraindications:

* **Determine your skin type and specific needs.**

Additional Recommendations:

The peeling process, although it varies depending on the type and intensity of the treatment, generally follows these steps:

* **Choosing the right type of peel.**

1. Cleansing: The skin is thoroughly cleansed to remove any impurities or makeup.

* **Make sure the treatment is appropriate for your medical history.**

Important Considerations for a Safe and Effective Peel

* **Skin diseases such as herpes or eczema.**

Before undergoing a peel, it is essential to consult with a beauty professional to:

* **Allergies to peel ingredients.**

4. Hydration: Skin is intensely hydrated to soothe and restore balance.

* **Pregnancy or breastfeeding.**

5. Sun Protection: It is essential to apply broad-spectrum sunscreen after the peel, as your skin will be more sensitive to the sun.

* **Open wounds or skin infections.**

1. Application of the Exfoliating Agent: The exfoliating product is carefully applied to the skin, following the professional's instructions.

* **Follow the professional's instructions before, during and after the procedure.**

2. Neutralization: In some cases, a neutralizer is applied to stop the action of the exfoliating agent.

* **Drink plenty of water to keep your skin hydrated.**

In conclusion, peeling has become an invaluable tool on the path to radiant and renewed skin.

BOTULINUM TOXINS IN AESTHETICS: AN IN-DEPTH ANALYSIS

Botulinum toxins, popularly known as Botox®, have revolutionized the field of aesthetics, offering a noninvasive alternative to combat wrinkles and fine lines. However, it is crucial to fully understand how they work, the ingredients used, and the procedures involved in order to make informed decisions about their use.

* **Follow a skincare routine appropriate for your skin type.**

AUTHORIZED BUTULINUM TOXINS

* **Use a broad-spectrum sunscreen daily.**

* **Avoid direct sun exposure for at least one week after the peel.**

Botulinum toxins are neurotoxic proteins produced by the bacterium Clostridium botulinum. Although highly toxic in large quantities, in aesthetic applications they are used in controlled, minimal doses to achieve a therapeutic effect.

Ingredients used in botulinum toxin procedures Botulinum toxin procedures generally involve the following ingredients:

Its mechanism of action is based on the temporary inhibition of the release of acetylcholine, a neurotransmitter essential for muscle contraction. By blocking acetylcholine, botulinum toxins relax facial muscles, smoothing out wrinkles and expression lines.

What are botulinum toxins?

1. Botulinum toxin: The main ingredient, present in various brand names such as Botox®, Dysport®, Xeomin® and Azzalure®.

Botulinum Toxin Procedures: Step by Step

1. Initial Consultation: The first step is a consultation with a qualified aesthetic physician to evaluate the patient's suitability for botulinum toxin treatment.

The patient's medical history and aesthetic goals will be reviewed, and a detailed physical examination will be performed.

3. Injection: Botulinum toxin is injected into specific points on the face using very fine needles. The number and location of injections will depend on the area being treated and the patient's aesthetic goals.

4. Aftercare: It is recommended to avoid touching or rubbing the treated area for the first few hours after the injection. Keep your head upright for at least 4 hours, and avoid strenuous physical activity for the first 24 hours.

3. Local anesthetic: In some cases, a topical local anesthetic may be

applied to minimize discomfort during the injection.

2. Preparation: The treatment area is cleaned and disinfected. A topical local anesthetic may be applied if necessary.

4. Preservatives: Some products may contain preservatives to extend their shelf life.

2. Diluent: This is used to adjust the concentration of botulinum toxin to the patient's required dose. The most common diluent is sodium chloride (physiological salt).

Botulinum toxins are mainly used to treat:

* **Neck wrinkles:** Horizontal bands on the neck ("turkey neck").

* **Hyperhidrosis:** Excessive sweating in the armpits, hands and feet.

* **Expression wrinkles:** Horizontal lines on the forehead ("frown lines"), vertical lines between the eyes ("crow's feet"), lines around the mouth ("perioral lines").

Areas of application of botulinum toxins in aesthetics

2. Side effects: Side effects are generally mild and temporary and include injection site discomfort, redness, swelling, and bruising. In rare cases, more serious side effects may occur, such as drooping of the eyelid or difficulty swallowing.

3. Contraindications: Botulinum toxin treatment is not suitable for everyone. It is not recommended for pregnant or breastfeeding women, people with allergies to the product's components, or those with certain medical conditions.

4. Cost: The cost of botulinum toxin treatment may vary depending on the region, the doctor's experience, and the amount of product used.

In conclusion, botulinum toxins represent a valuable tool in the field of facial aesthetics, offering a noninvasive alternative to combat wrinkles and expression lines. However, it is essential to approach this treatment with knowledge and responsibility, consulting with a qualified medical professional to ensure your safety and obtain the best possible results.

Important considerations before treatment

1. Results: The results of botulinum toxin treatment typically last between 3 and 6 months. Maintenance treatments are required to maintain long-term results.

2. Safety: Botulinum toxins are safe when administered by a qualified medical professional and following established guidelines.

* **Migraine:** Prevention of chronic migraine episodes.

A Journey to Youth: Exploring the World of Facelifts

Among them, facelifts have become a popular option to combat the visible signs of aging and rediscover the In the tireless pursuit of eternal youth, cosmetic procedures have gained a prominent place in today's society.

LIFTING

A facelift, also known as a facial lift, is a surgical procedure designed to **rejuvenate the face** by removing excess skin and tightening facial muscles. This procedure addresses sagging skin and wrinkles, especially those that occur on the forehead, cheeks, neck, and jawline.

Types of facelifts:

1. Full Facelift: This is the most extensive procedure and covers the entire face, from the forehead to the neck. Deep wrinkles are eliminated, the skin is tightened, and facial muscles are repositioned for overall rejuvenation.

2. Forehead Lift: Focuses on the upper part of the face, addressing horizontal forehead wrinkles, drooping eyebrows, and a droopy upper eyelid.

What are the different types and what results can be expected?

There are several types of facelifts, each with its own characteristics and specific objectives:

What is a facelift?

facial vitality. But what exactly are facelifts?

4. Cheek Lift: Combats sagging cheeks and nasolabial bags, restoring volume and definition to the central face.

6. Mini facelift: It is a less invasive version of the full facelift, ideal for patients with moderate signs of aging.

7. Liquid Lift: It is not a surgical procedure, but a rejuvenation technique that uses facial fillers to redefine the contour of the face and reduce wrinkles.

5. Neck Lift: Addresses sagging, loose skin on the neck, eliminating horizontal wrinkles and redefining the neck contour.

3. Brow lift: Lifts drooping eyebrows and opens the gaze, rejuvenating the upper part of the face.

Considerations to keep in mind:

Before opting for a facelift, it's crucial to consult with a board-certified plastic surgeon to evaluate your case and determine if this procedure is right for you. Factors such as your overall health, lifestyle habits, and realistic expectations should be considered.

Additional recommendations:

* **Lead a healthy lifestyle:** A balanced diet, regular exercise, and adequate sun protection are key to maintaining healthy skin and delaying the signs of aging.

Recovery is usually an outpatient procedure and requires special care in the first few days, such as rest, cold compresses, and medication. The final results are gradually seen over the weeks following the procedure, revealing a more youthful and smoother face.

It's important to note that facelifts are not a permanent solution to aging. Over time, your skin will continue its natural aging process, so the results may last for several years, but they are not permanent.

The facelift procedure is performed under general or local anesthesia in an operating room. The duration varies depending on the type of facelift, but generally ranges from 2 to 4 hours.

Procedure and recovery:

Surgeon's instructions during recovery are critical to achieving the best results.

In conclusion, we affirm that facelifts offer an effective alternative to combat the visible signs of aging and rediscover the vitality of the face. However, it is crucial to approach them with information, responsibility, and realistic expectations to achieve a satisfactory experience and lasting results. Remember that beauty tips.

* **Realistic Expectations:** It is important to have realistic expectations about the procedure and understand that results may vary for each individual.

POSTOPERATIVE CARE: METICULOUSLY FOLLOW THE FACIAL IMPLANTS

In the dynamic and fascinating world of facial aesthetics, implants have emerged as a revolutionary tool, challenging the boundaries of natural beauty and offering patients the opportunity to sculpt their features in a personalized way. Join us on a journey to discover the secrets of these procedures, exploring their types, applications, benefits, and important considerations.

1. Permanent facial implants:

* **Chin implants:** Designed to increase the projection and definition of the chin, creating a more balanced facial profile.

Redefining Facial Aesthetics: A Dive into the World of Beauty

Types of Facial Implants:

FACIAL IMPLANTS resides in inner and outer harmony, and that youth is not defined solely by physical appearance.

* **Nasolabial groove implants:** Reduce the appearance of deep expression lines that form around the nose and mouth.

* **Facial fillers:** Injectable substances such as hyaluronic acid or polycaprolactone that are used to fill wrinkles, furrows and fine lines, restoring youth and radiance to the face.

* **Tightening threads:** Their function is to tighten the skin of the face and neck, combating sagging and improving facial definition.

2. Resorbable facial implants:

* **Cheek implants:** Add volume and definition to the cheekbones, rejuvenating the face and enhancing its features.

Applications of Facial Implants:

* **Fill in furrows and fine lines:** Reduce the appearance of wrinkles, expression lines and nasolabial folds.

* **Facial rejuvenation:** Restore youth and vitality to the face, combating sagging and improving skin texture.

Benefits of Facial Implants:

Facial implants provide a number of benefits to patients, including:

* **Cheekbone, chin and lip augmentation:** To create a more harmonious and defined face.

* **Defining facial features:** Emphasize and define features such as cheekbones, chin, and jawline.

* **Correction of facial asymmetries:** Balance facial proportions and correct congenital or acquired asymmetries.

Facial implants offer a wide range of applications to improve facial aesthetics, including:

* **Minimally invasive:** Most procedures are outpatient and minimally invasive, with a quick recovery.

* **Improved self-esteem:** Satisfactory results can improve self-confidence and self-esteem.

Important Considerations:

* **Customized Results:** Implants are tailored to each patient's specific needs and desires.

* **Long-lasting results:** Permanent implants offer long-term results, while resorbable implants provide temporary improvements that can be repeated.

1. Consultation with a specialist: It is essential to consult with a board- certified plastic surgeon or dermatologist to determine if facial implants are right for you and to discuss your expectations and goals.

2. Follow-up and maintenance: It is important to follow the specialist's recommendations to ensure proper healing and long-term care of the implants.

In conclusion, facial implants have become an invaluable tool in the field of aesthetics, offering patients the opportunity to redefine their features, improve their appearance, and boost their self-esteem. However, it is crucial to approach these procedures with caution, consulting with a qualified specialist to ensure optimal results and a satisfactory experience.

FACELIFT THREADS

Rejuvenating the Face with Minimally Invasiveness: A Look at the

1. Natural results: An experienced surgeon will be able to achieve natural

and harmonious results that adapt to the patient's facial anatomy.

Facelift threads

3. Procedure and recovery: Procedures are performed under local or general anesthesia, depending on the complexity. Recovery is usually quick, with minimal discomfort.

2. Selecting the right implant: The type of implant used will depend on the area to be treated, the desired result, and the patient's lifestyle.

What are facelift threads?

Facelift threads are medical devices implanted under the skin to lift, tighten, and reposition sagging facial tissue. These threads are made from biocompatible and absorbable materials, such as polydioxane or polycaprolactone, ensuring their safety and adaptability to the body.

In the dynamic world of aesthetics, the quest for youth and facial harmony has driven the development of increasingly less invasive techniques with more natural results. Among these alternatives, facelift threads have gained a prominent place, offering an effective solution to combat sagging skin and reverse the signs of aging.

* **Anchor threads:** Designed to fix and reposition deep structures of the face, such as muscles and ligaments, providing a long-lasting tightening effect.

* **Collagen-stimulating threads:** They promote the natural production of collagen in the skin, improving its elasticity and combating sagging in the long term.

Facelift thread implantation is an outpatient procedure typically performed under local anesthesia. The procedure typically takes between 30 minutes and an hour, depending on the complexity of the treatment and the area being treated.

General steps:

* **Suspension threads:** Their main function is to lift and tighten sagging facial tissues, such as cheeks, cheekbones, eyebrows and facial oval.

Thread implantation procedure:

There are several types of facelift threads, each with specific characteristics and applications:

Types of facelift threads:

2. **Marking points:** The doctor marks strategic points on the face where the threads will be placed.

4. **Thread insertion:** Threads are inserted under the skin using very fine needles, following a specific pattern to achieve the desired effect.

5. **Anchoring and tensioning:** The threads are anchored at attachment points and carefully tensioned to achieve the lifting effect.

3. **Anesthesia:** Local anesthesia is applied to minimize discomfort.

1. **Cleaning and preparation:** The area to be treated is cleaned and disinfected.

6. **Completion:** A light bandage or compression is applied to the treated area.

* They are patients with good general health.

Facelift threads are an excellent option for patients who:

What are the benefits of facelift threads?

* They present mild to moderate sagging in different areas of the face.

Facelift threads offer several advantages over other facial rejuvenation methods:

* They are looking for a natural and minimally invasive facial rejuvenation.

* **Versatility:** They can be used in different areas of the face, such as cheeks, cheekbones, eyebrows, facial oval, neck and neckline.

* Avoid intense physical activities during the first few days.

Who are facelift threads indicated for?

* Do not touch or rub the treated area.

* **Quick recovery:** Patients can return to their usual activities in a short period of time, usually the day after the procedure.

What is the post-procedure care?

* **Long-lasting effects:** Facelift threads provide long-lasting results that can range from 1 to 2 years, depending on the type of thread used and the patient's habits.

It's important to follow your doctor's recommendations to optimize results and minimize the possibility of complications. Some general precautions include:

* **Minimally invasive:** The procedure requires no incisions or sutures, minimizing recovery time and the risk of complications.

* They want to avoid more complex surgical procedures.

* **Natural results:** The threads achieve a subtle and natural lifting effect, improving facial harmony without altering the natural expression of the face.

Follow a healthy diet and stay properly hydrated.

In conclusion, facelift threads have become an effective and popular tool in the field of facial aesthetics, offering a safe and minimally invasive alternative to combat sagging skin and reverse the signs of aging. If you are considering this treatment, it is important to consult with a physician specializing in aesthetic medicine for a personalized evaluation to determine if this technique is right for your needs.

Botulinum toxin is another biological medication used in aesthetic and dermatological clinics that has gained a certain degree of approval among its users and has been shown to be suitable for injection under the skin of the face with wrinkles, which are a clear sign of aging after the age of 40. It is a simple procedure with a quick recovery time of just a couple of weeks. However, its use can cause moderate, but not serious, side effects in some patients.

Unlike hyaluronic acid, which fills the channels between skin cells with collagen, Botox is a muscle relaxant that temporarily paralyzes the muscles. Its effects last four to six months.

* Avoid direct sun exposure.

* Sleep on your back for the first week.

ACNE

Side effects include pain and bruising in the treated area, difficulty swallowing, drooping eyelids, throat irritation, cough, and rhinitis. In these cases, a few drops may be recommended, along with avoiding excessive alcohol and eating a natural diet. According to the beauty salon, the price of a botulinum injection session for wrinkles around the eyes is around $250 or €250, while those for cheekbones and the mouth area can be $200 or €200. Dermatology nurses are authorized to perform this procedure.

In grades III and IV, pimples that have become inflamed or infected, such as pustules, nodules, and cysts, can often cause pain.

Lesions can be grade III (pustules and nodules) or grade IV (nodules and cysts). These are deeper lesions, develop much more slowly, and leave significant scarring when they disappear.

Comedonal acne is a type of acne in which the predominant lesions are open comedones (blackheads) and closed comedones (pimples). Inflammatory acne, the appearance of redder, more painful "bumps" is known as papules, or nodules if they are deeper.

There are several etiological factors related to the appearance of acne, ranging from genetic and hereditary factors, healthy eating habits, psychological and emotional states, significant hormonal changes such as those that occur during pregnancy and menstruation, certain medications, and the improper use of some cosmetics.

Its appearance in the outermost layer of the skin has shown that in comedones, this microorganism secretes chemotactic factors and possesses chemotactic activity. This attracts polymorphonuclear leukocytes, which, upon entering the follicle, can phagocytose P. acnes and trigger the release of hydrolytic enzymes.

Acne is an inflammatory disease, caused by multiple factors, that affects the sebum-producing glands located on the face, back, chest, shoulders, and even the upper arms.

As we see in our following chart, these can be grade I, also called comedones and papules, or grade II, which present papules and pustules like deep acne. Here, acne is mild or moderate, where the patient may have oily skin and pimples, which appear as whiteheads or blackheads on the face, back, or chest. Most pimples will not cause any other symptoms.

In Facial Aesthetics, we often encounter patients suffering from acne, which in dermatology refers to an inflammatory disease of the pilosebaceous unit. It is one of the most common dermatological pathologies, affecting almost 80% of adolescents between the ages of 13 and 18.

Avoid excessively fatty foods, leave it for one day at a time

- If there is excess sebum and too many dead skin cells, pores become clogged. Bacteria (especially the Propionibacterium acnes species) can then become trapped inside the pores and multiply, causing the skin to swell and redden—the beginning of acne.

Another factor that can influence the appearance of acne is the foods that cause acne due to their composition. Foods that cause pimples are primarily foods rich in sugar and fat, such as chocolate, dressings, fatty meats, fried foods, sausages, fast foods, frozen ready meals, and excessive consumption of bread, cookies, candy, sweets, milk, and yellow cheeses, mild soap made specifically for people with acne.

Avoid touching your face with your hands or resting it on objects that tend to accumulate sebum and skin residue, such as the telephone receiver.

Depending on the degree of severity on the skin, the main acne lesions are:

To treat these papules and eliminate acne from the face, you should follow some tips such as:

• Do not pop the beans while they are ripening or drying.

Nodules: more advanced lesions, larger and located deeper in the dermis.

Wash your face twice a day (no more) with warm water and a whitish or yellowish in color.

• For medication, consult a dermatologist who will prescribe antibiotics that can help alleviate the effects of acne:

• Oral antibiotics (taken by mouth) such as tetracycline, doxycycline, minocycline, erythromycin, trimethoprim, sulfamethoxazole, and amoxicillin.

Papules: Red, swollen lesions due to inflammation.

Change your pillowcase regularly.

• Pustules: lesions filled with purulent material, containing pus

• Topical antibiotics (applied to the skin) such as clindamycin, erythromycin, or dapsone.

INTERNATIONAL NOMENCLATURE OF COSMETIC INGREDIENTS

The manufacture of has an international body to ensure that the ingredients that are used or patented comply with the proven approaches for the health of the general public and repeat customers of spa and aesthetic clinics.

Known as the International Nomenclature of Cosmetic Ingredients or INCI, for its acronym in English: International Nomenclature of Cosmetic Ingredients, is a naming system. This list includes waxes, oils, pigments, chemicals, and other ingredients in soaps, cosmetics, among others, based on scientific names and in other languages, such as Latin and English. INCI names often differ from IUPAC systematic names or common references. The language used is English, to name most cosmetic ingredients, in the INCI nomenclature. As the official list indicates, the universal name must appear on the labels of cosmetic products in most countries. Initially, the CTFA (USA) names were used.

The INCI names of the ingredients are the Latin binomial names of genus and species, in the USA the common name known to consumers in that country is also placed in parentheses. In the United States, under the "Food, Drug, and Cosmetic Act and the Fair Packaging and Labeling Acta, certain information is required to appear on the of the cosmetic industry. In Canada, the regulatory standard follows the "Guideline is the Cosmetic Regulations". Ingredient names must meet these requirements using INCI names. In Venezuela, the nomenclature of chemical compounds is regulated by the Ministry of Popular Power for Health and Social Protection, while the quality control in labels and nomenclature of products must be approved by the National Autonomous Service of Standardization, Quality, Metrology and Technical Regulations. The nomenclature, with exceptions, obeys the IUPAC, and secondly, standards based on the INCL In Spain, the Spanish Agency for Medicines and Health Products, on its public page the list of INCI names.

Microdermabrasion

Among the cosmetology therapies we find dermabrasion, which is a skin exfoliation procedure that is based on the application of a device that rotates rapidly to refine the outer layers of the skin. This technique was developed in Europe and the device is designed with painless diamond tips, softening the blackheads of the pores allowing their extraction to be easier.

EFFECTS.

Among its effects, it reduces the hyperpigmegtation or coloration of the skin with spots or Other imperfections. A side effect of this therapy is the burning reaction, redness and swelling of the treated skin, but this indicates the beginning of another cycle of skin cell replacement with a more youthful and smoother result. An evolved term that allowed the advancement in the first devices is Microdermabrasion, which is an appropriate method to stimulate at a microscopic or very small level, it is a non-invasive aesthetic procedure that removes the superficial layers of the skin. The result obtained is similar to the softest peels, so the patient can return to their activities immediately. Its main purpose is to stimulate renewal in a natural way, helping to eliminate scars and reduce wrinkles in a suitable session plan once every 0 to 15 days, depending on the patient's condition, the tolerance of their skin type, preferably not very sensitive or mixed.

The characteristic of this procedure is the degree of depth of the skin layers to which it can reach as the epidermis, but even the dermis; which is the middle layer. The skin consists of a protective outer layer (epidermis) and an inner layer of living tissue (dermis). The upper part of the epidermis is made up of dead cells that contain keratin, the corneal scleroprotein that also makes up hair and nails.

To achieve hair regeneration, collagen production is increased by applying a gel based on this substance that will restore elasticity to the skin.

CHAPTER 4 BODY TREATMENTS

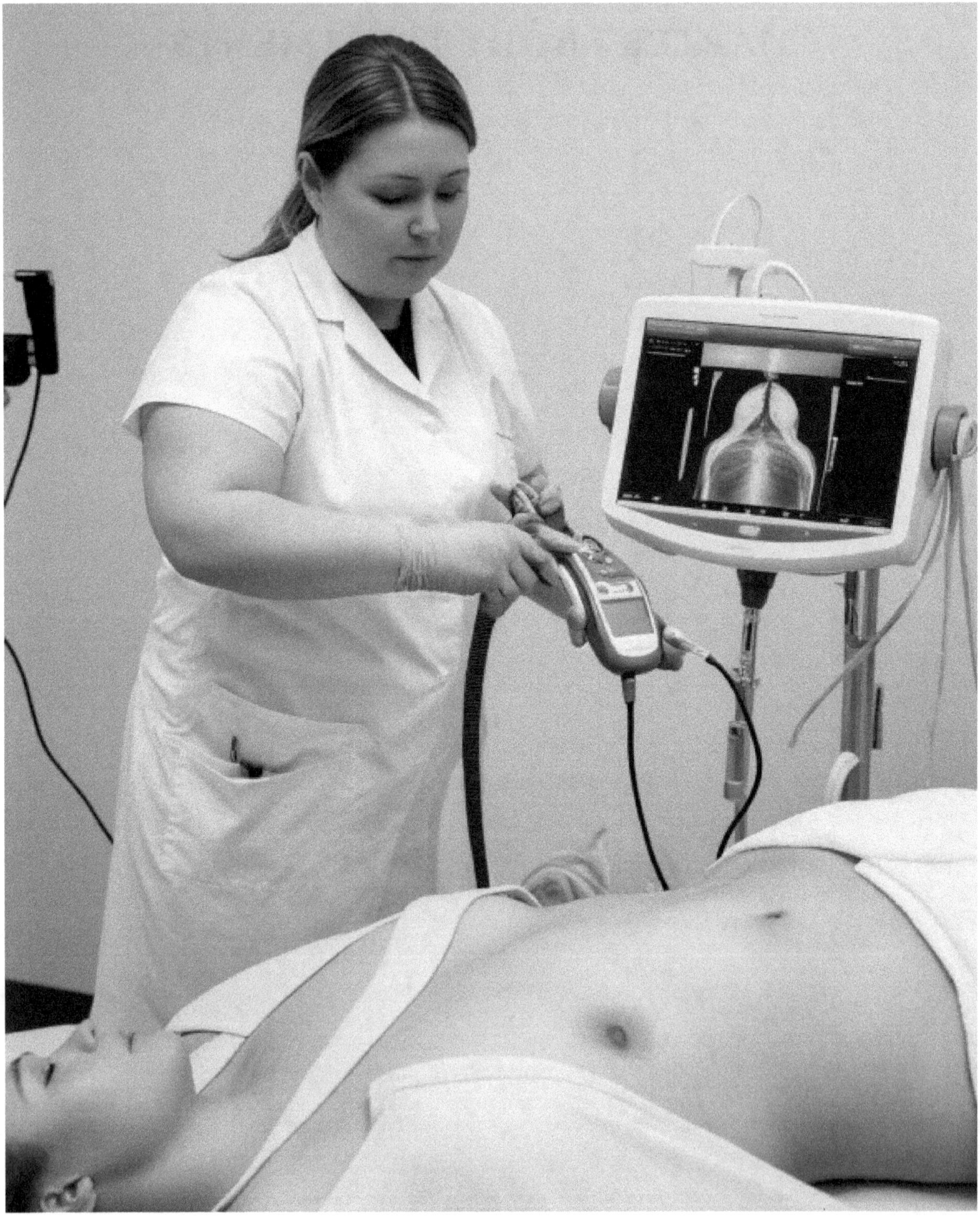

TYPES OF BED POSITIONS

For the esthetician, the treatment protocol consists of a series of stages: skin examination, skin preparation (hygiene, special peeling, and steam bath), a core treatment based on the application of slimming and lipolytic cosmetics, or the application of techniques such as ultrasound and slimming massage with drainage maneuvers. In this chapter, we will break down each of these for better understanding. In massage therapy, there are three supine positions, each of which establishes several support points or areas of the body where we will work specific muscles and bones according to the natural blood pressure of the circulatory system. Their use refers to the application of aesthetic massages, physical therapy, surgery, and hospital stays in nursing. The term "decubitus" derives from the Latin word "decumbere," which means to lie down, to recline, to lie down. There are three basic positions, so to speak, that primarily influence the fixed points of each individual's circulatory system and their specific ailments. They are part of the theory of body mechanics, which studies the balance and movement of bodies applied to human beings and is conceptualized as the discipline that deals with the proper functioning of the musculoskeletal system in coordination with the nervous and circulatory systems.

- Supine or dorsal decubitus: This type of decubitus where the patient lies face up, lying on their back.

- Lateral decubitus: This can be divided into right lateral decubitus or left lateral decubitus, and refers to the massage therapist's or esthetician's intention to work on a specific area, taking into account the organs. In physical therapy, it also refers to pain or a therapy applied to rehabilitate a patient's mobility, circulation, and stability.

- Prone or Ventral Position: In this position, the patient lies face down, resting on the ventral wall and abdomen. Therefore, the stretcher used must have a special opening for the face and breathing.

After the COVID-19 pandemic, the prone position became popular as a medical recommendation made by an Italian doctor for patients hospitalized in intensive care units.

In addition to these positions, horizontal surface inclinations are also used in nursing and medical practice:

- Inclined Decline Position: Also known as the Trendelenburg position with the patient's feet pointing upwards, this position is used in respiratory physiotherapy. The bed maintains a central axis, and the patient is strapped in by each limb, thus encouraging the return of venous blood to the heart through the inferior vena cava.

● Prone Reclining Position: In this position, the patient remains with their head up and their feet down.

Other accepted positions during hospitalization include the antishock position, a variation of the reverse Trendelenburg position where the patient raises their legs parallel to each other for a reasonable period of time, while the rest of the body, up to the head, remains down.

FOUR-HAND MASSAGE

A Sensory Journey: Exploring the Charm of Four-Hand Massage

In the realm of wellness and relaxation, four-hand massages stand as a unique sensory experience. Unlike traditional massages, where a single therapist works on the body, this technique involves two expert practitioners who synchronize their movements to offer a doubly pleasurable and therapeutic experience.

Origin and History: A Legacy of Wellness

The origins of four-hand massages date back to ancient Eastern cultures, where the practice of massage was considered a healing and revitalizing art. In Thailand, for example, traditional Thai massage, also known as "Nuad Phrommathep," could be performed by two or more therapists at the same time, who would combine their movements to stimulate the body's vital energy.

In the West, the popularity of four-hand massages began to surge in the late 20th century, driven by the growing demand for deeper and more personalized wellness experiences. Since then, this technique has gained followers around the world, positioning itself as an incomparable luxury and relaxation option.

Procedures and Techniques: A Synchronized Dance of Hands

Four-hand massages are characterized by the synchronization and coordination of two therapists working in unison on the client's body. Each therapist focuses on a specific body part, utilizing a variety of massage techniques such as:

* **Efflorescence:** Gentle, long strokes to stimulate blood and lymphatic circulation.

* **Petrissage:** Deep kneading to release muscle tension.

* **Friction:** Firm, targeted strokes to treat contractures and trigger points.

* **Percussion:** Rhythmic tapping to stimulate circulation and vitality.

* **Vibration:** Vibrating movements to relax and release stress.

Throughout the massage, therapists alternate roles and adapt their techniques to the client's specific needs, creating a fluid and personalized experience. Constant communication between therapists is crucial to maintain synchronization and ensure a safe and pleasurable experience.

Benefits for Body and Soul: A Symphony of Well-being

Four-hand massages offer a wide range of benefits for the body and soul, including:

* Physical: Relief of pain and muscle tension: The combination of techniques and pressure applied by two therapists simultaneously helps release deep-rooted muscle tension, relieving pain and improving flexibility.

* Improved blood and lymphatic circulation: Synchronized movements stimulate blood and lymphatic circulation, helping to eliminate toxins and oxygenate tissues.

* **Reduction of stress and anxiety:** The release of endorphins and deep muscle relaxation contribute to reducing stress, anxiety, and cortisol levels.

** * **Improved Sleep:** Four-hand massage can help regulate sleep patterns and promote deeper, more restful rest.

Emotional:

* **Sense of Well-being and Harmony:** The immersive sensory experience and synchronized movements generate a feeling of deep peace and well-being.

* **Release of Negative Emotions:** Four-hand massage can help release trapped emotions in the body, promoting emotional catharsis.

* **Strengthening the Emotional Bond:** The shared experience between the client and the two therapists can strengthen the emotional bond and trust.

Considerations and Tips: A Mindful Experience

To make the most of the benefits of four-hand massage, it is important to consider a few aspects:

* **Communicate Needs and Preferences:** Before beginning the massage, it is essential to inform the therapist of any physical condition or personal preferences to ensure a safe and enjoyable experience.

* **Choose a trusted massage center:** It is advisable to look for a massage center with certified and experienced professionals in the four-hand massage technique.

* **Create a relaxing environment:** A calm and quiet environment, with dim lighting and soft music, will contribute to the relaxation experience.

* **Let yourself be carried away by the experience:** It is important to relax, disconnect from the outside world, and allow yourself to be transported by the synchronized movements and the feeling of well-being generated by the four-hand massage.

A Magic Touch: A Gift for Body and Soul

Four-hand massages represent a unique and incomparable wellness experience. The synchronization of two expert therapists, the variety of techniques, and the depth.

BODY MASSAGE PROTOCOL

Among the oldest forms of therapy known to man are massage and somatotherapy. Its origins are in the East, but today it is widely used in the West Oriental massage is designed to relieve tiredness, heaviness, stiff shoulders, and headaches. It takes care of the nerves, joints, muscles and the endocrine system. Among the most important benefits of massage maneuvers there are numerous effects such as the activation of important physical and biochemical reactions. Stimulates the metabolism with reactivation, general toning of the skin. with these, the formation of keratin is stimulated thanks to the attention to the nutritional conditions and the elimination of cellular debris. Better stimulation and oxygenation of the tissues is also promoted.

The most suitable massage maneuvers are the following:

• Effleurage: It is the route of the body; it consists of Slow movements and light frictions made with the palms of the hands, semi-flexed according to the part to be massaged. The contact must be felt with the entire palm of the esthetician hand.

• Friction: It consists of passing the open hand with the fingers together. On the surface to work we apply strong pressure, with energy to produce color in the area. Frictions can be made in different directions.

• Kneading: It is applicable to regions of muscle mass, it aims to tighten deep tissues. This maneuver favors the supply of blood, improves venous protection, thus freeing the muscles from deep tensions.

• Percussion: It is a more stimulating movement that consists of a series of repeated, rhythmic or slower strokes that produce immense stimulation, accelerating its vitality, while its circulation increases the speed of the venous current.

• Vibration: It is practiced with the tips of the fingers with the palms of the hands; the skin receives rapid and continuous shaking which tones up its general condition.

• Pressure: It is done with the fingertips on the different points to be treated. It causes a better b" potency to the muscle fiber. Pinching: It consists of pinching the skin, we take the skin between the thumb and the Other fingers. It is usually done on the back of back and legs.

• Rotation: They are applied with both hands making a movement of the muscle mass, on the axis of the hole, they are loose and natural movements on the body circulations.

• Knuckle: Manipulation performed with the thumb and the knuckles of 4 fingers, flexing each knuckle. A small circle is made, it is worked deeply and its purpose is to relax the muscles, it also helps to eliminate adipose tissues, such as cellulite.

• Typing: It is done with the tips of the fingers slightly curved and quickly, one finger after the Other. It is a widely used maneuver in facial treatment.

ANTI-CELLULITE AND REDUCING COSMETICS

This topic specifically deals with the protocols of body treatments for alterations of the subcutaneous and connective tissue, such as localized obesity and cellulite. In the case of localized obesity, its external signs are manifested in the buttocks, abdomen, extremities with an excessive accumulation of adipose tissue and its causes are genetic factors, hormonal alterations and psychological factors of woman. On the other hand, cellulite is defined as an alteration of the connective tissue where two fundamental phenomena occur: viscosity of fundamental substance and hypertrophy of adipose cells where the skin becomes soft and spongy to the touch.

There are three types of cellulite: hard where there are undulations of the tissue and there is pain when pressing, soft cellulite is the one that becomes spongy to the touch, and edematous cellulitis which is common together with circulatory disorders where there is sometimes edema influenced by mechanical and vascular factors.

The fatty subcutaneous tissue plays an essential role in lipid metabolism. Any alteration in this lipid reserve, either by excess or by defect must be treated from a medical point of view. A person is considered overweight when they exceed the desirable weight by more than 10%, and obese if they exceed 20% of that desirable. The cutaneous needs in the treatment of obesity are based on reducing the accumulation of localized adipose tissue and favoring lymphatic circulation and venous return

Anti-cellulite cosmetics combines different active principles fundamentally associated with three types of actiom lipolytic, venotonic and depolymerization. In the event that cellulite is edematous, an attempt Will be made to improve microcirculation, for which anti-cellulite cosmetics that contain antiedematous venotonic substances in their formulation such as ruscus, horsetail, horse chestnut, arnica and guraná will be applied. In cellulite with localized fat accumulation, cosmetics with lipolytic action such as L-carnitine, protein and iodinated derivatives are used mainly.

In the case of reducing cosmetics, they base their action on lipolytic active principles whose function is to mobilize the lipids of the skin tissue. They also contain venotonic and antiedematous substances that promote vascular permeability and the mobilization of excess fluids. The reducing cosmetics are applied with active and deep massages that favor the mobilization of fat. Occlusive techniques favor the penetration of reducing cosmetics and favor the elimination of liquids.

FACIAL MASSAGE PROTOCOL

The set of tasks for the performance and care of a facial massage treatment are as follows.

1. Apply moisturizer all over the face.
2. Perform circular movement, from the neck we Will make the circular movements and go up towards the area behind the ears.
3. Then with the fingers we make a stretch towards the chin area.
4. On the chin we make circular movements and stretch.
5. Then in the buccinator muscle of the lips we place the fingers from side to side, one above and the Other below, and stretch. Then do circular friction and stretch again.
6. Placing the four fingers on the masseter muscle, make circular movements up to three repetitions and stretch.
7. Place the thumb at the level of the Wing of the nose, make a circular motion and stretch up to the superciliary muscle on the opposite side.
8. Before going up, make a zigzag along the Maso-Genian line and stretch with the Other hand.
9. Then work the eyes from the outer corner to the inner, passing through the nostrils, between the eyebrows and the temple.
10. Then make circular movements again with the four fingers at the level of the Wing of the nose and stretch towards the opposite muscle until reaching the superciliary.
11. After the external corner to the internal one passed through the nostrils, between the eyebrows and the temple.
12. Then we zigzag at the level of the periorbital wrinkles, we stretch towards the Wing of the nose, three downwards and three upwards, covering the entire orbicularis oculi muscle, always from the external to internal commissure. This step serves to restore the collagen in that area.
13. Perform zigzag friction in the area of the forehead where the lines of expression are marked.

Also with the ring finger we pass a line for what are expression lines.

14. At the end one makes the hands interlock in the chin area, raises them by turning the hand downwards and raises again. This step stretches the skin muscles of neck, all the muscles of chin. It is done very slowly.
15. The face should not be left with residues, it should be moisturized but not shiny.

The steps to be followed by the beautician in case a deep facial or makeup removal is necessary, are the following:

1. Remove make-up from the patient's eyes and lips.
2. Apply cleansing milk to the rest of the face.
3. Tone up by applying astringent.
4. Exfoliate.
5. We apply ozone steam for 10 to 15 minutes.
6. We perform the extraction of comedones on the client's face.
7. Tone with rose water and dry skin.
8. A gauze to cover the face.
9. We apply high frequency, place for 10 to 15 minutes.
10. We apply a soothing or moisturizing mask and leave it for 20 minutes.
11. We perform a facial massage either with aromatherapy oils or a moisturizing and nourishing cream.
12. We apply sunscreen.

BODY MASSAGE PROTOCOL

The massage can be practiced with the patient lying on the floor or on a table. The surface on which the person lies should be neither too soft nor too hard.

Once the massage is given, and also before practicing it, it is a good measure to cover the parts of the clients body that have been treated or that are going to be massaged to avoid an unpleasant sensation, in a room with a comfortable temperature.

When the subject is prone and has an arched back, place a cushion under the knees. If, on the other hand, it is in the prone position, it will be fine to place it under the abdomen.

The use of some kind of ointment, which can be scented with different natural essences such as pine, mint, eucalyptus, lemon, orange favors the fluidity of the movements.

Before practicing a massage it is necessary to warm your hands if they are cold, remember that you must match your breathing to that of the patient and that you must always keep your hands in contact with the other's body. The pressure should come more from the masseur's weight than from his strength.

When a part of the right side of the body such as a leg or an arm is massaged, it is advisable to also massage the same part on the Other side, since the sensation that the patient perceives must be unity and globalist.

Avoid jumping continuously from one area to another, rather try to proceed with fluid and continuous movements. Repeat the route several times trying to provide small but pleasant variations from time to time.

When you are giving a massage you do not have to think about anything else, initially it is the technique that supports the task, but then this will have to be relegated to oblivion little by little if you want to achieve a true loving contact.

Avoid massaging and massage if you have little time to practice or receive a truly effective body massage, it is essential to have at least 30 to 40 minutes.

RADIO FREQUENCY PROTOCOL

They are electromagnetic radiation that oscillate simultaneously in the electric and magnetic field, although it is a system of therapeutic use known in surgery for many years. Radio frequency generates an electric field that changes from positive to negative, which causes a rotational movement of the molecules that generate heat. The two types of radio frequency used are bipolar; that causes a superficial heating of the skin, and the unipolar that causes a heating of the deepest part of the dermis acting on the adipose tissue. Since the radiofrequency device has both unipolar and bipolar heads, we can deliver the energy to different depths and thus treat different types of cellulite and also facial laxity and Other areas.

Among the benefits of radiofrequency, it produces a deep heating that affects the skin and subcutaneous fatty tissue, a heating that goes from the inside out, which Will favor lymphatic drainage which allows to reduce fluids and toxins, increases the circulation of the area which allows to improve the metabolism, both of the subcutaneous fatty tissue and the general appearance of the skin. It also promotes the formation of new collagen, allowing all the tissue to acquire firmness thanks to the reorganization of the fibrous septa. And finally, after the controlled thermal injury with tissue retraction, there is an inflammatory response that Will be accompanied by fibroblast migration, which Will further reinforce the collagen structure, resulting in rejuvenation of the treated area. The immediate effect of radiofrequency is the retraction of collagen.

It is recommended to take into account contraindications such as pregnancy, people with metal prostheses, patients with heart disease and tissue diseases such as cancer and people who are overweight.

The radiofrequency treatment protocol is as follows:

1. Prepare the area and the client.
2. We divide the abdomen into quadrants.
3. We work per section for 5 to 7 minutes.
4. We use a lot of conductive gel in each area.
5. We apply radio frequency in constant circles.
6. Remove the conductive gel with a paper towel.
7. We use soothing gel to finish.

CAVITATION PROTOCOL

It consists of a treatment in which small bubbles are generated in a controlled way that destroy the fat cells without damaging the blood system, all through a device, which works thanks to the cavitation gel with which circular movements are made. In this way, we achieve that the fat found in different areas of our body is transformed into a liquid state and thus is eliminated from our body through the urinary tract. They can produce small bruises or hematomas, this because of the infiltration that occurs in the treatment. It is applied with duration of 60 minutes in 10 sessions once a week.

The benefits bring magnificent results without the need for surgery without the need for sick leave. On the other hand, it reaffirms itself activating cells that give rise to the creation of new cells that do not have fat, with greater elasticity, eliminating unwanted cellulite.

Contraindications

in this treatment are overweight, autoimmune diseases, auditory pathologies, patients with liver or kidney problems, as well as pregnancy and lactation. Others are people with pacemakers and acute skin lesions.

The steps to follow as a treatment protocol are:

1. Prepare the area and the clients
2. Divide the abdomen into quadrants.
3. We work each zone for 10 to 8 minutes.
4. Apply conductive gel to each area in a generous amount.
5. We place the cavitation at about 90 degrees from the skin.
6. We help each Other with a towel.
7. We remove with a paper towel.

REDUCING MASSAGE PROTOCOL

The steps to follow as a reducing treatment protocol are:

1. Prepare the work area.
2. Weigh the patient and take his measurements in the area to be reduced.
3. Massage with orange oil.
4. Use passive gymnastics using the positive and negative electrodes.
5. Leave to act for a period of 20 to 30 minutes.
6. Clean the worked area.
7. To finish we apply the firming cold gel.

THERMOTHERAPY

It is an application of heat for therapeutic purposes. There are several ways to apply this heat and generally that is sought is a sedative and relaxing effect. This technique uses different forms of heat as treatment, whether in solid, semi-liquid or gaseous form. For it to be considered as thermotherapy it is necessary that the temperature is higher than the physiological one the organism has. As for the maximum temperature, it depends on the thermal sensitivity of the patient. It is applied for a period between 10 to 30 minutes.

Among the benefits of thermotherapy is that it stimulates the circulation of vitamins and oxygen in the tissue, thanks to an improvement in blood supply. In addition, the pores of the skin open and allow the detoxification of the tissues. The increase in temperature helps to promote the elimination of localized fat in the abdomen. It allows improving the contour and promotes an increase in metabolism. Also the contraindications to this treatment, no significant side effects are mentioned. But some care must be taken into account when the area to be treated is inflamed and in case of malignant processes or tumors.

VACCINATION THERAPY

Vaccination therapy is a deep massage technique that is used together with a high-tech device that, through a suction system and two rollers, pulls the skin and stimulates blood and lymphatic circulation in its depth. To obtain expected results, a minimum number of sessions ranging between 10 and 20, twice a week is necessary and the total duration of the treatment is variable depending on the area to be treated. Each session with a duration of 25 to 30 minutes in small areas such as the face, arm, abdomen for 45 to 60 minutes. It is in larger areas such as trochanters (cartridge belts) and for comprehensive treatments from 90 minutes.

The benefits of this treatment are that with these cutaneous gymnastics, it restructures the connective tissue, facilitates the elimination of toxins and liquids, and improves the appearance of orange-type skin by increasing local micro-circulation. It also allows to restore the tone of the tissue of the whole body. The treatment applied to the face also helps to reduce wrinkles and reduce localized volumes, naturally toning the tissues. In addition to its use in case of cellulite, it is a complement to liposculpture. Finally, its contraindications refer to people in case of pregnancy, type 1 and 2 diabetes, in coagulation problems and cancer. It is also avoided in case of hernias and you know if they are suffering from a feverish state.

ULTRASOUND THERAPY

Exploring the Body: A Guided Journey Through Ultrasound and Sonography

In the vast universe of medicine, ultrasound and sonography stand as indispensable tools for exploring the interior of the human body. While these techniques share the same physical principles, they differ in their applications and objectives. Join us on a journey to discover the secrets hidden by this dynamic duo in the medical and aesthetic fields.

Delving into Sound: What is Ultrasound and Sonography?

Ultrasound: Ultrasound, also known as diagnostic ultrasound, is a technique that uses high-frequency sound waves to generate real-time images of the interior of the body. These waves bounce off tissues and organs, creating echoes that are captured and processed by a device called a sonogram. The resulting images, known as sonograms, provide valuable information about the structure, movement, and function of different parts of the body.

Ultrasound: Ultrasound, on the other hand, is a more general term that encompasses both sonography and other applications of high-frequency sound waves, such as ultrasound therapy or ultrasonic cleaning. In a medical context, the term "ultrasound" is often used interchangeably with "sonography," although technically it refers to the physical phenomenon itself.

An Arsenal of Uses in the Medical Field

Ultrasound, with its ability to visualize the interior of the body without radiation, has become an essential tool in various fields of medicine:

Obstetrics and Gynecology: Ultrasound is essential for monitoring pregnancy, allowing the developing fetus to be viewed, assessing its growth, and detecting possible abnormalities. It is also used to diagnose gynecological conditions such as ovarian cysts, uterine fibroids, or ectopic pregnancies.

Cardiology: Echocardiography provides detailed information about the heart, its valves, and blood flow. It can detect cardiac abnormalities, assess heart function, and guide procedures such as catheter or valve placement.

Radiology: Abdominal ultrasound is used to examine organs such as the liver, pancreas, gallbladder, and kidneys. It can detect tumors, cysts, and gallstones, among other pathologies.

Urology: Urinary tract ultrasound helps diagnose problems with the prostate, bladder, kidneys, and urethra. It is also used to guide procedures such as prostate biopsies or catheter placement.

Traumatology: Musculoskeletal ultrasound can evaluate muscles, tendons, ligaments, and joints for injuries, inflammation, or joint effusions.

Neurology: Transcranial Doppler ultrasound is used to evaluate cerebral blood flow and detect potential vascular problems.

**Beauty Through Technology: Ultrasound in Aesthetics

Ultrasound has also found its place in the field of aesthetics, offering a non-invasive alternative to traditional procedures:

Facial Diagnosis: Facial ultrasound allows for the analysis of skin structure, including wrinkle depth, fat distribution, and tissue elasticity. This information is valuable for determining the most appropriate aesthetic treatment.

Therapeutic Ultrasound: Low-intensity ultrasound waves are used to stimulate collagen and elastin production, improving skin texture and tone, reducing sagging, and combating wrinkles.

Ultrasound Lipolysis: This technique uses high-intensity ultrasound to eliminate localized fat in specific areas of the body, such as the abdomen, thighs, or buttocks.

Important Considerations

While ultrasound and sonography offer a wide range of benefits, it is important to keep in mind some considerations:

Safety: Ultrasonography is a safe and noninvasive technique that does not use radiation. However, in some cases, such as pregnancy, it may be necessary to limit the amount of ultrasound exposure time.

Accuracy: The accuracy of ultrasound depends largely on the experience and skill of the ultrasound operator.

Complexity: Interpreting ultrasound images can be complex and requires specialized training.

Limitations: Ultrasonography cannot visualize all body tissues, such as bones or air in the lungs.

In conclusion, ultrasound and sonography are invaluable tools in the fields of medicine and aesthetics, offering a window into the human body without the need for invasive procedures. Their ability to accurately diagnose.

They are a type of waves whose vibration is above 20,000 Hz, that is, they emit a wave that oscillates more than 20,000 times in a time of one second. The equipment emits vibratory and sound waves that are not perceptible by the human ear. These waves are applied through a head, which moves through the areas to be treated, whether facial or body, in pulses or continuously, depending on the case, it is a treatment that does not involve pain or discomfort. It is done in 8 to 10 sessions.

Ultrasound eliminates varicose veins, reduces the appearance of acne, eliminates cellulite, tones the skin, and helps a wound heal better. It also serves to dissolve the accumulated fat through the waves that it emits on the adipose tissue, eliminating cellulite over time. As always, possible contraindications such as cases of people with pacemakers, cancer, and pregnancy should be analyzed, It means in addition to people with skin hypersensitivity disorders. In addition, its wave should never be applied on delicate areas of the body such as ears, testicles, the brain, etc.

SHOCK WAVE

A journey toward beauty and wellness in aesthetic medicine

In the dynamic world of aesthetic medicine, shock waves have emerged as an innovative and effective alternative for various treatments, offering remarkable and long-lasting results. Unlike traditional methods, shock waves are noninvasive, making them an attractive option for those seeking to improve their appearance without undergoing surgery.

What are shock waves?

Shock waves are high-energy acoustic waves that are transmitted through a medium, such as water or body tissue. Initially developed for use in renal lithotripsy (the fragmentation of kidney stones), shock waves have found a niche in aesthetic medicine due to their ability to stimulate the production of collagen and elastin, proteins essential for the health and appearance of the skin.

How do shock waves work in aesthetic medicine?

Upon penetrating the skin, shock waves generate microvibrations that trigger a series of beneficial effects:

* **Stimulation of collagen and elastin production:** Shock waves activate fibroblasts, cells responsible for the production of collagen and elastin, proteins that provide firmness and elasticity to the skin.

* **Improved blood circulation:** Shock waves increase blood flow to the treated area, promoting oxygenation and cellular nutrition.

* **Reduction of inflammation:** Shock waves have an anti-inflammatory effect, helping to reduce swelling and redness.

* **Breakdown of fat cells:** In some cases, shock waves can help eliminate localized fat cells.

In what procedures are shock waves used?

Shock waves have become a versatile tool in aesthetic medicine, with applications in a wide range of treatments:

1. Facial Rejuvenation:

* **Wrinkle and Fine Line Reduction:** Shock waves stimulate collagen and elastin production, helping to blur wrinkles and fine lines, especially on the forehead, between the eyebrows, and around the eyes.

* **Facial Sagging Improvement:** Shock waves tighten the skin and improve elasticity, combating sagging in areas such as the face, neck, and décolletage.

* **Photoaged Skin Treatment:** Shock waves help improve skin texture and tone, combating damage caused by sun exposure.

2. Body:

* **Cellulite Reduction:** Shock waves help break down fat cells and improve blood circulation, reducing the appearance of cellulite on the thighs, buttocks, and abdomen.

* **Stretch marks:** Shock waves stimulate collagen production, which can help improve the appearance of stretch marks on the thighs, buttocks, and abdomen.

* **Treatment of body sagging:** Shock waves tighten the skin and improve elasticity, combating sagging in areas such as the arms, thighs, and abdomen.

3. Other treatments:

* **Erectile dysfunction:** Shock waves can improve blood circulation in the penis, which could help treat erectile dysfunction.

* **Scars:** Shock waves can help soften and improve the appearance of scars.

What are the benefits of shock waves?

Shock waves offer several advantages compared to other treatment methods:

* **Non-invasive:** No surgery or incisions are required, minimizing recovery time and the risk of complications.

* **Effective:** Shock waves have proven effective in various clinical studies.

* **Long-lasting results:** Treatment results can last up to a year or more.

* **Safe:** Shockwave therapy is a generally safe procedure with a low risk of side effects.

What are the side effects of shockwave therapy?

Shockwave therapy side effects are typically mild and temporary and include:

* **Redness**

* **Swelling**

* **Minor discomfort**

Rarely, bruising or muscle soreness may occur.

Who are ideal candidates for shockwave therapy?

Shockwave therapy is a good option for people seeking a noninvasive and effective treatment to improve their appearance.

DERMOSCOPE

The Dermiscope: An Essential Tool in the Arsenal of Medical Aesthetics

In the dynamic world of medical aesthetics, technology plays a crucial role in offering patients increasingly precise and personalized results. Among the innovative tools that have transformed dermatological practice, the **dermiscope** stands out as an indispensable ally for the diagnosis and treatment of various skin conditions.

What is a dermiscope?

The dermiscope, also known as a dermatoscope or epiluminescent light microscope, is a portable device that allows visualization of skin structures in greater detail than the human eye. Through a magnifying lens and a lighting system, the dermiscope magnifies the image of the skin up to 40 times, revealing subtle characteristics that might go unnoticed with the naked eye.

What are the uses of the dermiscopy in medical aesthetics?

The dermiscopy has become a fundamental tool in the field of medical aesthetics, with applications that cover a wide range of procedures and treatments:

1. Accurate diagnosis of skin lesions:

* **Early detection of skin cancer:** The dermiscopy allows the identification of vascular patterns and structures that may indicate the presence of melanomas and other types of skin cancer in their early stages, increasing the chances of successful treatment.

* **Differentiation of benign and malignant lesions:** Detailed analysis of the skin with the dermiscopy helps differentiate between benign lesions, such as moles or seborrheic keratoses, and potentially malignant lesions, such as melanomas, avoiding unnecessary biopsies and allowing for appropriate management.

* **Pigmentation and Vascularization Assessment:** The dermiscope allows for precise observation of melanin distribution and vascular patterns in the skin, providing valuable information for diagnosing conditions such as melasma, vitiligo, or rosacea.

2. Guide for Aesthetic Procedures:

* **Treatment Area Selection:** The dermiscope facilitates the precise selection of the treatment area for procedures such as the removal of dark spots, wrinkles, or varicose veins, ensuring greater efficacy and minimizing the risk of side effects.

* **Lesion Depth Assessment:** By visualizing the layers of the skin in greater detail, the dermiscope allows the specialist to determine the depth of lesions, such as scars or stretch marks, guiding the selection of the most appropriate treatment technique.

* **Treatment Response Monitoring:** The dermiscope allows for detailed monitoring of skin evolution after aesthetic procedures, assessing the response to treatment and adjusting it as needed.

3. Improved communication with the patient:

* **Shared visualization of lesions:** The dermiscope allows magnified images of their skin to be shown to the patient, facilitating understanding of the diagnosis and treatment plan.

* **Greater transparency and information:** The use of the dermiscope fosters transparency and trust between the patient and the specialist, allowing a better understanding of skin conditions and available options.

Procedure for using the dermiscope:

1. **Skin cleaning and preparation:** The area to be examined is properly cleaned and prepared to optimize visualization.

* **Gel or oil application:** A conductive gel or oil is applied to the skin to facilitate light transmission and improve image quality.

* **Dermiscope positioning:** The dermiscope is placed in contact with the skin, maintaining constant pressure and an appropriate distance.

* **Observation and Analysis:** Skin structures are meticulously observed and analyzed, looking for patterns, colors, and shapes that may indicate the presence of a lesion.

* **Documentation of Findings:** The observed findings are documented through photographs or videos for later analysis and follow-up.

In conclusion, the dermisoscope has become an indispensable tool in the field of medical aesthetics, offering more accurate diagnoses, guiding aesthetic procedures more effectively, and improving patient communication. Its widespread use has contributed to raising the standards of care in aesthetic clinics, providing patients with personalized care and optimal results.

LASERS AND AESTHETIC EQUIPMENT

The Magic of Light: Exploring the World of Lasers in Medical Aesthetics

In the dynamic world of medical aesthetics, lasers have emerged as revolutionary tools, offering a wide range of safe and effective treatments to improve physical appearance and address various dermatological conditions. Their precision, versatility, and ability to interact with tissues at the cellular level make them indispensable allies for dermatologists, plastic surgeons, and aesthetic physicians.

Types of Lasers and Their Applications:

Delving into the world of lasers, we find a wide variety of types, each with specific characteristics and applications in the field of medical aesthetics:

1. Ablative Lasers:

* **Erbium-YAG Laser:**

* **Uses:** Facial rejuvenation, removal of wrinkles, stretch marks, and scars.

* **Procedure:** The laser emits short pulses of energy that vaporize the superficial layers of the skin, stimulating the production of collagen and elastin for smoother, more even skin.

* **CO2 Laser:**

* **Uses:** Removal of warts, moles, and actinic keratoses.

* **Procedure:** The laser emits a fine beam of light that vaporizes skin lesions with great precision.

2. Non-ablative Lasers:

* **Vascular Laser:**

* **Uses:** Removal of varicose veins, telangiectasias (enlarged veins), and vascular spots.

* **Procedure:** The laser targets the hemoglobin in the blood vessels, gradually coagulating and eliminating them.

* **Diode Laser:**

* **Uses:** Permanent hair removal.

* **Procedure:** The laser emits infrared light that targets the hair follicle, preventing future growth.

* **Nd:YAG Laser:**

* **Uses:** Facial rejuvenation, scar and stretch mark removal.

* **Procedure:** The laser heats the deep layers of the skin, stimulating collagen and elastin production, improving texture and elasticity.

3. Fractional Lasers:

* **Fractional Er:YAG Laser:**

* **Uses:** Facial rejuvenation, reducing enlarged pores, acne treatment.

* **Procedure:** The laser fractionates the energy into small beams that penetrate the skin, stimulating collagen and elastin production and improving overall texture.

* **Fractional CO2 Laser:**

* **Uses:** Deep facial rejuvenation, wrinkle and scar removal.

* **Procedure:** Similar to the fractional Er:YAG laser, but with greater penetration depth, ideal for treating fine lines and deeper wrinkles.

Procedures and Considerations:

Laser procedures in medical aesthetics are performed by trained professionals in safe, clinical settings. The duration and number of sessions will depend on the type of laser used, the condition being treated, and the patient's individual needs.

Important Considerations:

* **Preparation:** A pre-assessment is essential to determine the appropriate laser type and treatment for the patient's condition.

* **Aftercare:** Physician instructions should be followed to ensure proper recovery and avoid complications.

* **Results:** Results are typically progressive and visible over time, depending on the treatment and the patient's condition.

In conclusion, lasers have transformed the landscape of medical aesthetics, offering a range of safe, effective, and minimally invasive treatments to improve physical appearance and address various dermatological conditions. Their precision, versatility, and ability to interact with tissues at the cellular level make them indispensable tools for healthcare professionals seeking to provide cutting-edge aesthetic solutions to their patients.

LIPOSUCTION

Sculpting Your Body with Precision

Liposuction has become one of the most popular cosmetic procedures in the world, appealing to those seeking to sculpt their bodies and eliminate stubborn fat deposits. But what exactly is liposuction? What are its uses and specific procedures? In this article, we'll explore this cosmetic procedure in depth, along with its benefits, risks, and important considerations.

What is Liposuction?

Liposuction is a minimally invasive surgical technique that uses a thin tube called a cannula to extract localized body fat deposits. These fat deposits, often resistant to diet and exercise, can accumulate in areas such as the abdomen, thighs, hips, buttocks, upper arms, back, and chin. **Uses of Liposuction:**

Liposuction is not a weight-loss technique, but rather is used to:

* **Remove stubborn fat deposits:** It is ideal for problem areas that do not respond to non-invasive measures such as diet and exercise.

* **Define body contour:** Liposuction can help sculpt and define areas such as the abdomen, thighs, waist, and arms, creating a slimmer silhouette.

* **Improve self-esteem:** By removing unwanted fat, liposuction can improve a patient's confidence and body image.

Types of Liposuction:

There are different liposuction techniques, each with its own characteristics:

* **Traditional Liposuction:** Uses a cannula connected to a suction pump to extract fat.

* **Ultrasonic Liposuction (Vaser Hi-Def):** Uses ultrasound to liquefy fat before extraction. * **Laser-Assisted Liposuction (Smartlipo):** Uses laser energy to melt fat before suctioning it out.

* **Tumescent Liposuction:** Injects a tumescent solution to numb the area and facilitate fat extraction.

Liposuction Procedure:

1. **Consultation with the Plastic Surgeon:** The first step is a consultation with a board-certified plastic surgeon to evaluate your case, determine if liposuction is right for you, and discuss your expectations.

2. **Anesthesia:** Local or general anesthesia is administered, depending on the area being treated and the extent of the procedure.

3. **Incisions:** Small incisions are made in the skin to insert the cannula.

4. **Fat Extraction:** The cannula is carefully moved to aspirate localized fat.

5. **Incision Closure:** The incisions are closed with sutures or stitches.

Recovery after Liposuction:

* **Swelling and Bruising:** It is normal to experience swelling and bruising in the treated area for the first few days.

* **Pain:** Pain is usually mild and can be managed with over-the-counter pain relievers.

* **Compression Garments:** Compression garments are recommended to help reduce swelling and improve skin adhesion to the new contour.

* **Rest:** It is important to avoid strenuous activities for the first week and follow your surgeon's instructions for proper recovery.

Risks and Complications:

As with any medical procedure, liposuction carries some risks, such as:

* **Infection:** It is important to choose a qualified surgeon and a clinic with proper hygiene measures to minimize the risk of infection.

* **Bleeding:** Excessive bleeding is uncommon, but can occur.

* **Nerve Damage:** In rare cases, the cannula can damage nerves, causing numbness or tingling.

* **Unwanted Results:** It is important to discuss your expectations with your surgeon and ensure that liposuction is the right procedure for you.

Important Considerations:

* **Suitable Candidates:** Liposuction is not for everyone. Ideal candidates are people in good health, with a stable weight and localized fat deposits.

* **Realistic Expectations:** It is important to have realistic expectations about the results. Liposuction is not a solution for obesity and does not eliminate cellulite.

* **Surgeon Selection:** Choose a board-certified plastic surgeon with experience in liposuction and who has a safe, modern operating room.

* **Costs:** The cost of liposuction varies depending on the surgeon, clinic, and area being treated.

In conclusion, liposuction can be a powerful tool for body sculpting.

CHAPTER 5 HAIR REMOVAL

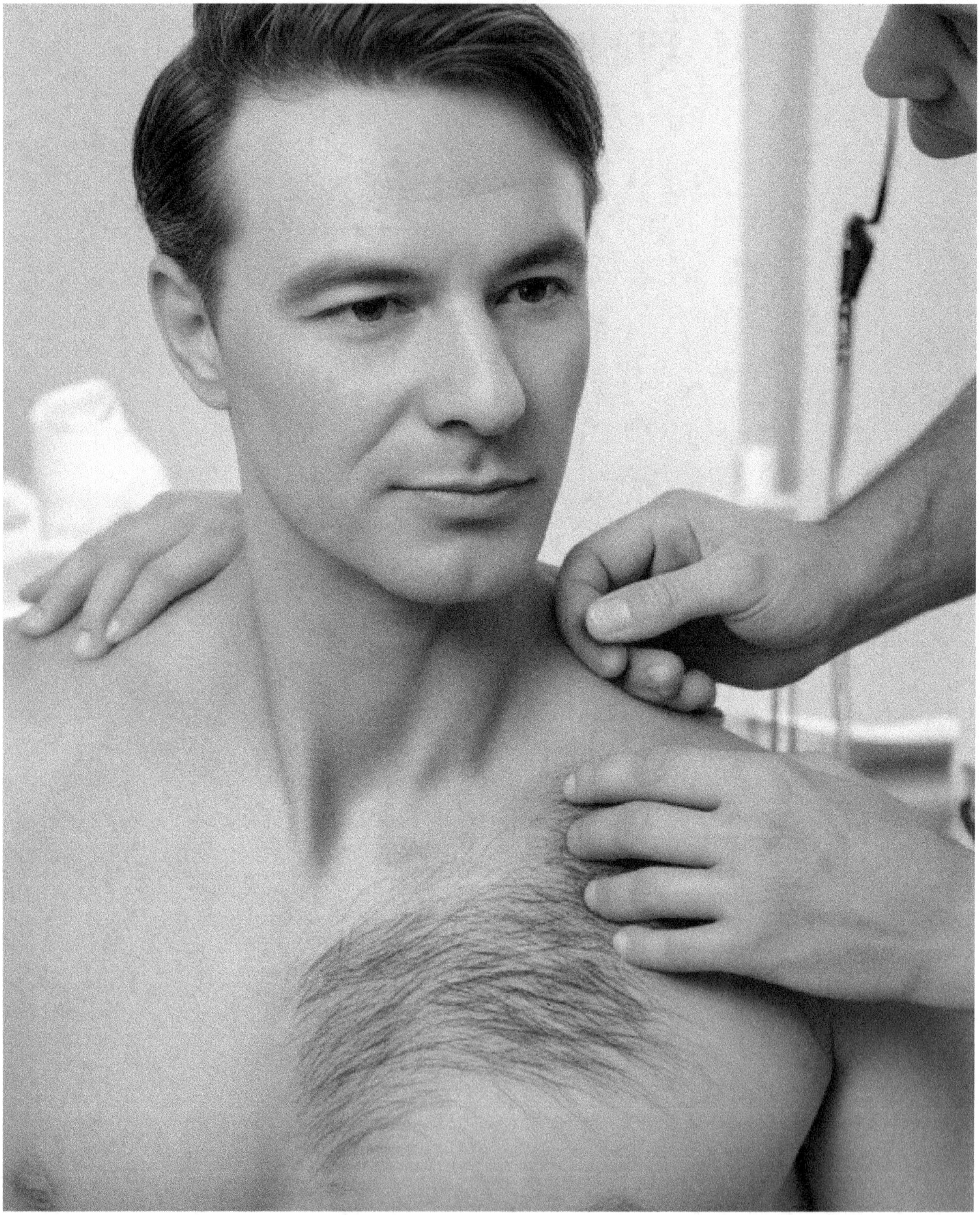

From our feeding up to the blood vessels present in a papilla located within the follicle, which extends a little at the root of the hair. A small muscle, the arrector pili or erector hair, attaches to each hair follicle. The muscle contracts under the control of the sympathetic nervous system, causing the hair to stand on end. Most mammals have tactile hairs that grow, in many cases, on the upper part of the lip and on the eyebrows, with the roots located on highly innervated erectile tissue. Paraffin wax is a high molecular mass saturated hydrocarbon mixture by refining petroleum. Currently most commercial waxes come from petroleum. Waxes are used to make candles, matches, wax paper, and cosmetics. They are also used to make rubber antioxidants, electrical insulators, paper baths, printing inks, textile finishes, leather coatings, and food containers. This range of products requires waxes with different melting points, as well as different loss, hardness, tensile strength, water resistance and ductility.

Hair development in humans begins in the embryo and in the sixth month the fetus appears covered with very fine hair (lanugo). In the first months of life the lanugo falls off and is replaced by thick hair on the head (hair) and eyebrows, and fine and fuzzy on the rest of the body. At puberty, thick hair appears in the armpits and pubes in both sexes, and in men it begins to grow on the upper part of the lip and chin, giving rise to the beard. The speed of its growth varies with the age of the person and with the length. When it is short, it grows about 2 cm per month, but the growth rate is halved when it is long. The greatest growth occurs in women whose age ranges between 16 and 24 years of age- Disorders in the structure of the hair or hair follicle cause abnormal growth or early or abnormal hair loss. Dry or dull hair is due to the effect of different chemicals.

Too frequent use of perms, shampoos, or lotions, especially those that contain alcohol or alkalis, can cause it. The cause of severe baldness is not known, but in many cases it has been attributed to a tumor in the adrenal cortex or to disorders of the pituitary, thyroid, or ovary. The early appearance of gray hair is associated with states of anxiety, intense emotions, deficiency diseases and hereditary causes. Alopecia or baldness is mainly due to hereditary causes. Certain forms of baldness can, however, be due to Other causes: premature alopecia, in which the hair of a young person falls without first turning gray, can be caused by seborrhea; Alopecia areata, in which it falls irregularly, is believed to be due to inflammation, nervous disorders or local infections, especially in states of psychological stress. Diffuse hair loss, a normal phenomenon, can reach abnormal proportions after fevers above 39.4 0 C during illnesses that cause a weakening of the body or after surgery. In reality, no hair regenerator prevents hair loss or facilitates hair growth. However, a drug called minoxidil has been investigated and appears to have some success in tests on men with hereditary baldness, who had suffered hair loss ten years earlier.

Hair follicle infections are also the source of many diseases. Tinea favus, caused by the fungus Achorion schoenleinii, is characterized by the formation of small crusts around the mouth of the follicles that often resemble a honeycomb. Another type of ringworm is caused by a fungus of the genus Trichophyton. These diseases are successfully treated by waxing (removing hair from affected follicles), cleaning with soaps or oils that remove scabs, and application of fungicides. Hairy areas, especially the head and pubis, are exposed to annoying infections from small insects and mites such as lice and crabs.

HAIR CHARACTERISTICS

As future professionals in the area of aesthetics, it is essential to acquire prior knowledge of all these issues, useful to our professional work.

Hair is a continuation of the epidermis; It is made up of cornfield cells, is flexible and comes out obliquely from the skin. It consists of a stem formed by dead cells, arranged in the shape of an elongated cylinder. The root is housed within the hair follicle. Hair is a skin appendix with a protective function in all mammals. It consists of pods or envelopes that cover this area.

It is where the vital functions take place in the epilation techniques that act on the hair bulb The race, age, sex and skin area to which we refer determine the characteristics of the hair. During fetal development until the eighth month the hair is called lanugo, at puberty terminal hair develops.

In the cortex the melanin granules are located, which determine the color of the hair and the keratin fibers that give it resistance. The cortex is affected by chemical depilatory techniques. The sebaceous gland accompanies the hair forming the pilo-sebaceous follicles. It produces sebum, which is shed into the follicle.

Hair growth is cyclical, and different phases can be differentiated, where the root has great metabolic activity. The anomalies that are associated with the hair to be considered in waxing are hypertrichosis and hirsutism. In both cases, electric and laser hair removal can be applied.

The shape of the hair is one of the most important and exact hereditary characteristics. The almost black hair of Papuans, Melanesians, and Africans grows from a curved follicle that continues in a spiral with a flat cross-section. The hair of the Chinese, Japanese, and Native Americans is straight, thick, long, and almost always black. It grows from a straight follicle, with a circular cross section, and has an easily distinguishable medulla. The hair of the Ainu, Europeans, Indians, and Semites is wavy. It grows from a straight follicle but with a certain tendency to roll up; the cross section is oval and the color varies greatly from one individual to another, from light blond to black.

TYPES OF HAIR FOLLICLES

Navigating the World of Hair Follicles: A Complete Guide for Aesthetic Clinics

In the intricate world of aesthetics, hair follicles occupy a central place, being the cornerstone of healthy, lush hair. Understanding their types, characteristics, and associated procedures in aesthetic clinics is essential to effectively address various hair conditions and achieve optimal results.

Types of Hair Follicles: A Detailed Classification

1. **Anagenic Follicles:** The protagonists of active growth. They represent approximately 3% of the follicles on the head and are characterized by their constant activity, producing new hair during a phase that can last between 2 and 6 years.

2. **Catagenic Follicles:** In transition to resting state. After the anagen phase, the follicles enter a phase of involution that lasts approximately 2 to 3 weeks, during which hair stops growing and prepares for hair loss.

3. Telogen Follicles: These are the home of resting hair. They represent approximately 90% of the follicles on the head and house hair that is in the resting phase, which can last between 3 and 4 months. Eventually, this hair falls out to make way for a new growth cycle.

Aesthetic Procedures to Address Hair Conditions

1. Hair Transplant: A revolutionary technique to combat baldness. It involves extracting healthy follicles from a donor area (usually the back or sides of the scalp) and then implanting them in the affected areas. This procedure allows for permanent and natural repopulation of thinning areas.

2. Scalp Micropigmentation:** Creating the illusion of greater density. This technique involves implanting pigments into the scalp to simulate the presence of hair, especially in areas with sparse hair. It offers long-lasting, natural-looking aesthetic results.

3. Scalp Mesotherapy: A nutritive cocktail to strengthen hair. Mesotherapy involves injecting microdoses of vitamins, minerals, and other nourishing active ingredients directly into the scalp. Its goal is to stimulate hair growth, combat hair loss, and improve overall hair health.

4. Platelet-Rich Plasma (PRP): Harnessing the regenerative potential of the blood. PRP is obtained from the patient's own blood and injected into the scalp, stimulating blood circulation, revitalizing hair follicles, and promoting hair growth.

5. Hair Laser: Combating hair loss from the root. Hair laser uses low-power light to stimulate hair growth, reduce inflammation, and improve blood circulation in the scalp. It is a noninvasive and safe procedure that can help slow hair loss and promote hair growth.

**Important Considerations in Aesthetic Clinics

When choosing an aesthetic clinic for a hair procedure, it is crucial to consider:

1. Experience and Reputation: Look for clinics with experienced and highly trained professionals in hair aesthetic medicine procedures.

2. Cutting-Edge Technology: Ensure the clinic has the latest equipment and technology to ensure optimal results.

3. Personalized Diagnosis: Obtain an accurate and personalized diagnosis of your hair condition to determine the most appropriate treatment.

4. Follow-up and Support: Look for clinics that provide close follow-up and support throughout the entire process, from the initial consultation to recovery.

Conclusion: A Comprehensive Approach to Hair Health

Hair follicles are essential elements for healthy and vibrant hair. Understanding their types, characteristics, and the various procedures available at aesthetic clinics allows you to effectively address different hair conditions and restore hair vitality. Remember that choosing a specialized clinic and seeking a personalized diagnosis are key to achieving optimal results and achieving your desired image.

HAIR REMOVAL AREAS OF THE BODY

Hair removal began in ancient times and primitive blades were used to shave the heads of enslaved people such as eunuchs in the Middle East and Egypt. Today depilatory techniques cover a large number of options from the simple shave, depilatory creams, waxes, lasers, and many more. If we look at the areas of the body, we see that surely we all like to have hair in our hair, to style it, wash it regularly and give it other care, but the rest of the hairs or hair follicles of the skin become a real nuisance when they grow in non-stop excess throughout life.

Women out of vanity or pretense sometimes tend to be more careful than men, who see in their abundant body hair a symbol of virility. However, most people don't think the same way and in waxing rooms we see people of every conceivable criteria.

DEPILATORY TECHNIQUES CLASSES

The term "depilation" is generally used in reference to any technique aimed at removing superfluous hair. However, the esthetician must clearly distinguish between epilation and epilation.

• Depilation: Includes techniques aimed at eliminating the aerial part of the superfluous hair, that is, it acts on the hair shaft. Shaving, abrasion, and depilatory creams are included here. They suppose a temporary solution, never definitive. These techniques are for personal use, they are called "homemade" and are never used in beauty salons.

• Epilation: These are techniques aimed at eliminating the hair by acting more deeply from the hair bulb. The aesthetic professional must indicate in the patient's file data such as treatment and products applied, existence of possible skin lesions, date of the next appointment and others. This is intended to have a record of the evolution of the client.

CHEMICAL DEPILATORY TECHNIQUES. It is a treatment that is not carried out at a professional level, but its characteristics must be known in order to advise clients. They are based on the destruction of the hair shaft.

In this technique of products in whose composition there are keratolytic agents that can destroy hair are thiols and alkali metal sulfides. Before its application, it should be tested on a sensitive area of the body such as the wrist or the bend of the arm.

PHYSICAL DEPILATORY TECHNIQUES. There are various aesthetic techniques for hair removal within the professional field. Physical techniques will be discussed first. The plucking or avulsion consists of pulling the hair shaft in order to also extract the bulb. There are variants on the material used: tweezers, electric razors or adhesive films or waxes.

Hot waxes: They are made up of four of compounds such as adhesive agents, plasticizers, softeners and aromatic additives. on their melting point or they range from 38 to 45 0 C. They are quite effective and are in high demand on a professional level. It should be warned of possible side effects on sensitive skin.

Warm waxes: They do not contain beeswax, so they are not waxes themselves. In their they have derivatives of rosin and resins in an excipient, such as mineral and vegetable oils.

Cold waxes: They are impregnated with a molten mixture of glucose, honey, synthetic resins, molasses, zinc oxide and mineral and vegetable Oils. They do not need a melter since the dough is left at room

ELECTRIC DEPILATION. It consists of the destruction of the area of the hair follicle Where the germ cells are located, in order to prevent new hair from growing. with these methods a definitive hair removal is achieved. The foundation of the technique lies in the application of electric current.

According to the voltage frequency, they are classified as:

• Needle hair removal, it is a very aggressive and complicated depilatory method.

• Electrolysis uses a low voltage direct current. • Thermolysis uses a low voltage, high amperage and high frequency.

• Flash system is a variant of the high frequency ones Where the frequency is increased and decreased in less application time.

LASER DEPILATION. Photoepilation is based on exposing the hair to light energy that is transformed into heat, leading to atrophy of the hair follicle. That is, hair removal occurs by photothermolysis. Its greatest advantage is that it does not cause pain, or infections and does not leave scars.

DEPILATORY SELECTION CRITERIA

The duration of the hair should be considered in coming out again or it Stops doing it permanently. Among the techniques that are Common to use in beauty salons we find:

• Mechanical techniques: avulsion by tweezers, or wax with all its modalities.

• Some chemical techniques such as growth retardants.

• Electrical techniques: hair removal with a needle or tweezers.

CONTRAINDICATIONS IN THE APPLICATION of AESTHETIC TREATMENTS:

- Avoid handling on tumor lesions of the skin. Aesthetic treatments are contraindicated in infectious processes, in order not to contribute to the generation of infection.
- In vascular disorders that lead to stagnation of blood.
- Certain skin lesions are contraindicated.

HAIR REMOVAL PROTOCOL

Before performing any depilatory method, the must check if the client has any skin lesions that contraindicate the treatment. In this case, the steps to follow are the following:

Apply biosecurity measures.

Have the materials and products ready to be applied.

Prepare the patient by offering the best care and information about the treatment and fill out the patient file.

Process:

Clean the area to using alcohol gel.

Place the powder with the wooden Stick we apply the wax, being careful not to

Then we place the cloth on the waxed area and in the opposite direction to the growth of the hair, we pull with a quick projected pull as far as to pull the skin so that it hurts less.

When finished, clean with the Oil and then apply the gel or the growth retardant gel.

SCALP DISEASES

The scalp is the skin that covers the top of your head. Unless your hair falls out, hair grows on your scalp. Different skin problems can affect Your scalp. Dandruff is a of the skin. The scales are Yellow or White. Dandruff can make Your scalp itch. It usually after and is more Common in men. Dandruff is usually a symptom of seborrheic dermatitis or seborrhea, a skin condition that causes redness and irritation.

Specific issues in hair

- Scalp
- Seborrheic dermatitis
- Psoriasis compared to seborrheic dermatitis of the scalp

Ringworm of the head

- Ringworm of the scalp

Children

- Cradle cap
- Childhond seborrheic dermatitis

Teenagers

- Dan

Treatments and therapies. Most of the time, using an anti- dandruff can help control dandruff. If that doesn't work, contact Your healthcare provider. There is a type of seborrheic dermatitis that can affect babies, cradle cap. It usually lasts for a few months and then goes away on its own. In addition to the scalp, it can sometimes affect Other parts of the such as the eyelids, armpits, groin, and ears.

Washing Your baby's hair every day with a mild and gently scrubbing the scalp with Your fingers or a soft brush can help. For severe cases, the doctor may some or cream.

Other names: Seborrheic dermatitis, Seborrheic eczema, Seborrhea. Other problems that can affect the scalp include:

- Ringworm of the scalp: A fungal infection that causes itchy red on the head.

It can also leave bald areas. It usually affects children.

•Scalp psoriasis: Causes itchy patches or thick, red skin with silvery scales that cause pain- half of people with psoriasis have it on their scalp.

HAIR MESOTHERAPY

Hair Mesotherapy: Revitalizing Your Hair from Within

In the dynamic world of aesthetics, the quest for beauty and rejuvenation is not limited to the face or body. The health and vitality of hair also play a crucial role in personal image, and this is where hair mesotherapy emerges as an innovative and effective technique to combat various hair problems.

What is hair mesotherapy?

Hair mesotherapy is a minimally invasive treatment that involves injecting small amounts of medical and natural active ingredients directly into the scalp. These active ingredients penetrate the deep layers of the skin, stimulating hair growth, combating hair loss, improving blood circulation, and nourishing the hair follicles.

What are the uses of hair mesotherapy?

Hair mesotherapy is used to address a wide range of hair problems, including:

* Hair loss:** Stimulates hair growth, reduces hair loss, and strengthens hair follicles.

* Baldness:** Helps slow the progression of baldness and can stimulate new hair growth in bald areas.

* Dandruff:** Regulates sebum production and combats scalp flaking.

* **Dry and brittle hair:** Moisturizes and nourishes hair, improving its appearance and texture.

* Oily hair:** Regulates sebum production and reduces scalp oiliness.

* Gray hair:** Can delay the appearance of gray hair or slow its rate of appearance.

What are the ingredients in a hair mesotherapy formula?

The hair mesotherapy formula varies depending on the clinic and the specific problem being treated. However, some of the most common ingredients include:

* Vitamins:** B1, B2, B3, B5, B6, B7, H (biotin), E, and C.

* Minerals:** Zinc, iron, copper, magnesium, and calcium.

* Amino acids:** Cysteine, arginine, glutamine, and aspartic acid.

* Hyaluronic acids:** Moisturize the scalp and stimulate collagen production.

* Plant extracts:** Ginkgo biloba, rosemary, cinchona, ginseng, and aloe vera.

How is the hair mesotherapy procedure performed?

The hair mesotherapy procedure is generally performed as follows:

1. **Initial consultation:** The doctor or aesthetician assesses the condition of the patient's hair and scalp to determine if mesotherapy is the right treatment and to formulate the appropriate active ingredient blend.

2. **Cleansing:** The scalp is thoroughly cleansed to remove any impurities or residue.

3. **Application:** The specialist uses an injection gun with very fine needles to apply small amounts of the active ingredient blend to the scalp, following a specific pattern.

4. **Massage:** The scalp is gently massaged to stimulate absorption of the active ingredients.

How many hair mesotherapy sessions are needed?

The number of hair mesotherapy sessions required will depend on the problem being treated and the patient's individual response. In general, 6 to 10 sessions are recommended, spaced 15 to 30 days apart.

What are the side effects of hair mesotherapy?

The side effects of hair mesotherapy are usually mild and temporary and may include:

* **Redness**

* **Swelling**

* **Itching**

* **Mild discomfort**

Rarely, more serious allergic reactions may occur. It is important to inform your doctor about any allergies or pre-existing medical conditions before starting treatment.

What are the advantages of hair mesotherapy?

Hair mesotherapy offers several advantages, such as:

* **Effectiveness:** It is an effective treatment for various hair problems.

* **Minimally invasive:** It does not require surgery or anesthesia.

* **Fast results:** Visible results can be seen in just a few sessions.

* **Fast recovery:** The patient can return to normal activities immediately after treatment.

* **Safety:** It is a relatively safe procedure with a low risk of side effects.

What are the disadvantages of hair mesotherapy?

The disadvantages of hair mesotherapy include:

* **Cost:** The treatment price may vary depending on the clinic and the number of sessions required.

* **Mild discomfort:** May cause redness.

HAIR TRANSPLANT

Hair Transplant: Everything You Need to Know

Hair transplant, also known as hair transplant, is an increasingly popular surgical procedure used to restore hair growth in areas where there has been permanent hair loss. This treatment has evolved considerably over the years and offers effective solutions for those experiencing baldness or thinning hair. In this article, we will explore in detail what hair transplant is, the different types available, when it is indicated, possible side effects, and the specific procedures involved.

What is Hair Transplant?

Hair transplant is a surgical procedure in which hair follicles are transplanted from areas with dense hair (donor) to areas where hair is sparse or has disappeared completely (recipient). The hair follicles are usually extracted from the back or sides of the scalp, where hair tends to be more resistant to loss, and are implanted in bald areas or where the hair is thinner. This process allows the transplanted hair to grow naturally and permanently.

Types of Hair Transplants

There are different techniques used in hair transplant procedures, each with its own advantages and considerations. The most common types of hair transplants include:

1. **Follicular Unit Extraction (FUE)**: In this method, hair follicles are extracted one by one from the donor area using specialized tools. This minimizes scarring and allows for a faster recovery. FUE is ideal for those who wish to avoid a visible linear scar in the donor area.

2. **Strip Technique (FUT)**: In contrast to FUE, the strip technique involves extracting a strip of tissue from the donor area, from which the hair follicles for transplantation are obtained. Although it leaves a linear scar, it can be hidden by the surrounding hair and allows for the transplantation of a larger number of follicles in a single session.

3. **Robotic Technique**: Some clinics use robotic systems to assist in the hair follicle extraction and implantation process. These systems can offer greater precision and speed compared to manual methods.

Indications for Hair Transplantation

Hair transplantation is indicated for people experiencing permanent hair loss or thinning hair in specific areas, such as the top of the head, hairline, or receding hairline. It is important to have realistic expectations about the results of the procedure and discuss any concerns with an experienced hair surgeon.

Side Effects of Hair Transplantation

While hair transplantation is generally safe and effective, like any surgical procedure, there may be some potential side effects, including:

1. **Swelling and Pain**: It is common to experience some swelling and discomfort in the treated area after the procedure. This is usually temporary and can be relieved with medication prescribed by your doctor.

2. **Scarring**: Both the FUE and FUT techniques may leave scarring in the donor area. However, with FUE, the scars are small and punctate, while with FUT, the scar is a longer line. Healing may vary depending on each individual's healing capacity.

3. **Infection**: There is a minimal risk of infection after the procedure, especially if postoperative care instructions are not properly followed. All physician recommendations should be followed to reduce this risk.

4. **Temporary Hair Loss**: It is possible to experience temporary hair loss around the treated area after the procedure. This is normal, and hair usually grows back within a few weeks or months.

Specific Hair Transplant Procedure

The hair transplant procedure generally follows these steps:

1. **Initial Consultation**: During the initial consultation, the surgeon will assess the condition of the hair and discuss the patient's expectations. Details of the procedure will also be discussed, and all questions will be answered.

2. **Preparation**: Before the procedure, the patient may be advised to avoid certain medications and supplements that may increase the risk of bleeding. The hair in the donor area may be trimmed to facilitate the extraction of hair follicles.

3. **Follicle Extraction**: On the day of the procedure, hair follicles are extracted from the donor area using the chosen technique (FUE or FUT).

4. **Recipient Site Preparation**: Small incisions are made in the recipient area where the hair follicles will be placed.

5. **Follicle Implantation**: The hair follicles are implanted. The procedure is carefully performed on the recipient sites one by one, ensuring a natural hair growth pattern.

6. **Postoperative Care**: After the procedure, detailed instructions will be provided on how to care for the treated area. This may include applying topical medications and avoiding activities that may damage the transplanted follicles.

7. **Follow-up**: Follow-up appointments will be scheduled to monitor the progress of hair growth and address any patient concerns.

In conclusion, hair transplantation is an effective option for those who wish to restore hair growth in areas where there has been permanent hair loss. With different techniques available, patients can find an approach that best suits their needs and preferences. However, it is important to understand the potential side effects and follow all doctor's recommendations before and after the procedure to ensure optimal results. If you are considering hair transplantation, consult with an experienced hair surgeon to discuss your options.

CHAPTER 6 ANATOMY

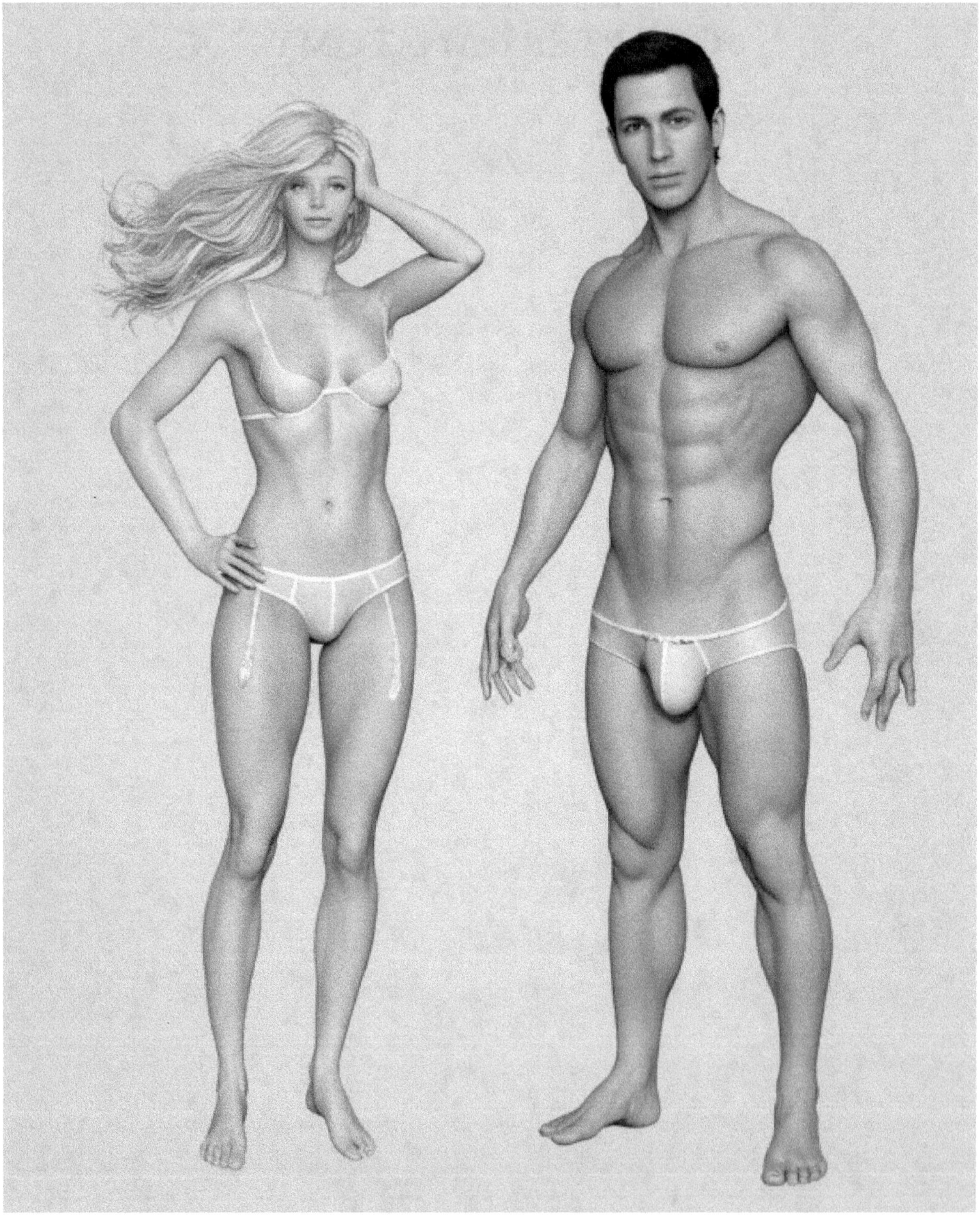

Anatomy, a term derived from the Greek anatomē, meaning "dissection," is a branch of the natural sciences concerned with the structural organization of living beings. It is a very ancient science, with origins dating back to prehistory. For centuries, anatomical knowledge has been based on the observation of dissected plants and animals. However, a proper understanding of structure implies an understanding of the function of living organisms. Consequently, anatomy is almost inseparable from physiology, which is sometimes called functional anatomy. Anatomy, which is one of the basic life sciences, is closely related to medicine and other branches of biology.

It is convenient to subdivide the study of anatomy into different aspects. One classification is based on the type of organism being studied; in this case, the main subdivisions are plant anatomy and animal anatomy. Animal anatomy is further subdivided into human anatomy (see below) and comparative anatomy, which establishes the similarities and differences between different types of animals. Anatomy can also be divided into biological processes, for example, developmental anatomy (the study of embryos) and pathological anatomy, or the study of diseased organs. Other subdivisions, such as surgical anatomy and artistic anatomy, are based on the relationship of anatomy to other activities under the general heading of applied anatomy. Yet another way of subdividing anatomy depends on the techniques used, such as microanatomy, which is based on observations obtained with the aid of a microscope.

Consequently, physiology is inseparable from anatomy, to the point that it is sometimes called functional anatomy. Anatomy, which is one of the basic life sciences, is closely related to medicine and other branches of biology. The skin provides valuable information about a person, such as possible internal disorders and our hygiene habits. It is very important both for our external appearance and our external relationships.

SKIN ORGAN

The skin is the organ that surrounds our body, covering the entire organism, it is a protective barrier between the internal and external environment. It has an undoubted aesthetic value, and constitutes the raw material on which the aesthetic professional works. For this reason, it is essential to acquire in-depth knowledge of its structure, function and alterations in order for us to be able to select and apply the most appropriate treatment. The outer layer or border of ourself as an external medium, is not simply an envelope that covers our body. It is an organized and constantly renewed system that a multitude functions, so many that it is classified as an organ, which is reason why the skin is also referred to as a cutaneous organ. The skin provides valuable information the such as possible internal disorders and our hygienic habits. It is very important both in Your external image and your external relations hip s. The characteristic capacity of the skin gives it an aesthetic function as a presenting organ through which the appearance is exposed to Others. two layers are differentiated in the skin:

- The epidermis is the most and is made up of cells to form a protective barrier-
- The dermis, consists of cells and fibers included in a fundamental substance.
- It's located under the dermis and is the fatty tissue.

The cell types to be highlighted in the epidermis are: keratinocytes or epithelial cells, and melanocytes. Keratinocytes constitute a protective barrier, they divide and migrate to higher layers forming the different epidermal strata. Then they will fall, while Other keratinocytes rise, thus ensuring cell renewal. Melanocytes make melanin, for skin and hair color. The epidermis consists of four layers of cells, except in the palms of the hands and the soles the feet which there are five when the lucid layer appears.

These epidermal strata are:

- basal stratum.
- stratum spinosum
- Stratum granular
- stratum lucid
- Stratum corneum.

In the epidermis, cell renewal is constant. The loss of dead cells of the stratum corneum is compensated by the division of the cells of the stratum basalis, renewing the other strata. Epidermal keratinization comprises the migration of cells to higher strata, the transformations that the cell during its journey, and cell desquamation. During the ascent, the cell is transformed into a cornecyte. The changes that occur are morphological, that is, cellular and biochemical organelles flatten and related to the synthesis of keratin. Keratin is a protein that has a function, waterproofs the skin and provides resistance to mechanical factors. The process by which melanin is formed in is called melanogenesis.

Melanin is a pigment that determines the color of skin and hair. Melanocytes synthesize melanin that is transferred to neighboring keratinocytes, which will transport and destroy it. Finally we have the granulocytes, they are blood cells characterized by the ways of coloring the organelles of their cytoplasm, in light microscopy. It is known as polymorphonuclear leukocytes, due to the variable forms of nucleus that it can present- However, this term can be misused since it is only correct for neutrophils and not for basophils, nor for eosinophils. There are three types of granulocytes in human neutrophils, eosinophils, and basophils.

PHYSIOLOGY

** Physiology in Aesthetic Clinics: A Journey Through the Human Body

Introduction:

The world of aesthetics has become an increasingly dynamic field, where science and beauty intertwine to deliver harmonious and lasting results. In this context, physiology plays a fundamental role, providing the scientific foundation for understanding the mechanisms that govern the functioning of the human body and its relationship to aesthetics.

*What is physiology?

Physiology is the science that studies the normal functioning of the human body, focusing on the structure and function of organs, tissues, and cells. It explores how these components integrate to maintain homeostasis, the internal balance essential for life.

*Physiology in Aesthetic Clinics:

In the field of aesthetic clinics, physiology becomes an invaluable tool for understanding the processes that affect the skin, hair, the body in general, and its aging. This knowledge allows aesthetic professionals to:

* Accurately diagnose:** Identify the underlying causes of aesthetic problems such as acne, spots, wrinkles, cellulite, or hair loss.

* Design personalized treatments:** Based on an understanding of each patient's individual needs, considering their medical history, lifestyle, and aesthetic goals.

* Select appropriate techniques:** Choose the most effective procedures and products for each case, taking into account the physiology of the skin, muscles, and the body as a whole.

* Optimize results:** Maximize the effectiveness of treatments and minimize the risk of side effects, understanding the mechanisms of action of each technique and product.

Classifications of physiology in aesthetic clinics:

To facilitate its application in the field of aesthetics, physiology is divided into different specialized areas:

1. Skin Physiology:**

Studies the structure, function, and composition of the skin, including:

* Epidermis:** The outermost layer, responsible for the protective barrier and pigmentation.

* Dermis:** The middle layer, rich in collagen and elastin, which provides elasticity and firmness.

* Hypodermis:** The deepest layer, composed of adipose tissue and responsible for thermal insulation.

2. Physiology of Aging:**

Investigates the biological mechanisms that determine skin aging, such as:

* Free radicals:** Unstable molecules that damage cells and accelerate aging.

* Glycation:** Abnormal binding of sugars to proteins, which affects elasticity and collagen.

* Loss of collagen and elastin:** Essential proteins for skin firmness and smoothness.

3. Body Physiology:**

Examines the functioning of the body in general, including:

* Endocrine System:** Regulates hormonal balance, which influences the health of the skin, hair, and the body in general.

* Circulatory System:** Supplies oxygen and nutrients to tissues, essential for cellular health and rejuvenation.

* Lymphatic System:** Removes toxins and waste, contributing to detoxification and overall well-being.

4. Hair Physiology:**

Examines the structure, growth, and life cycle of hair, including:

* Hair Follicle:** The structure where hair is produced.

* Growth Cycle:** The different phases of hair: anagen (growth), catagen (transition), and telogen (resting).

* Factors that affect hair:** Stress, diet, genetics, and hormones.

In conclusion, physiology is a fundamental pillar in aesthetic clinics, providing a scientific framework for understanding the processes that affect the beauty and well-being of the human body. By mastering this area, aesthetic professionals can offer personalized, effective, and safe treatments, maximizing results and meeting their patients' needs.

AESTHETIC DENTISTRY

*** Exploring Aesthetic Dentistry: Enhancing Smiles with Precision and Artistry*

In the field of modern dentistry, the pursuit of beauty and function go hand in hand. Aesthetic dentistry, often referred to as cosmetic dentistry, is a specialized branch that focuses on improving the appearance of teeth, gums, and the overall aesthetics of the smile. Beyond mere vanity, aesthetic dentistry plays a crucial role in boosting confidence, improving oral health, and restoring self-esteem. This comprehensive guide delves into the definition, different types of treatments, and broad applications of aesthetic dentistry within the field of dentistry.

** Understanding Aesthetic Dentistry

Aesthetic dentistry encompasses a variety of procedures intended to enhance the visual appeal of a person's smile while maintaining or improving their oral health. It involves a combination of artistry and scientific precision to achieve natural-looking results that blend perfectly with the patient's facial features. Unlike traditional dentistry, which primarily focuses on addressing functional problems such as cavities or gum disease, cosmetic dentistry prioritizes aesthetics without compromising functionality.

** Key Goals of Cosmetic Dentistry:

1. **Improving Smile Appearance**: Cosmetic dentistry aims to correct dental imperfections such as discoloration, misalignment, gaps, and irregular shapes to create a more harmonious and attractive smile.

2. **Restoring Confidence**: By improving smile aesthetics, cosmetic dentistry helps people regain confidence in their appearance, leading to improved self-esteem and overall well-being.

3. **Preserving Natural Teeth**: Many cosmetic procedures focus on preserving as much of the natural tooth structure as possible while achieving the desired cosmetic results, promoting long-term oral health.

4. **Personalization**: Each patient's smile is unique, and cosmetic dentistry offers personalized treatment plans tailored to individual needs and preferences, ensuring optimal results.

** Types of Cosmetic Dental Treatments

Cosmetic dentistry encompasses a wide range of treatments, each designed to address specific concerns and deliver aesthetically pleasing results. These treatments can be broadly classified as follows:

** 1. Teeth Whitening

Teeth whitening, also known as bleaching, is one of the most popular and affordable cosmetic dental treatments. It involves the use of bleaching agents to lighten the color of teeth, effectively removing stains and discoloration caused by aging, smoking, or the use of coloring substances such as coffee or red wine. Professional teeth whitening performed by a dentist produces superior results compared to over-the-counter products, delivering brighter, more even teeth in a relatively short period of time.

2. Dental Veneers

Dental veneers are thin, custom-made shells, usually made of porcelain or composite resin, that are bonded to the front surface of the teeth. Veneers are used to correct a variety of cosmetic problems, including discoloration, chipped or cracked teeth, gaps between teeth, and minor misalignments. They provide a durable, natural-looking solution to improve the appearance of a smile while preserving the underlying tooth structure.

3. Dental Crowns

Dental crowns, also known as caps, are tooth-shaped prostheses that are placed over damaged or decayed teeth to restore their strength, function, and appearance. Crowns can be made of a variety of materials, including porcelain, ceramic, metal alloys, or a combination of these materials. They are commonly used to cover severely discolored or misshapen teeth, protect weak teeth from further damage, and support bridges or dental implants. 4. Dental Bonding

Dental bonding involves the application of a tooth-colored composite resin material to repair minor imperfections such as chips, cracks, or gaps in the teeth. The resin is sculpted and shaped to blend seamlessly with natural teeth, resulting in a more uniform and aesthetically pleasing smile. Dental bonding is a cost-effective and minimally invasive alternative to procedures such as veneers or crowns, and offers immediate results with little to no discomfort.

5. Orthodontic Treatments

Orthodontic treatments, including braces and clear aligners such as Invisalign, are commonly used.

Orthodontic procedures are used to correct misaligned teeth and malocclusions (bite problems). While primarily aimed at improving dental function and oral health, orthodontic procedures also contribute to improving the aesthetics of the smile by properly aligning teeth and closing gaps. Advances in orthodontic technology have led to the development of more discreet and comfortable options for patients seeking to straighten their teeth without the visibility of traditional metal braces.

6. Gum Contouring

Gum contouring, also known as gum reshaping or tissue sculpting, involves the surgical removal of excess gum tissue to improve the symmetry and proportion of the gums to the teeth. This procedure is often performed to treat a "gummy smile," in which an excessive amount of gum tissue is visible when smiling, or to correct uneven gum lines. Gum contouring can dramatically improve the overall appearance of a smile and create a more balanced and harmonious aesthetic.

** Applications of Aesthetic Dentistry

Aesthetic dentistry finds widespread applications in various dental specialties, addressing both aesthetic problems and functional impairments. Some of the key applications include:

1. Restorative Dentistry

Aesthetic principles are integral to restorative dentistry, which focuses on repairing and replacing damaged or missing teeth. Whether restoring a single tooth with a crown or bridge, or reconstructing a complete smile with dental implants, aesthetic considerations play a crucial role in achieving natural-looking results that blend seamlessly with the remaining dentition.

2. Prosthodontics

Prosthodontics is a dental specialty that deals with the restoration and replacement of missing teeth and oral structures. Aesthetic dentistry techniques are essential in the design and fabrication of various prosthetic devices, including dentures, bridges, and implant-supported restorations, to ensure optimal fit, function, and aesthetics for the patient.

3. Periodontics

Periodontology focuses on the prevention, diagnosis, and treatment of gum disease and other conditions affecting the supporting structures of the teeth. Aesthetic periodontal procedures, such as gum contouring and grafting, are performed to improve the appearance of the gums and enhance the overall aesthetics of the smile, particularly in cases of excessive gingival display or gum recession.

4. Endodontics

Endodontics deals with the diagnosis and treatment of diseases of the dental pulp and root canals. While primarily concerned with preserving tooth health and function, endodontic procedures, such as root canal therapy, can also have aesthetic implications, particularly in cases where tooth discoloration or damage affects the appearance of the smile.

5. Orthodontics

Orthodontics focuses on the diagnosis and treatment of misaligned teeth and malocclusions. Aesthetic considerations are paramount in orthodontic treatment planning, as patients often seek orthodontic intervention not only to improve dental function but also to achieve a more attractive and confident smile.

In conclusion, cosmetic dentistry represents the union of art and science in the pursuit of smile perfection. By combining advanced dental techniques with an artistic eye for detail, cosmetic dentists can transform smiles and improve the lives of their patients. From teeth whitening and veneers to orthodontic treatments and gum contouring, the field of cosmetic dentistry offers a wide range of solutions to address virtually any cosmetic problem. As the demand for beautiful smiles continues to grow, cosmetic dentistry remains at the forefront of innovation, delivering natural-looking results that inspire confidence and radiate happiness.

TREATABLE DISEASES

Within the immune system, lymph is a part of the blood plasma that crosses the walls of the capillaries, diffuses through the interstices of the tissues and, after being loaded with substances produced by the activity of the cells, enters the lymphatic vessels through which it circulates until it is into the venous

Primary immunodeficiencies are generally congenital and range from and controllable abnormalities to deficiencies so severe that they become a battle incompatible with life extension. Secondary immunodeficiencies can be controlled or inhibited by inducing prompt treatment for malnutrition. They can also treated with minimal doses of toxic drugs such as those used in cancer treatments in alternative medicine and botany. According to recent advances (1980 and 1996), but not complementary, they can be benign or serious, that is, they are related to B lymphocytes as is the case in autoimmune diseases, or to T lymphocytes as occurs in cases of diseases terminal diseases such as leukemia and AIDS that require more invasive healing methods such as bone marrow transplants. Acute leukemia is a form of leukemia that is frequently diagnosed in children and Young adults.

Its symptoms are irregular fevers, spjntaneous from the gums, mucous membranes or under the skin, and rapidly evolving anemia. In recent years it has shown that the combination of chemotherapies, ionizing radiation and a diet in anticancer agents such as green leafy vegetables, carotenes and fruits such as pineapple and soursop have improved the cure rate between 50% and 90% of patients treated.

Current medicine classifies Six components whose cellular activity directly interferes in the immune defense process of Our nutrients within the bloodstream. From these components, three are different than cells, and the other three are a type of soluble protein. The three categories of immune cells are: granulocytes, monocytes or macrophages, and Granulocytes are the most abundant cells with nuclei in the blood and they ingest the antigens that penetrate the then use their powerful enzymes to destroy them, thus representing the cells that will communicate the acquired immunity to the system, once they re-enter to attack us.

Monocytes make up a small percentage of all cells which, when they are located in the tissues of the organs and out of the are transformed into macrophages, developing powerful tentacles to trap external allergens. Lymphocytes are the most cells of the immune system. There are the of B lymphocytes that are responsible for the humoral or serological immunity that produce immunoglobulins, and those of the T type that are for cellular balance by directly attacking antigens and producing cytokines, destruction that becomes more effective When the person is already have been to antigen before. The remaining three cells are immunoglobulins, cytokines, and complement proteins that combine with one type of antigen and contribute to its destruction.

It has been known that the side effects of antihistamines are almost zero and harmless, however their long-term suppressive action of beta-carotene can be harmful for patients with recurrent allergies, so it is recommended to accompany the diet with foods high in this content like the orange ones, which are carrots, squash and tangerines. The organs that are part of the immune system are the tonsils, which is a mass of lymphoid tissue with nodules located in the throat which has a function of protecting the pharynx from bacteria that enter through the digestive system. It is in the thymus, located at the level of the Sternum that plays an important role until adolescence of the individual, also formed by lymphatic tissue and that is assumed as a constructor of T lymphocytes since in adulthood it is filled with fat and its function is probably replaced by bone marrow from skeletal bones. Finally, we find the spleen, which is a spongy organ located behind the stomach and just below the diaphragm and is composed of two types of tissue: the so-called White pulp that produces lymphocytes that are released into the bloodstream to attack infections and the red pulp that It is responsible for eliminating broken cells with the help of macrophages in addition to being a reserve of iron similar to that of the liver with bile. An overactive spleen is associated with the appearance of anemia due to an irregular function on the red cells.

The lymphatic system, recognized for being located on the left side of the circulatory system, is formed by circulatory capillaries and ducts in which digested lipids from the intestine are collected and transported to the to eliminate and destroy toxic substances and to the spread of diseases. Its main function is the destruction of the material that results from the degradation of the proteins made up of amino acids, which thus form the lymph, which flows through the lymphatic capillaries to finally eliminate through muscular movements. Hence the importance of avoiding a sedentary life and doing physical exercise such as walking, running in the open field, or practicing a of preference.

The ailments or ailments that are considered treatable by botanical medicine and by medicine because they originate from poor nutrition are many and we will expose them below. Among the most Common autoimmune diseases we find those caused by few allergies that cause skin itching or itching that is suffered by redness of the epidermis, tachycardia and even sudden diarrhea episodes. This group of diseases are produced by the foods we eat and their treatment is based on controlling the foods that have the allergen that triggers the immediate symptoms. In the case of food allergies in general, they can produced by canned foods, shellfish, some sausages, some noodles and nuts such as peanuts or peanuts.

In a similar way, it happens to infants and adults who suffer from lactumen, a disease characterized by allergy or metabolic reaction to the ingestion of milk with lactose, which is already controllable through specific brands that manufacture products visibly different of cells, and the Other three are a type of soluble protein. The three categories of immune cells are: granulocytes, monocytes or macrophages, and Granulocytes are the most abundant cells with nuclei in the blood and they ingest the antigens that penetrate the then use their powerful enzymes to destroy them, thus representing the cells that Will communicate the acquired immunity to the system, once they re-enter to attack us. Monocytes make up a small percentage of all blcxyd cells which, When they are located in the tissues of the organs and out of the are transformed into macrophages, developing powerful tentacles to trap external allergens. Lymphocytes are the most cells of the immune system. There are the of B lymphocytes that are responsible for the humoral or serological immunity that produce immunoglobulins, and those of the T type that are for cellular balance by directly attacking antigens and producing cytokines, destruction that becomes more effective When the person is already have been to antigen before. The remaining three cells are immunoglobulins, cytokines, and complement proteins that combine with one type of antigen and contribute to its destruction.

It has been known that the side effects of antihistamines are almost zero and harmless, however their long- term suppressive action of beta-carotene can be harmful for patients with recurrent allergies, so it is recommended to accompany the diet with foods high in this content like the Orange ones, which are carrots, squash and tangerines. The organs that are part of the immune system are the tonsils, which is a mass of lymphoid tissue with nodules located in the throat which has a function of protecting the pharynx from bacteria that enter through the digestive system.

It is in the thymus, located at the level of the Sternum that plays an important role until adolescence of the individual, also formed by lymphatic tissue and that is assumed as a constructor of T lymphocytes since in adulthood it is filled with fat and its function is probably replaced by bone marrow from skeletal bones. Finally, we find the spleen, which is a spongy organ labeled with the indication: Without lactose. Another group of patients who are already Offered a range of for the treatment of their disease are celiacs or allergic to gluten, which is a nutrient present in Wheat, rye, legumes and foods made with flours. processed. These patients are prepared a diet rich in vegetables, fruits and gluten-free foods since eating these foods directly can cause terrible diarrheal episodes as in the case of lacto allergies. Finally, we find the phenylketonurics who basically must avoid sweets such as powdered soft drinks, chewing gums and sweeteners that contain the artificial amino acid phenylalanine that acts against the cells themselves, producing similar reactions to those already mentioned in the person who consumes them. .

The treatments with antihistamines prescribed by a doctor are since there are only 25 plants with this property and they are Of European origin. (See chapter Of blog articles). Children and Young with type I diabetes or insulin-dependent IDDM mellitus, which is to have an autoimmune linkage mechanism. Its symptoms are marked thirst, weight loss and fatigue due to the failure of main Source Of energy which is glucose. It constitutes 10 to 15% Of the cases and is of rapid evolution.

Type 2, or non-insulin- is adult diabetes and usually appears in over 40 years Of age and has a Slow evolution. Blood and urine testS allow its diagnosis since it does not symptoms. Another autoimmune disease with 10% mortality among women and men who suffer from it during the first 3 years is myasthenia gravis, which is a non-hereditary autoimmune disease, in which the lymphocytes in the blood produce antibodies that destroy the receptors, as acetylcholine located in muscle cells.

Its symptoms are the loss of motor reflexes of the extremities in various degrees of severity. Acetylcholines role is to transmit signals between nerves and muscles, so when its receptors are destroyed, muscle contraction cannot be induced. A diet similar to the muscle diet presented in this book would be reasonable, including such as White Wine or beer, Soy in all its forms and derivatives, lemon, and whole grains and cereals.

Within the group of diseases produced in the organs of the immune system are tonsillitis which is an inflammation produced by a viral or bacterial infection, or irritation of external origin. When there is an increase in the volume of a lymph node in the area below the shoulders, or the groin, it is called adenopathy and it can be caused by bacteria or viruses that overload the node. The ears are also located near specific glands, so its relationship with infections, balance problems and drug use is closely associated with the discomfort that as a side effect arises both in young and in adults. Another Epstein-Barr virus infection is infectious mononucleosis that is transmitted through saliva when sharing food, kissing and sputum, so you should be aware of mouth sores and affects the production of lymphocytes and red blood cells, in adolescents and young adults that makes it susceptible to inflammation in various parts of the due to cell growth in addition to weakness.

In the group of various dermatoses or skin allergies, an extensive number of diseases are mentioned, ranging from those with genetic inheritance such as psoriasis, also known as caracha, scabies or scab, is a chronic skin disease that It affects 2% of World population and is distinguished by Slight pinkish scaly lesions on fair skin that appear on the chest and back. Similar to this is anthrax, popularly known as fish eye, which are produced by the bacteriurn Bacillus anthracis and affect humans and cattle and are skin ulcers presented with a black center that are surgically removed and antimi obial drugs.

Epidermitis, seborrhea of the scalp also causes dandruff due to the increase and alteration of the secretion of sebum or fatty matter produced by the glands and its treatment is Aesthetic conditions such as erythema of the face of the malar area, which is the one in the Shape of a butterfly on the rosy cheeks, forehead and nose that in some cases evolves as acne, which is an eruptive disease of the follicles of the sebaceous glands that secrete a A purulent Cyst that leaves spots and scars on the surface of the skin, which is why the recipes for treatment or natural masks in the next chapter of this book are recommended.

A carelessness in the cleanliness next to that of the face together with a high fat diet can unleash the well-known purulent abscesses. Personal hygiene and diet play an important role in avoiding these types of skin eruptions, as well as avoiding tap water in areas where parasites are detected. Congenital or moles are by the accumulation of pigments in the skin and at any age of the person and are mostly benign, but if itching and burning are experienced they should be examined by an oncologist to rule out psoriasis, anthrax or cancer of skin.

Herpes is a group of skin diseases caused by human pathogenic viruses that appear on the face and lips accompanied by flu and colds, and of which type 1 , 2, and the varicella-zoster It presents with vesicles of liquid that dry in 5 days and its most serious cases are treated with Soy products. infection of the eye, called dendritic keratitis, can irreversibly damage the cornea, requiring a transplant. In the Summer season, during beach walks, it is currently more common than usual with climatic changes, severe sunburn and ultraviolet radiation that makes it necessary to use sunglasses, a hat and sunscreen for protection. to skin that should not be longer than 4 hours. For its treatment, also consult Our section on masks in the chapter on sexual reproduction.

Sweating is important for the natural elimination of body toxins through the skin and through physical exercise, but When we must remain in work areas or carry out work outside, we can avoid bad humoral or body odors through frequent ingestion. of aromatic herbal teas such as cinnamon, vanilla and pepper in meats, in addition to the use of flavored talcum and box moisturizers. TO finish briefly outlining the diseases associated with the functioning of the immune system, we point out those of greater severity such as arthritis and rheumatic fever, which are characterized by the appearance of fever with inflammation of the joints of the limbs such as legs and arms, also associated with scarlet fever. which is a fever accompanied by angina pain. All these diseases are recommended to be followed with the recommendations presented in the chapter on our circulatory diet since they also present symptoms associated with other organs such as the heart.

Other serious diseases associated with the lymphatic and endocrine systems are Addison's disease, which occurs due to insufficient hormonal secretions of the kidney glands, where it is necessary to include iodized table salt in the diet and of the collagen such as the White of bird eggs. Regarding multiple sclerosis patients who require natural immunomodulators to control myelin attacks, it is recommended to include a diet high in cereals such as oats and flaxseed in addition to the inclusion of White vegetables such as turnip.

In the case of cancer of any type, it is due to the proliferation of abnormal cells in the tissues of the organs and of important endocrine glands of the body, for which we recommend following this shifted immune diet or in combination with the foods listed in the menus. In addition of the endocrine diet, to the listed antioxidant-rich foods and cleansing herbs such as cats claw in Your diet.

HERPES

This is another viral skin condition affecting 1 in 3 people in the general population: Herpes. Its name comes from the Greek word herpein, meaning "to crawl," a generic term for various types of skin rashes caused by the most important human pathogenic viruses. Its main representatives are:

Ø Herpes simplex virus type 1. SIMPLEX. Two types are known. Herpes virus type 1 causes fever blisters in association with various febrile infectious diseases (colds, flu, pneumonia). The blisters appear around the lips and in the mouth (also called cold sores); on the nose, face, and ears, and on the oral and pharyngeal mucosa. During the period between rashes, the virus has been isolated in the neuronal cell bodies of the facial nerve: this is its reservoir. There is no curative treatment; oral and topical medications such as Acyclovir can be used to relieve pain, itching, and inflammation.

Ø Herpes type 2 or genital herpes: Herpesvirus type 2 causes genital herpes. This is a sexually transmitted disease of increasing importance. It is occasionally accompanied by headache and fever. It begins with moderate local itching followed by a progressive eruption of vesicles. These rupture, form scabs, and eventually dry up. This entire process can last from one to three weeks. New vesicle eruptions often appear when the previous eruption is drying up. Another route of transmission is congenital: the newborn of an infected mother becomes infected during birth, contracting the systemic disease, which is often fatal. This serious risk requires these children to be delivered by cesarean section. Genital herpes has been treated topically since 1982 and as a systemic treatment since 1984. Herpesvirus type 2 is the cause of cervical cancer: the viruses lodge in the mucosal cells and, years later, eventually cause the transformation, sometimes cancerous, of these cells.

Viruses can also infect the central nervous system, especially in weakened or immunosuppressed patients, such as those with cancer, causing severe encephalitis. Early treatment can prevent death or serious brain damage.

Varicella-Zoster Herpes (VZ). Recurrence of the varicella-zoster virus, which was not completely eradicated by the immune system during childhood chickenpox and remains lodged in the nerve ganglia. In situations of immunodeficiency, the virus reactivates and causes the infection known as shingles. The skin innervated by the nerve containing the virus suffers a blistering eruption, accompanied by intense pain and altered sensation. Initially, the blisters are filled with clear fluid, then become cloudy, and finally rupture and form crusts that dry out after 5-10 days. The pain caused by the herpes zoster virus can be intense and last for several weeks. After recovery, neuralgia may persist in the affected area. High-dose treatment can reduce symptoms, and appropriate analgesic treatment is also necessary. Severe cases can be treated with corticosteroids (cortisone). Persistent neuralgia can be treated with nerve stem blocks or surgery. In patients undergoing chemotherapy for neoplastic diseases, the development of shingles can be fatal. Vaccines are being tested in Japan for children being treated for leukemia; preliminary results appear promising. A herpes infection of the eye, called dendritic keratitis, can cause irreversible damage to the cornea. Ø Other important herpesviruses are the Epstein-Barr virus, which causes infectious mononucleosis, and cytomegalovirus, which can cause birth defects when it infects pregnant women.

Natural treatments recommend relieving certain discomforts that occur during the course of this disease, such as burning skin by applying compresses of cold water and apple cider vinegar, taking antihistamines to control itching, and also sleep aids such as black tea, chamomile, and ground nutmeg to prevent insomnia. Over-the-counter creams and astringent lotions such as calamine help dry out blisters in the first week when applied sparingly to the area where the herpes infection develops.

PSORIASIS

Psoriasis is a chronic, recurring skin disease characterized by the appearance of erythematous, scaly plaques and papules on the skin's surface. It affects 2% of the world's population. The lesions are usually slightly raised above the normal skin surface and clearly distinguishable from normal skin; their color ranges from red to reddish brown. They are usually covered by small, grayish-white scales that adhere to the underlying rash and,

If removed, they leave an erythematous surface with hemorrhagic dots. The extent of the disease can vary from a few small lesions to widespread involvement of most of the skin surface. It typically affects the elbows, knees, scalp, and chest.

The etiology of the disease is unknown, although very rapid epidermal cell proliferation has been observed (three to four days compared to the normal three weeks). It almost never occurs in people with black skin pigmentation, and a family history is noted. Various topical preparations may be helpful, and the rash sometimes resolves with sun exposure. A successful treatment for severe chronic psoriasis was introduced in 1979. It involves first covering the skin with a dye that absorbs ultraviolet light and then exposing the area to ultraviolet light. Because this technique increases the incidence of mild skin cancers, it is reserved only for severe cases of psoriasis.

LIPOMA

A lipoma is a tumor containing fatty tissue. These noncancerous lumps develop under the skin and appear pale or colorless. Lipomas usually feel soft and movable. Lipomas generally do not cause symptoms. However, a lipoma that includes several blood vessels or nerves may feel soft or painful. The exact cause of lipomas remains unknown. Some genetic conditions, such as Gardner syndrome, may increase the chance of developing a lipoma. Lipomas do not require medical treatment unless they are painful, bothersome, or prevent the person from living a normal life.

Treatment options for lipomas include:

Ø liposuction

Ø drainage

Ø steroid injection

Ø surgical excision

A cold or viral infection can cause swollen lymph nodes. Lymph nodes are small glands that filter harmful substances from lymphatic fluid, which is the clear liquid that flows through the lymphatic vessels. These small, bean-shaped lymph nodes are an essential component of the immune system. They produce and store white blood cells that destroy disease-causing pathogens and debris.

Sometimes, lymph nodes swell in response to bacterial or viral infections. They may feel hard and painful. Swollen lymph nodes usually appear in the head, neck, armpits, or groin.

Several factors can cause swollen lymph nodes in people, such as:

Ø A cold or other viral infection

Ø Bacterial infections

Ø Tooth infection

Ø Ear infection

Ø Medical conditions that affect the immune system, such as rheumatoid arthritis or lupus

People who have swollen lymph nodes due to an infection may also experience other symptoms, such as runny nose, cough, sore throat, fever, headaches, and fatigue. In most cases, swollen lymph nodes heal on their own without medical treatment. If they don't, treatment should address the underlying cause, usually an infection.

A swollen lymph node that feels hard, rubbery, or immobile may indicate a more serious medical condition. Certain types of cancer, such as lymphoma, leukemia, and breast cancer, can affect the lymph nodes. Anyone concerned about swollen lymph nodes should consult a physician.

CYSTS

Another condition that aestheticians should recognize and refer to medical specialists is a cyst, which is a closed sac of tissue containing fluid or debris. Cysts can form anywhere on the body. Their texture varies depending on the material trapped inside the sac. A cyst can develop due to a blocked sebaceous gland or hair follicle. Cysts feel like soft blisters when they are near the skin's surface, but they can feel like hard bumps when they develop deep within the skin.

A hard cyst near the skin's surface usually contains dead skin cells or trapped proteins. Types of cysts include:

Ø Ganglion cysts, which are common in the wrists and hands

Ø Synovial cysts, which develop in the spine

Ø Pilar cysts, which appear on the scalp

Ø Mucous cysts, which can form on the feet, toes, or inside the mouth. Cysts rarely require treatment and usually stop growing and disappear on their own. In some cases, a black dot may develop near the center of a cyst. When this happens, a cyst may burst, releasing a white or yellow discharge.

An infected cyst that is red, swollen, or painful may require medical treatment, such as:

Ø Antibiotics

Ø needle aspiration

Ø corticosteroid injections

Ø a surgical procedure to remove the cyst. On the other hand, we also find dermatofibromas.

Dermatofibromas are hard, brown or red bumps found under the skin. They usually develop in exposed areas of the skin, such as the legs, arms, and back. Dermatofibromas do not develop into cancer. Generally, people with dermatofibromas do not experience other symptoms. However, in some cases, a dermatofibroma may cause itching, irritation, or sensitivity to the touch. Dermatofibromas develop when excess cells accumulate in the thickest layer of skin, called the dermis. The exact cause of dermatofibromas remains uncertain, but possible causes include:

Ø Trauma or injury to the skin

Ø Insect or spider bites

Ø Splinters

Dermatofibromas generally do not require treatment, but they tend to remain in the skin for the rest of a person's life. A doctor may be asked to surgically remove the dermatofibroma if it is unsightly or located in an uncomfortable area.

Other treatment options will only remove part of the dermatofibroma. These include:

Ø Freezing it with liquid nitrogen

Ø Corticosteroid injections

Ø Shaving the top layers of the growth

Ø Removing its core

Among the most common autoimmune diseases are those caused by food allergies, which cause everything from skin itching or itching accompanied by reddening of the epidermis, rapid heartbeat, and even sudden episodes of diarrhea. This group of diseases is caused by the foods we eat, and their treatment is based on controlling the foods that contain the allergen that triggers the immediate symptoms. In the case of those with general food allergies, these allergies can be caused by canned foods, seafood, some pork sausages, some noodles, and nuts such as peanuts.

A similar situation occurs with infants and adults suffering from lactumen, a disease characterized by an allergy or metabolic reaction to the consumption of milk containing lactose. This disease is now controllable through specific product brands that manufacture products visibly labeled with the following information: lactose-free. Another group of patients who are already offered a range of specially processed products for the treatment of their condition are those with celiac disease or those allergic to gluten, a nutrient present in wheat, rye, legumes, and foods made with processed flours.

These patients are given a diet rich in vegetables, fruits, and gluten-free foods, since eating these foods directly can cause terrible diarrheal episodes, as is the case with lactose allergies. Finally, we find phenylketonurics, who must basically avoid sweets such as powdered soft drinks, chewing gum, and sweeteners containing the artificial amino acid phenylalanine, which acts against the body's own cells, producing reactions similar to those mentioned above in the person who consumes them. Treatment with antihistamines prescribed by doctors is appropriate, since there are only 25 plants with this property, and they are of European origin. (See the blog article chapter.) Children and young people who suffer from type 1 diabetes or insulin-dependent mellitus (IDDM), which is believed to have an autoimmune mechanism. Its symptoms are intense thirst, weight loss, and fatigue due to the failure of the main energy source, glucose. It accounts for 10 to 15% of cases and progresses rapidly. Type 2, or non-insulin-dependent, is adult-onset diabetes and usually appears in people over 40 years of age and progresses slowly. Blood and urine tests allow for its diagnosis, as it produces no symptoms.

Another autoimmune disease with a 10% mortality rate among women and men who suffer from it during the first 3 years is myasthenia gravis. This is a non-hereditary autoimmune disease in which blood lymphocytes produce antibodies that destroy acetylcholine receptors located on muscle cells. Its symptoms include the loss of motor reflexes in the extremities, varying in severity. The function of acetylcholine is to transmit signals between nerves and muscles, so when its receptors are destroyed, muscle contraction cannot be induced. A diet similar to the muscle-building diet presented in this book would be recommended, including foods such as white wine or beer, soy in all its forms and derivatives, lemon, and whole-grain pasta and cereals. Within the group of diseases produced in the organs of the immune system are tonsillitis, which is an inflammation caused by a viral infection.

Swollen or bacterial lymph nodes, or irritation of external origin. When a lymph node located in the area below the shoulders or groin enlarges, it is called adenopathy and can be caused by bacteria or viruses overloading the node. The ears are also located near specific lymph nodes, so their relationship with infections, balance problems, and drug use is closely associated with the discomfort that arises as a side effect in both young people and adults. Another Epstein-Barr virus infection is infectious mononucleosis, which is transmitted through saliva when sharing food, kissing, and sputum. Therefore, one should be alert for mouth sores. It affects the production of lymphocytes and red blood cells in adolescents and young adults, making them susceptible to inflammation in various parts of the body due to cell enlargement and weakness.

The group of various dermatoses or skin allergies includes a wide range of diseases, ranging from those associated with genetic inheritance, such as psoriasis, also known as scabies, or mange. This chronic skin disease affects 2% of the world's population and is characterized by mild, pinkish, scaly lesions on light-colored skin that appear on the chest and back. Similar to this is anthrax, commonly known as fish eye, which is caused by the bacterium Bacillus anthracis and affects humans and cattle. These ulcers are skin lesions with a black center that are surgically removed and treated with antimicrobial drugs.

Epidermitis, a seborrhea of the scalp, also causes dandruff due to increased and altered secretion of sebum, or fatty matter, produced by the glands. It is treated with shampoos. Aesthetic conditions such as facial erythema in the malar area, which is the butterfly-shaped rash on the rosy cheeks, forehead, and nose, which in some cases develops into acne, an eruptive disease of the sebaceous gland follicles that secrete a purulent cyst that leaves spots and scars on the skin's surface, are why the treatment recipes or natural masks in this chapter are recommended. Neglecting facial hygiene, along with a high-fat diet, can trigger the well-known purulent abscesses. Personal hygiene and nutrition play an important role in avoiding these types of skin rashes, as well as avoiding tap water in areas where parasites are found. Congenital spots or moles are caused by the accumulation of pigment in the skin and appear at any age. Most are benign. However, if you experience itching and burning, you should be examined by an oncologist to rule out psoriasis, anthrax, or skin cancer.

Herpes is a group of skin diseases caused by human pathogenic viruses that appear on the face, back, shoulders, and lips, accompanied by colds and flu, including types 1, 2, and varicella-zoster. It presents with fluid-filled blisters that dry out within 2 to 4 weeks, and the most severe cases are treated with soy products. A herpes infection of the eye, called dendritic keratitis, can cause irreversible corneal damage, requiring a transplant. It should be treated for the first 72 hours with oral treatments, while immunosuppressed patients may be hospitalized and treated intravenously. It is a virus that rarely recurs, but it should be treated due to its ability to cause disability and intense pain in the blisters on the skin where it appears.

During the summer, severe sunburn and ultraviolet radiation burns are becoming more common than usual due to climate changes during beach walks. This requires the use of sunglasses, a hat, and sunscreen to protect the skin from exposure, which should not exceed 4 hours. For treatment, also see our section on masks in the chapter on sexual reproduction. Sweating is important for the natural elimination of toxins through the skin and through physical exercise, but when we must remain in work areas or perform work outdoors, we can avoid unpleasant humoral or body odors by frequently drinking aromatic herbal teas such as cinnamon, vanilla, and pepper on meats, in addition to using scented talcum powder, perfumes, and body moisturizers.

To finish briefly outlining the diseases associated with the functioning of the immune system, we point out the most serious ones such as arthritis and rheumatic fever, which are characterized by the appearance of fever with inflammation of the joints of the limbs such as legs and arms, also associated with scarlet fever, which is a fever accompanied by angina pain. All of these diseases are recommended to be followed with the recommendations presented in the chapter on our circulatory diet, as they also present with symptoms associated with other organs such as the heart. Other serious diseases associated with the lymphatic and endocrine systems are Addison's disease, which occurs when hormonal secretions from the kidney glands are insufficient. It is necessary to permanently include iodized table salt in the diet and collagen products such as egg whites. For patients with multiple sclerosis who require natural immunomodulators to control myelin damage, it is recommended to include a diet high in grains such as oats and flaxseed, in addition to white vegetables such as turnips. In the case of cancer of any type, it is due to the proliferation of abnormal cells in the tissues of the body's organs and important endocrine glands. Therefore, we recommend following this immunological diet in rotation or in combination with the foods listed in the endocrine diet menus, in addition to the antioxidant-rich foods listed and purifying herbs such as cat's claw in the following diets.

Our nails are the flat, horny, protective coverings that appear on the upper part of the final segment of human fingers. Nails are made of dead cells that contain a fibrous protein, keratin. Each nail has a base or root, which is the part that penetrates the skin; a body, which has an outer and inner side attached to the skin; and the edge, the free end. The skin below the root and the body is called the nail matrix. It is thin and covered with vascularized papillae, and because the horny material is transparent, these give the nail its characteristic color. Near the base, there are fewer papillae and they are less vascularized; it is the whitest part and, due to its peculiar shape, is called the lunula. Nail growth is due to cell division at the base and on the inner surface of the nail body.

In conclusion, we can affirm that skin diseases affect millions of people worldwide. Understanding the classification and specific symptoms of these conditions is the first step to obtaining a proper diagnosis and treatment. Consultation with a dermatologist is essential in these cases.

HANDS AND FEET

Nails are protective coatings, flat and horny, which appear in the upper area of the final segment of human fingers. Nails are made up of dead cells that contain a fibrous protein, keratin. Each nail has a base or root, which is the part that penetrates the skin; a which has an outer face and an inner face attached to the skin; and the edge, the free end end. The skin Wow the root and is called the nail matrix; it is thin and covered with vascularized papillae, and the horny material is transparent, these give the nail its characteristic color. Near the base there are fewer and less vascular papillae; It is the

Whitest part and it causes of its peculiar is called the lunula. Nail growth is due to the division of cells at the base and on the inside of the nail

Pedicure

It is the treatment of the corneal skin conditions of the feet. A pedicurist or pedicurist, commonly called a callista, is the who the pedicure. A pedicure treatment is also a way to improve the appearance of the feet and the ones.

Starting you get a tub of warm water, a towel, and the necessary utensils; don't forget the pumice Stone, pliers, cuticle scissors and a file in good condition.

Choose the shade of nail polish that you are going to use, and have some cotton nearby. Try to have everything on hand so you don't have to run to get it in the middle of the Put all the utensils in a basket or container to make things easier for yourself.

Remove the Old nail polish. It is advisable to use a polish remover that does not contain acetone, as this substance could dry out Your and cause them to crack or hurt at the edges.

Get Your feet Wet. Soak Your feet for fifteen minutes in warm water with a special pedicure product, or add some scented Oil to the water. In addition to being relaxing, it Will soften Your feet to facilitate the removal of dry and dead skin.

Dry them very w ell. not forget to dry well between the toes, as it is a very susceptible for the development of bacteria and accumulation of dirt. Dry Your feet very well and run the corner of the towel between your toes.

Soften your feet. Smooth feet are as flawless polish. Regularly removing calloused skin will help prevent thickening of some areas of skin that may later crack. This softness on the feet requires a little effort and dedication. Try to avoid the unpleasant razor completely, as its use carries the risk of cuts and damage to the deep layers of the skin. Instead, use a metal-surfaced foot file or a pumice Stone. Rub them vigorously into areas of callused and dry skin, especially the heels and metatarsals. Doing this frequently, it will save you a lot of time on future pedicures.

Keep Your feet in Shape. Keeping Your nails in shouldn't be overlooked. Long nails can damage Your socks and even alter the way you walk

When you cut them, be careful not to overdo it a nail could bury itself. so don't leave them flush or file much. The Shape of the nail should be as a mirror of the natural curve of the cuticle. File the edges gently. If Your toenails have a bit of volume, you can use a file to even them out a bit.

If you want to remove the cuticles, do not cut them, you could hurt yourself, better push them gently towards the rest of the skin. This will be easier after your foot bath.

Soften Your feet. Smooth feet are as important as flawless polish. Regularly removing calloused skin will help prevent thickening of some areas of skin that may later crack. This softness on the feet requires a little effort and dedication. Try to avoid the unpleasant razor completely, as its use carries the risk of cuts and damage to the deep layers of the skin. Instead, use a metal-surfaced to file or a pumice stone. Rub them vigorously into areas of callused and dry skin, especially the heels and metatarsals. The removal of calloused skin will be smoother and easier after having thoroughly moistened Your feet.

Moisturize Your feet. After so much work, it's time to Your feet. Apply a special moisturizing for feet, so that they feel soft and smooth. Since the skin on Your feet is much thicker than that of any Other part of Your body, you Will need a very effective moisturizing The intensive action of the moisturizing cream for dry feet is ideal for this purpose.

Take the time to massage Your feet while you apply the cream. In addition to very relaxing, it Will stimulate circulation and help the cream to well into the skin.

Manicure

A manicure is a cosmetic beauty treatment for the nails and hands that is usually done at home or in a beauty salon. In a manicure, the edges of the nails are cut or filed, the hands are massaged, and nail polish is applied. Not only because of the delicacy that this job requires but the drying times. Finally, we can say that doing a basic manicure, with cleaning, care and makeup of the nail should last between 1 hour and 1 hour and a half maximum. The professional manicure is a highly requested aesthetic service because it allows us to keep our hands and nails completely neat and clean. In addition, the fact of cutting the nails helps to avoid deformations or ingrown nails. Manicure, like the rest of makeup in general, has its origin in Ancient Egypt. Initially the pharaohs used henna to paint their nails, both the color and the length indicated the level in this civilization. The French manicure in the 18th Century in Paris. Its Pink base and White tip design enchanted everyone, and it was extremely in the 1920s and 1930s. The manicure tips out there are:

BASIC MANICURE. The basic manicure is actually the foundation of all manicures.

- Permanent manicure. This of manicure or nail can used in all manicure.

- French manicure.

- Reverse French manicure.
- American manicure.
- Italian manicure.
- Russian manicure.

Nail diseases

The most Common nail diseases are onychomycosis (fungus), ingrown toenail (When the sides of the nail sink into the foot) and anonychia (total or partial lack of the nail).

Striated nails. Stretch marks can be. -Longitudinal: they are the most common, and one of the first reasons for consultation. The doctor out that they don't really have any pathological significance. They often appear with age, starting around the age of 60, and their origin is usually hereditary. There is no and effective treatment to end stretch marks, although some cosmetic firms have gels that form a small layer that optically provides uniformity to the nail. However, this product cannot change its nature.

-Transverse or 'Beau's Lines': They after an alteration in the growth of the nail. The causes can acute febrile processes, nutritional alterations or the use of cytotoxic drugs, but also due to serious diseases.

2. Soft and weak nails. They may be:

-Fine, Without consistency: It may due to chronic diseases, rheumatic diseases , etc. -They break easily or get a 'slit' (onychorresis). It often occurs from repeatedly putting Your hands in water, especially after an age.

Separation by layers. Called Lamellar Onicoschisis, it after the age of 50 or 60, for the Same reason mentioned above: an excess of hand washing. The remedy is to try to wash them less.

Yellow color. It can be due to the abuse of lacquers, fungal or bacterial infections, or also due to psoriasis. 5. Ingrown nails.

This is a pathology often associated with Young and its cause is eminently hereditary, like most nail-related diseases. It sticks into the meat, inflaming it. The solution is to wear a Shoe that is less tight and avoid those that end in a Do not trim the spikes of the big toe nail, you have to leave the edges and preferably cut it in a Square You can also soak a Cotton ball in antiseptic and place on these edges, between the nail and the flesh. The proper length of the protruding "white" part should 1 millimeter.

Fungi (Mycosis). Athlete's foot is a cutaneous mycosis of the foot. This disease, which is also called tinea is caused by species of the genus Trichophyton or by Epidermophyton floccosum. The symptoms are redness of the skin followed by the appearance of cracks between the fingers and watery discharge, accompanied by itching (itching) in all phases. It is very contagious and can be acquired by walking on damp floors such as those in bathrooms and swimming pools or sinks. The fungus can spread to other parts of the body. A very Common mistake is to think that all nail diseases are caused by fungi, although they are the most frequent cause. Even dermatologists themselves can sometimes find it difficult to diagnose mycosis in this part of the anatomy. Possible clues of a fungal infected

1. Distal color change (of the free or "White" part). often a yellowish or Whitish area may appear.

2. The nail separates, due to thickening in some areas of the nail.

3. Formation of a under the nail. All three causes can occurs isolation, and even these manifestations do not have to indicate fungi in all cases.

Microtrauma- Due to pressure with shoes or from doing some aggressive sports, such as running or playing tennis, sometimes the nails 'shed', or purple or yellowish streaks appear. The only is aesthetic and the problem by itself if we abandon that habit. The doctor denies that the origin is a lack of calcium. The small White spots are due to Slight micro-trauma near the cuticle, by gestures as surprising as putting Your hands in the pockets of tight jeans. On the Other hand, when we talk about large White spots, it can a symptom of kidney failure or cirrhosis.

Bitten nails (onychophagia). In addition to the aesthetic problems that it causes, nail biting can alter the Shape of the teeth or affect the health of the nails: they do not grow well due to the continuous nibbling to which they are and micro-traumas are created throughout the entire length. nail bed (the part that is under the nails), thus altering its anatomy. There is also damage around the nail, small wounds that cause the finger to swell and hurt.

. Lack of protein. Actually, if we follow a correct diet, it would not be necessary to take nutritional supplements to strengthen the nails, the problem is that currently we do not eat as well as we should. In that case nutricosmetics for weak hair and nails can help. Calcium, which has always been thought to intervene in the hardness of the nail, is not so important in it. On the other hand, proteins do have it: you have to take the right amount of them to show off healthy nails.

. Calluses A corn is thickened skin that forms on the top or side of a Most of the time it is caused by shoes that do not fit well. A callus is thickened skin on the hands or soles of the feet. Thickening of the skin is a protective reaction. Corns can be painful When pressure is put on them. Calluses are rarely painful. [n general, they form on the soles of the feet, under the heels or metatarsal region, on the palms, or on the knees.

CIRCULATORY SYSTEM

The blood circulatory system is of great because it is responsible for the transport of nutrients, oxygen and regulatory factors to all organs and tissues of the in order to function. In addition, it is also responsible for eliminating waste products, controlling the temperature. For the aesthetic professional, a knowledge of certain parts of this device is important, such as the situation of the vessels of the venous system, blood pressure, which direction the blood carries through the arteries and veins and the aesthetic problems related to this device, since through its intervention you can improve its functioning and sometimes avoid some problems.

It is made up of the heart, which is an organ that exerts the effect of a pump, pushing the blood with a certain flow and pressure. Blood vessels are the circuit by which blood circulates to every organ in the body. Microcirculation is the process by which the exchange of nutrients and oxygen takes place in the cells of the capillaries.

Massage can facilitate the venous return of blood to the heart using different techniques, manual and mechanical. Many of the alterations of the circulatory system can treated by aesthetic professionals. It is important to know the direction of the blood and its pressure in the vessels through which it passes when applying a massage. There are many massage techniques, both manual and mechanical that can be used to treat circulatory problems.

AESTHETIC PROBLEMS RELATED TO THE CIRCULATORY DEVICE

The different aesthetic problems that can be treated by the aesthetic professional to improve the health of their clients are listed below:

LYMPHATIC SYSTEM

The lymphatic system is a "drain" system for the body, located parallel to the blood circulatory system. Its function is to collect waste, through the lymphatic vessels, from the interstitial fluid that surrounds the cells, forming the lymph.

This is cleared in the lymph nodes and returned to the blood again. In addition to exercising a cleaning function, it also actively participates in the protective function, since they are the main defense centers, where lymphocytes are stored and multiplied.

The possibility of carrying out a lymphatic drainage massage allows us to intervene directly in this process because we can activate the lymph circulation. It different functions:

- Collects waste produced by cells or found in the interstitial fluid that surrounds them, such as proteins, cell debris, microorganisms and Others.

- Returns to the blood circulatory system, the plasma infiltrated in the tissues, thus preserving the protein concentration of the interstitial fluid, which if not carried out we would die.

- Performs fat absorption and transport tasks from the abdominal area.

This system not have any pump that drives the lymph through the vessels, as with the heart in the circulatory system, but rather through systems similar to those seen such as valves, muscle contraction and others. It is made up of a Wide network of vessels, called lymphatic vessels, which is why the lymph that passes through the lymphatic organs known as nodes is The Lymphatic System is a parallel system to the blood that is responsible for collecting the waste produced in the tissues, filtering them and returning them to the blood, to the venous system. The lymph nodes are responsible for cleaning the lymph and the maturation of cells as important as lymphocytes. For the future aesthetic professional, knowledge of the location of the lymphatic stream is to carry out their work as efficiently as possible.

Manual Lymphatic drainage is a type of massage that facilitates the circulation of lymph by acting directly on the blood vessels. The dysfunctions in the return of the flow of the lymph and the accumulations of this forming edema, represent affections related to this system and aesthetics.

LOCOMOTOR APPARATUS

The musculoskeletal system is divided into two different systems, the skeletal system and the muscular system, related to each other. The function of the locomotor system is to provide the individual with the necessary movements so that he can live, allowing him to relate to his environment and to meet his physiological needs. In turn, it is also in charge of maintaining the fundamental Structure Of the as well as protecting some vital organs. This device is made up of bones, muscles, joints and nerves, and can suffer disorders that will affect the system causing alterations and pathologies that can sometimes be treated through aesthetic treatments. Therefore, having a good knowledge of this device will allow you to know what are the aesthetic processes that can be carried out.

THE BONE SYSTEM

Also known as a skeleton, it is made up of more than two hundred articulated bones. Its main function is to an internal framework of the human body in addition to providing Bones are the Structures that make up the bone system. The functions performed by the examples as follows:

- They serve as support for the muscles insertion.
- They form the framework that and the organs.
- They constitute one of the main calcium reserves in the body, regulating its metabolism through continuous exchange with the blood.

Joints are structures that join bones the weight of the body while it out. In addition, they have a hard fibrous capsule that in turn is covered by a synovial fluid that acts as a lubricant. There are three of joints depending on their degree of mobility: immobile or synarthrosis, semi-mobile or amphiarthrosis, and mobile or diarthrosis.

THE MUSCULAR SYSTEM.

This system accounts for of body weight and is made up of muscles, which have the function of converting nervous or hormonal signals into mechanical movement. The number of muscles that we can find in the is approximately 600, with different and sizes and classified according to the function they perform. A knowledge of this system will allow to apply, with excellent results such as massages, lymphatic drainage or excitomotor currents to improve circulation and the feeling of fatigue or muscle pain. Although there are some contraindications to these treatments in cases of specific injuries. The functioning of the muscles is very similar to that of an engine since it consumes fuel in the form of adenosine triphosphate ATP cells and produces mechanical effects such as muscle contraction. The types of muscle tissue can by the function they perform, thus we have the following groups.

• Skeletal muscles: They are the most important as they account for 40% of mass, and are so called because the muscles are inserted into the skeleton. It is also known as striated muscle, due to its structure with transverse striations or voluntary because its contraction is voluntary and is controlled by the central nervous system in many cases.

• Smooth muscles: Their contraction is involuntary, that is, they are innervated by the autonomic nervous system. They have elongated cells, they do not form a homogeneous tissue, but rather with other tissues, giving rise to other organs.

• Cardiac muscle: There are Other groups that are not so interested in the field of aesthetics, such as the cardiac muscle, which to a of the muscle tissue for the movement of the from the embryonic state to the death of the individual. Here are the graphs of the main muscles of the face and body.

CHAPTER 7 NUTRITION

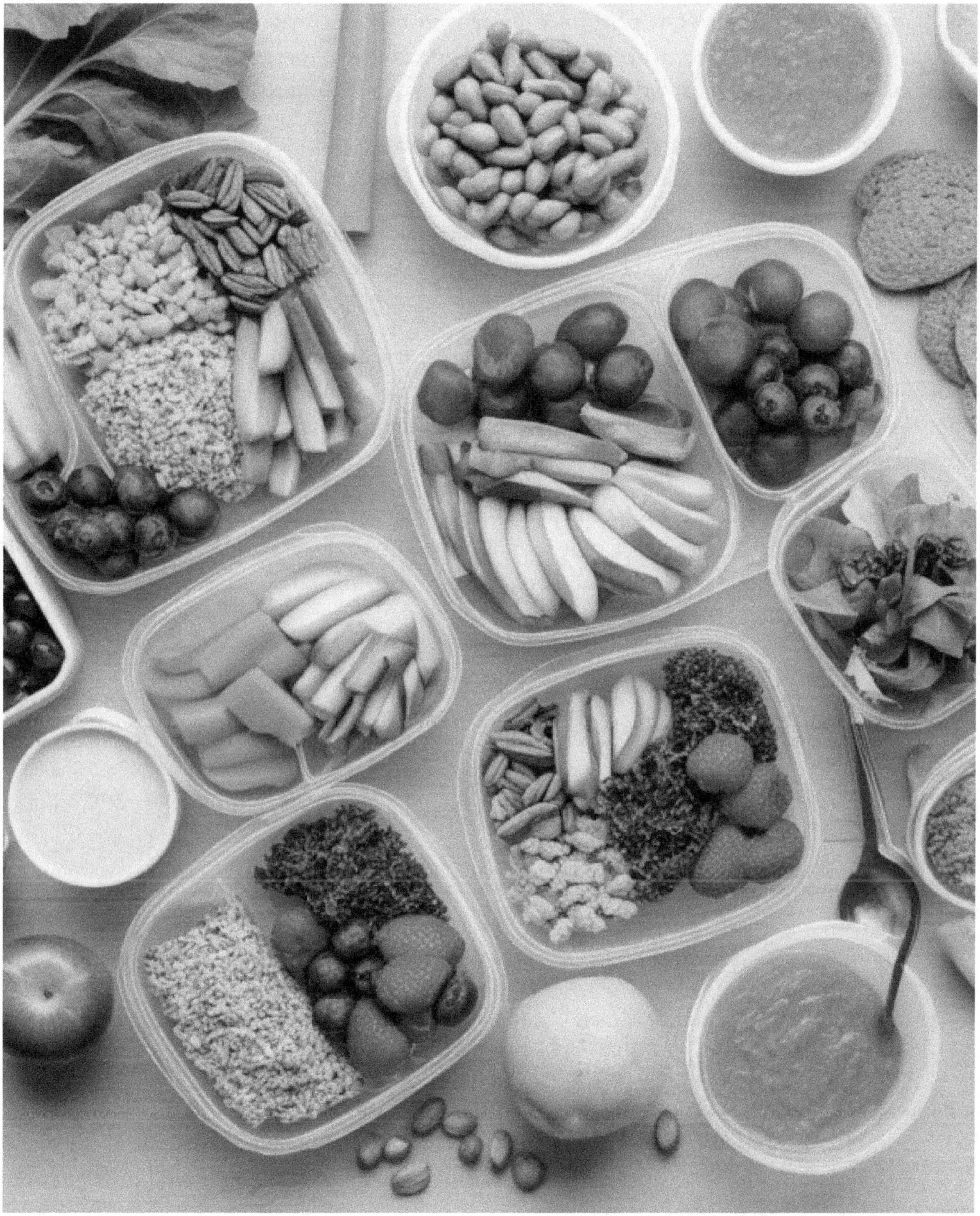

There are two types of functions performed by cells in they are anabolism, which refers to the accumulation and reserve of nutrients in the liver and other organs. Then they go hand in hand with catabolism that is for cellular oxidation after all substances are used and reduced.

It depends on several intrinsic factors that cannot be controlled, while extrinsic factors can control. They can be monitored with a nutritionist, aestheticist and endocrinologists.

The endocrine glands are specific organs located throughout the body that release substances called hormones. For example, the thyroid releases thyroxine, while the bone marrow absorbs calcium and releases calcitonin.

Nutrients are classified according to their required quantity and are divided into macronutrients, which are the ones that the requires in greater quantity to function and are proteins or amino acids and or lipofats. And we also find the micronutrients that are the ones that are required in the least amount and are vitamins and minerals.

Nutrients are classified according to their function in energy such as lipids and sugars used as fuel for the body, the plastic function of transforming proteins, and the regulatory function that is responsible for regenerating metabolism through vitamins and minerals.

Among the types of nutrients we find carbohydrates or also known sugars, are divided into:

- Simple - glucose, galactose (milk), fructose (fruit)
- Double - maltose (cereals), weeds (cane), lactose (milk)
- Complex - starches (starches and flours), pectin (peel of sorne fruits), cellulose (most Common plant stevia)

VITAMINS AND SUPPLEMENTS

Navigating the World of Vitamins, Minerals, and Supplements: A Guide to Health and Wellness

In the vast universe of health and wellness, vitamins, minerals, and dietary supplements play a fundamental role. These micronutrients, essential for the proper functioning of the body, are classified in various ways to facilitate their understanding and proper use. Join us on this journey to explore the different categories of these health allies, their benefits, and consumption recommendations based on specific symptoms.

Classification of Vitamins and Minerals:

1. Classification by solubility:**

* **Fat-soluble:** Vitamins A, D, E, and K. They are stored in the body's fatty tissues and are absorbed along with fat.

* **Water-soluble:** Vitamins B and C. They dissolve in water and are eliminated in urine.

2. Classification by Function:

* **Vitamins:** Organic compounds essential for metabolism, immune function, and overall health.

* **Minerals:** Inorganic chemical elements that are part of bone structure, body fluid regulation, and nerve function.

Dietary Supplements:

Dietary supplements are products that contain concentrated nutrients, such as vitamins, minerals, amino acids, herbs, and enzymes. Their purpose is to supplement the diet when the intake of these nutrients through food is insufficient.

Types of Supplements:**

* Vitamin supplements:** Provide concentrated amounts of specific vitamins.

* Mineral supplements:** Provide concentrated amounts of specific minerals.

* Herbal supplements:** Contain plant extracts with medicinal or nutritional properties.

* Other supplements:** May include amino acids, probiotics, enzymes, and other compounds.

Recommended Use for Specific Symptoms:**

1. Nutritional Deficiencies:**

* Symptoms of Vitamin B12 Deficiency:** Fatigue, muscle weakness, numbness or tingling in the hands and feet, memory and concentration problems.

* Symptoms of Iron Deficiency:** Anemia, fatigue, paleness, shortness of breath, headache, and dizziness.

* Symptoms of Vitamin D Deficiency:** Bone and muscle pain, muscle weakness, fatigue, sleep problems, and depression.

2. Disease Prevention:**

* Omega-3 Supplementation:** May help reduce the risk of heart disease, stroke, and some types of cancer.

* Calcium and Vitamin D Supplementation:** Important for bone health and osteoporosis prevention.

3. Enhanced Physical Performance:**

* Creatine Supplementation:** May help increase muscle strength and endurance during exercise.

* Protein supplementation:** Contributes to muscle growth and repair, especially after exercise.

Important to remember:**

* Consult a healthcare professional:** Before taking any supplement, it is essential to consult with a doctor or nutritionist to assess your need and safety.

* Appropriate dosage:** Do not exceed the recommended dose on the product label.

* Drug interactions:** Inform your healthcare professional about any medications you are taking to avoid interactions.

* Supplement quality:** Choose supplements from trusted, reputable brands.

In conclusion, vitamins, minerals, and dietary supplements can be valuable tools to complement your diet and improve overall health. However, it is crucial to consume them responsibly and under the supervision of a healthcare professional to avoid risks and optimize their use. By understanding the different categories of these micronutrients and their specific applications, we can make informed decisions and take full advantage of their wellness benefits.

THREE EATING PRACTICES

Veganism, the Paleo diet and the ketogenic diet are the three most prominent eating practices of recent years, and they continue to spread among fans of healthy eating. From social networks, blogs, bookstores and other channels of ideological promotion we it with insistent circumspection. We consider that their approaches are not absurd, but are based on studies and the experience of many different who not only lean to avoid excess of some foods for reasons of local climatic scarcity, immunological diseases or Others such as cancer colon, but also learn to replace the possible effect of nutrient deficiency there are other alternatives of menus to prepare throughout the day that promise to maintain a more stable health.

For example, veganism is here to stay, since unlike vegetarianism, it is allowed to include eggs and milk, veganism replaces them with milk and soy-based ice cream; and butter, jelly, and honey are not allowed. The vegan goes a little beyond his eating habits and in addition to avoiding meat, and fish, he does not the use of clothing such as wool or leather. It was in the year 1944 When the Vegan Society was born in Great Britain created by Donald Watson in Leicester, England has distinctive elements of their level or status. It is known that the first known vegetarian was the philosopher Pythagoras. Some celebrities who have been publicly recognized for their vegan habits are the Singer of the Beatles band Paul McCartney, Carlos Santana, Ellen Pink, actress Natalie Portman. Asian food stores stock several of these products, and like other regular diet plans are kept with increased portions of all kinds of cereals and natural fruits. Vegans could became seriously deficient in the amino acid tryptophan and vitamin B1 if they do not include strawberries and chia, or sesame seeds.

Contrary to the above, the Paleolithic diet or better known by its diminutive as "paleo" boldly states that the most suitable foods for humans are those that were available in the caveman era, these foods are meats, vegetables, fruits and fish. It was devised by a gastroenterologist named Walter in 1975. They prefer green fruits instead of ones, since they develop less fructose. The meat of all edible must be from a healthy animal that has been without disease, they leave vegetables in the background but include salads that are only garnished with olive oil and nuts.

Curiously, they eliminate sugary desserts and cereals considering their low-density protein for men. For this reason it is believed that paleophiles could find themselves with problems with triglycerides or harmful fat in the blood, problems with the flu due to low carbohydrates. When losing weight in this way hypothioroidism, ketosis, kidney problems and dizziness Crossfit is a therapy that is also associated with this diet.

Finally we find the keto diet, whose name comes from the metabolic process known as ketosis. Ketosis is a higher proportion of ketone bodies in the body, due to involuntary fasting or missing specific times for each meal such as breakfast. Acetone is a ketone body, which is in oxidative metabolism, and is present in normal human urine in very small amounts. A plate of sardines or tuna fillet, or cod fried in coconut or Olive Oil with few vegetables, cereals and lots of avocado salad is the watchword on the menu.

It was inspired by a clear scientific, there are various situations in which acetone in higher amounts in the urine, such as in pregnancy, in fasting situations, in alcoholic ketoacidosis and in ketoacidosis, to indicate the most frequent. All these situations have in Common an abnormal accumulation of ketones in the body, as a result of insufficient or inadequate use of carbohydrates. Instead of these, fatty acids are used as a metabolic source, whose final products, ketones, accumulate and, consequently, their presence becomes evident in the urine.

There are many celebrities in the United States who have joined this healthy eating movement. This diet came to leave behind all the myths and detractions of other diet plans such as Dukan and Atkins.

FOOD ADDITIVES

A Fascinating Journey into the World of Food Additives: Classification, Origin, and Uses in the Food Industry and Nutrition

In the dynamic world of the food industry, food additives play a crucial role in ensuring the quality, safety, flavor, and visual appeal of the products we consume every day. These often misunderstood and debated compounds provide a wide range of benefits, from preservation to enhancing organoleptic properties. Join us on a journey to explore the classification, origin, and recommended uses of food additives, demystifying their role in the food industry and nutrition.

Classification of Food Additives:** A Universe of Functions

Food additives are classified according to their primary function within food. This classification provides a better understanding of their impact on product characteristics and their appropriate use in the food industry. Below is an overview of the main categories:

1. Preservatives:** As the name suggests, preservatives aim to extend the shelf life of foods by inhibiting the growth of microorganisms such as bacteria, molds, and yeasts. Some common examples include:

* Potassium sorbate:** Used in cheeses, dried fruits, and baked goods.

* Sodium nitrite:** Found in cured meats such as sausages and ham.

* Sodium benzoate:** Used in soft drinks, sauces, and jams.

2. Antioxidants:** These compounds fight free radicals, unstable molecules that can damage cells and cause food spoilage. Common antioxidants include:

* Vitamin C (Ascorbic Acid):** Found in fruit, citrus, and vegetable juices.

* BHA (Butylated Hydroxytoluene):** Used in edible fats and oils.

* BHT (butylhydroquinone):** Used in cereals and baked goods.

3. Colorings:** Colorings are added to foods to intensify or modify their color, making them more visually appealing and palatable. Some common examples include:

* Tartrazine:** Found in sweets, beverages, and ice cream.

* Carmine:** Used in cheeses, sausages, and confectionery.

* Beta-carotene:** Used in margarines, cereals, and fruit juices.

4. Flavorings:** Flavorings add or intensify the flavor and aroma of foods, creating unique and pleasing sensory experiences. Some common examples include:

* Vainillin:** Found in dairy products, desserts, and baked goods.

* Monosodium glutamate (MSG):** Used in soups, sauces, and prepared dishes.

* Plant and spice extracts:** Used in a wide variety of foods to enhance their flavor.

5. Sweeteners:** Sweeteners provide a sweet taste to foods, often used as sugar substitutes or to reduce calorie content. Some common examples include:

* **Saccharin:** Found in diet drinks, candy, and chewing gum.

* Aspartame:** Used in low-calorie products, desserts, and dairy products.

* Stevia:** Used as a natural sweetener in yogurts, ice cream, and beverages.

6. Thickeners and stabilizers:** These additives modify the texture and consistency of foods, improving their palatability and appearance. Some common examples include:

* Agar-agar:** Found in jellies, jams, and desserts.

* Guar gum:** Used in ice cream, sauces, and dressings.

* Carrageenan:** Used in dairy products, cheeses, and desserts.

7. Acidity regulators:** These compounds control the pH of foods, influencing their flavor, texture, and shelf life. Some common examples include:

* Citric acid:** Found in carbonated beverages, fruit juices, and preserves.

* Soy bicarbonate:** Used in baked goods, pastries, and sauces.

* Soy citrate:** Used in cheeses, beverages, and dairy products.

8. Emulsifiers and stabilizers:** These additives help maintain the uniformity of mixtures by preventing the separation of their components. Some common examples include:

* Soy lecithin:** Found in chocolate, mayonnaise, and baked goods.

METABOLIC DISEASES

** Addressing Metabolic Diseases: A Nutritional Approach

Metabolic diseases have become one of the leading threats to global health, affecting millions of people worldwide. These conditions, which encompass a wide range of disorders, have a significant impact on quality of life and can lead to serious complications if not properly controlled.

The 9 Most Common Metabolic Diseases:**

1. Diabetes Mellitus:** A disease characterized by elevated blood sugar (glucose) levels due to a lack of insulin or resistance to its action.

2. Hypertension:** Sustained high blood pressure that damages blood vessels and increases the risk of cardiovascular disease.

3. Heart Disease:** An umbrella term that encompasses a range of heart conditions, such as heart attacks, strokes, and heart failure.

4. Obesity:** Excessive accumulation of body fat that increases the risk of various chronic diseases.

5. Metabolic Syndrome:** A set of risk factors that increase the likelihood of developing heart disease, type 2 diabetes, and stroke.

6. Hypothyroidism:** A condition in which the thyroid gland does not produce enough thyroid hormone, which can lead to various symptoms, such as fatigue, weight gain, and skin problems.

7. Hyperlipidemia:** High levels of cholesterol and triglycerides in the blood, which increases the risk of heart disease.

8. Chronic Kidney Disease:** Gradual deterioration of kidney function that can lead to kidney failure.

9. Gout:** A condition characterized by recurrent attacks of pain and inflammation in the joints, caused by the accumulation of uric acid in the blood.

Prevention Through Nutrition:**

The good news is that many of these metabolic diseases can be prevented or effectively managed through lifestyle changes, especially those related to diet. Nutrition plays a key role in reducing the risk of these conditions and improving overall health.

Nutritional Strategies for Prevention:**

1. Balanced Diet:** Eat a variety of nutritious foods from all food groups, including fruits, vegetables, whole grains, legumes, lean proteins, and low-fat dairy products.

2. Portion Control:** Moderate portion sizes to avoid excessive calorie consumption and control body weight.

3. Reduction in Saturated and Trans Fats:** Limit consumption of saturated and trans fats, which are found in red meat, full-fat dairy products, and processed foods, and replace them with healthy fats such as those found in olive oil, avocado, and nuts.

4. Increase Fiber:** Include an adequate amount of fiber in your diet, found in fruits, vegetables, legumes, and whole grains, to improve digestion, control blood sugar levels, and promote satiety.

5. Moderate Sugar Intake:** Reduce your intake of added sugars, found in sugary drinks, desserts, and processed foods, to prevent weight gain and the development of chronic diseases.

6. Adequate Hydration:** Drink enough water throughout the day to keep your body hydrated and promote proper organ function.

7. Regular Physical Activity:** Engage in regular physical activity, including at least 30 minutes of moderate exercise most days of the week, to improve cardiovascular health, manage weight, and reduce the risk of chronic diseases.

Additional Recommendations:**

* Consult a professional nutritionist or dietitian:** Get personalized guidance on a healthy eating plan tailored to your individual needs and health goals.

* Read nutrition labels:** Pay attention to the nutritional information on food labels to make informed purchasing and consumption decisions.

* Plan meals:** Planning meals in advance helps you make healthy choices and avoid the temptation of processed or non-nutritious foods.

* Cook at home:** Preparing meals at home allows you to control the ingredients and quality of the food you eat.

* Eat regularly:** Having regular meals and snacks throughout the day helps maintain an active metabolism and prevent overconsumption of food at any one time.

Metabolic diseases are a reality in today's world, but they are not incurable.

PREBIOTICS AND PROBIOTICS

** *Navigating the Microbiome: Prebiotics and Probiotics, Allies for Gut Health*

In the fascinating world of nutrition, the study of the gut microbiome has taken a leading role. This complex ecosystem, made up of trillions of microorganisms, plays a fundamental role in our overall health, from digestion to the immune system. Among the protagonists of this microscopic universe are **prebiotics** and **probiotics**, two allies that, although often confused, offer unique benefits for our well-being.

Prebiotics: Food for Beneficial Bacteria

Prebiotics are non-digestible compounds of plant origin that act as food for the beneficial bacteria that reside in our gut. They function like fertilizers, stimulating the growth and activity of these bacteria, which perform vital functions for our health.

Where do prebiotics come from?

Prebiotics are found naturally in a wide variety of foods, especially those rich in fiber:

* Fruits:** Apples, bananas, blueberries, oranges, strawberries.

* Vegetables:** Asparagus, onions, garlic, artichokes, broccoli.

* Legumes:** Lentils, chickpeas, beans.

* Whole grains:** Oats, quinoa, brown rice.

* Nuts:** Almonds, walnuts, pistachios.

What are the benefits of prebiotics?

* They improve digestion:** They help break down food and absorb nutrients efficiently.

* They strengthen the immune system:** They stimulate the production of immune cells and fight harmful bacteria.

* They promote gut health:** They help prevent constipation, diarrhea, and other digestive diseases.

* They reduce the risk of chronic diseases:** They may help prevent diabetes, heart disease, and some types of cancer.

How to increase your prebiotic intake?

* Eat more fruits and vegetables:** Aim for at least 5 servings a day.

* Include legumes and whole grains in your diet.**

* Opt for fermented foods:** Yogurt, kefir, sauerkraut, and kimchi are excellent sources of prebiotics.

* **Consider prebiotic supplements:** If your diet doesn't provide enough, supplements can be considered under the supervision of a healthcare professional.

Probiotics: Reintroducing Beneficial Bacteria

Probiotics are live microorganisms that are consumed in sufficient quantities to provide a health benefit to the host. They act as an army of beneficial bacteria that enter our gut to restore the balance of intestinal flora.

Where do probiotics come from?

Probiotics are found naturally in some fermented foods:

* Plain yogurt:** No sugar or additives.

* Kefir:** A fermented milk-based beverage.

* Sauerkraut:** Fermented cabbage.

* Kimchi:** Fermented vegetables typical of Korean cuisine.

* Miso:** Fermented soybean paste.

* Tempeh:** Fermented soybeans.

What are the benefits of probiotics?

* They improve digestion:** They help break down lactose, combat constipation, and promote bowel regularity.

* They strengthen the immune system:** They fight harmful bacteria and stimulate the production of immune cells.

* They treat and prevent digestive diseases:** They can help relieve irritable bowel syndrome, Crohn's disease, and ulcerative colitis.

* They improve mental health:** They can help reduce anxiety, depression, and other mental health problems.

* They aid in recovery from illness:** They can be beneficial during and after antibiotic treatment.

How to increase your probiotic intake?

* Eat foods rich in probiotics:** Include them in your daily diet.

* Take probiotic supplements:** Consult with a healthcare professional to determine the appropriate type and dosage.

** Key Differences between Prebiotics and Probiotics

Prebiotics:

* Are non-digestible compounds.

* They feed the beneficial bacteria present in the gut.

* They do not permanently colonize the gut.

Probiotics:

* Are live microorganisms.

* They enter the gut to restore intestinal flora.

DIETARY FIBER VS. GLUTEN

** *Gluten: A Guest Not Always Welcome at Our Tables*

Gluten, a protein present in wheat, barley, rye, and their derivatives, has gained prominence in recent years, not only for its role in the production of bread, pasta, and other food products, but also for its impact on some people's health.

What is gluten and how does it affect us?

Gluten is a protein composed of two main fractions: **gliadin** and **glutein**. These proteins give gluten its ability to form an elastic network that retains gases during fermentation, giving rise to the characteristic texture of bread and other baked goods.

However, for some people, gluten can be a chain of health problems. Among the most common gluten-related conditions are:

* Celiac disease:** An autoimmune disease in which the immune system attacks gluten, damaging the lining of the small intestine. Symptoms include diarrhea, fatigue, weight loss, and abdominal discomfort.

* Non-celiac gluten sensitivity:** A condition in which people experience digestive discomfort or other symptoms after consuming gluten, but do not have intestinal damage.

* Wheat allergy:** An allergic reaction to wheat, which can include symptoms such as hives, bloating, difficulty breathing, and, in severe cases, anaphylaxis.

Classification of dietary products

In response to the growing demand for gluten-free alternatives, the food industry has developed a wide range of dietary products. The classification of these products is based on their gluten content:

1. Gluten-free products:**

* Contain less than 20 parts per million (ppm) of gluten.

* They bear a "gluten-free" certification seal issued by a recognized entity.

* Examples: Gluten-free flours (rice, corn, quinoa), gluten-free breads, gluten-free pastas.

2. Low-Gluten Products:**

* They contain between 20 and 100 ppm of gluten.

* They must have clear labeling indicating their gluten content.

* Examples: Some cereals, cookies, or products made with low-gluten flours.

3. Products Containing Gluten:**

* They contain more than 100 ppm of gluten.

* They must include gluten in the list of ingredients.

* Examples: Wheat bread, traditional pasta, beer.

Origin and Uses of Gluten in the Food Industry

Gluten has been used for thousands of years in the production of various food products due to its unique properties:

* Structure Formation:** Gluten provides shape and texture to breads, pastas, and other baked goods.

* Gas Retention:** Gluten's ability to trap gases during fermentation is crucial for the bread's volume and airiness.

* Improving Cohesion:** Gluten provides cohesion to doughs and pasta, preventing them from crumbling during handling and baking.

Specific Uses of Gluten in the Food Industry:

* Bakery:** Gluten is essential for breadmaking, providing its characteristic structure and texture.

* Pasta Making:** The gluten network in pasta gives it firmness and elasticity, allowing it to retain its shape during baking.

* Meat Products:** Gluten is used as a binding agent in some meat products, improving their texture and cohesion.

* Sauces and Dressings:** Gluten can act as a thickener in sauces and dressings, providing a creamier texture.

Gluten Consumption Recommendations

For most people, gluten is a safe component of the diet. However, if you have any of the gluten-related conditions, it is important to follow your doctor or nutritionist's recommendations regarding its consumption.

* Read food labels carefully:** Look for "gluten-free" or "low-gluten" products if you need to avoid it.

* Consult a healthcare professional:** If you suspect you may have gluten sensitivity or celiac disease, consult a doctor or nutritionist for a personalized diagnosis and advice.

* Explore alternatives:** There are various gluten-free flour and product options that can help you maintain a varied and nutritious diet.

In conclusion, gluten is a protein with an important role in the food industry and nutrition. While it is safe for most people, for some it can trigger health problems.

VEGETABLES

It is within this group that vegetables are found. They are not only those of tubers, but there are also those of Other characteristics. The human is made up of four chemical elements which are oxygen (65%), nitrogen (3%), hydrogen (10%) and carbon (18%). In addition to Other minerals such as calcium, sulfur, potassium and phosphorus, of which, according to carried out with laboratory rats, When they were eliminated from the diet, there were serious deficiencies in the functioning of some organs.

Surely you have ever heard of cabbage, carrots, garlic and many more. Well, these are also vegetables and we must recognize that they are not only part of the diet of vegetarians. Undoubtedly, the considerable amount of some of the main vitamins, minerals, sugars, dietary fibers and fats that these contain are sufficient reasons to include them in our plate from any breakfast or lunch in which we have the urgent need to eat some food that leaves us the feeling of fullness.

It is even known that the amount of calories they have, with to that of the proteins in meats, are lower; ideal characteristic in the case of people who avoid being overweight.

What are the advantages of including them in Our diet?

Among these also called are a wide variety of options from their edible leaves, stems, bulbs and firstly, there are green leafy vegetables that have vitamins such as E, which is considered to help the blood, muscular, as well as sexual system and which is in vegetable oils, in addition to vitamin K, which has an relationship with coagulation of the blood. of the B complex vitamins, in a quantity comparable to that of grains, cereals and legumes; green leaves have vitamin B5 and B6, which help in the metabolism of fats and proteins.

It also has vitamin C and folic acid and minerals such as the antacid magnesium and iron that influence the amount of red blood cells and diseases such as anemia. The most important are lettuce, which is eaten Without seasoning to improve digestion and bile irrigation. Cabbage is another leafy vegetable with many immunological as it contains nitrogen, as well as spinach and watercress or Swiss chard contain vitamin A. In another group are stem vegetables. The best known is celery, which is a soft-stemmed vegetable whose young leaves are also edible. Natural are attributed to it to expel digestive gases, evacuate urine regularly and to improve liver diseases such as jaundice and best of all, its phosphorus content helps the brain to maintain concentration.

Other vegetables are chives and parsley as well. Next are those of that go from carrot, turnip, radish, cassava and Sweet potato; among the best known. They contain vitamins such as A, which in carrots is an excellent nutrient to improve and maintain eyesight, controls diarrhea and revitalizes the in general. Turnip and radish have beneficial properties for liver and kidney function. Caloric are attributed to sweet beets, that is, they give energy due to their protein content, with vitamins A and , B6, Biotin; which should in the daily content of our diet, and fiber.

On the other hand, there are tubers such as potatoes and Sweet whose nutritional value is mainly found in the so it can be and preserved in water to use as a condiment with Stews. In addition, the best known for their economy are cassava, yam, Otoe and the Vine, which do not have a high vitamin content, compared to the improved potato species that are marketed, but have a starch and protein content- which intervene in the synthesis of enzyme chains in metabolism. Another tuber a little less used but quite necessary for the is Ginger, which is a small and fleshy root with a Slight spicy flavor that is used in some Asian and is a peculiar ingredient in recipes. It serves as a hot tea for coughs and as well as helps to avoid dizziness, and in the female reproductive system it relieves menstrual discomfort.

A product of nature that must also be included among the bulbs or roots are fungi, which in its various edible and are mushrooms and champignons. These have vitamin D and proteins useful in the functioning of the body due to their acidic and extra meaty taste.

The bulbs are other vegetables such as the onion that is the most cleansing of the vegetables due to its rubefacient properties as well as it prevents diseases of the nervous, urinary, and skin systems. As well as eliminates parasites from the intestines and tones the brain.

It has vitamins A and B. Its apparent vegetable is garlic, which is an excellent muscle and nerve regulator, which is Why it is Widely used in cooking to prevent heart disease. In addition, it is made to having a Slight anti-infective capacity such as those of the ears.

Lastly, there are flower vegetables. Broccoli, Kohlrabi, Cabbage, and Cauliflower are the ones that are classified like this. These last two have the possibility of irritating the digestive system in people with nutrition, so they should preferably be accompanied with other high-fiber vegetables such as carrots and beets, and minerals such as garlic, always. They have vitamin B6, Biotin which are important in the daily metabolism of amino acids, as well as minerals such as calcium, chlorine that help in the maintenance of blood clotting and nerve transmission, and iodine that improve the functioning of the glands. thyroid that control metabolism and growth.

THE FRUITS

They are the female organs into a fleshy set from the stems of woody shrubs, bushes and Woody plants. When ripening, most of the fruits change their green color to more Yellow and reddish tones, obtaining great softness and sweetness.

The botanical families of the plants of the vegetable kingdom that produce edible fruits are varied, thus being able to find in a family a plant that bears fruit and another of the Same family that only flourishes. Thus, through the pollination of flowers, they continue to be through the field of science applied in agricultural farms around the World for export.

How many kinds of fruits are there?

We have all ever felt an affinity for a particular fruit, even When they are mixed into the Wide variety of products derived from sugars and desserts.

The classification of the fruits themselves has not yet been within the group of researched Works, but for Your understanding, in this work the fifty best known have organized according to their botanical relationship, consistency and flavor on the palate.

ACID FRUITS: Pineapples, Passion Fruit, Lemons, oranges, Grapefruits, Tangerines, Green apples. Ascorbic acid or vitamin C is a nutrient that is present in greater amounts in citrus fruits than in Other vegetable planté. The body cannot store this vitamin, as it happens with proteins and vitamin A, so it must consumed daily for good health. This acts within the together with the collagen protein that is responsible for body structures such as bones and teeth. Its deficiency is associated with diseases such as scurvy and hemorrhages.

MILKY FRUITS: Papayas, Mamones, Bananas or Bananas, Bananas, Mangos, Maméis, Cacaos (Chocolate), Guavas, Soursop, Breadfruits, Nonis. They are fruits rich in antacids that are produced in tropical areas from which their latex is also extracted and given various industrial uses. It contains papain, an enzyme that directs proteins in metabolism. Another of the fruits of the milky tree are bananas, which have a high content of water, regular carbohydrates and only a of fat, protein and fiber. The Guineo or banana is a fruit that is also rich in which serves to maintain the acid-base and fluid balance as well as the nerve transmission in which blood pressure intervenes. Mango is a fruit that in its green State is rich in lactic acid sugars, ideal for people with digestive and intestinal fermentation problems. Maduro is a tasty fruit rich in sugar and fiber. Mamey and cocoa are foods with pulp rich in nitrous acids that are of nitrogen trioxides which, mixed with mineral salts, stabilize the le vel of White blood cells in the immune system, which is discussed later.

FRUITS of CLIMBING: watermelons, Melons, cucumbers and pickles. They belong to the Same family of vines whose fruits have a hard and fleshy shell. They are poor in nutrients but provide sugars, minerals and fiber in addition to their purifying properties of the levels of harmful sterols such as cholesterol and astringents that is distinguished by its occasional bitter taste in relation to the taste system and the tongue.

SEMI-ACID SWEET FRUITS: Red apples, Tomatoes, Plums, Chinese suckers, Peaches, Apricots, Peaches, Cherries, Pears, Kiwis or Berries, Strawberries, Raspberries, There are many qualities of this group of fruits. Apples, due to their medium level of acidity, benefit the body with their ability to neutralize the level of cholesterol and have vitamin C, as well as chlorine and that balance the cellular fluid. Grapes have an intense cleansing capacity from the stomach to the liver and intestines, toning the heart nucleus due to its moderate acidity level. This aged fruit is converted into raisins that keep its nutritional content intact in sugars, fiber and calories that make it ideal for a snack meals. Similar to this is the tomato which is a Source of minerals such as chlorine and and vitamins A and C that help purify the of purulent substances in the gallbladder. Plums, suckers, peaches, apricots, and cherries are a group of the same plant family and are distinguished by their vitamin C content. The pear, in addition to vitamin C, has some of the B complex as well as small amounts of phosphorus and iodine that influence the acid- base and thyroid balance, which is Why it is attributed its ability to regulate blood pressure. Finally, or kiwis also have sugars, vitamin C and levels of folic acid that improve the metabolism of nucl eic acids.

DRY AND FATY FRUITS: Avocados, walnuts, Almonds, Hazelnuts, Chestnuts, Coffees, Palm Coconuts, Nances, Loquats, Olives, Olives, Sunflowers. This is a group of fruits that are very rich in protein and fat. Starting with the avocado, which is a fruit rich in healthy, unsaturated fats that do not raise the cholesterol if eaten in moderation. Regenerative qualities of the respiratory, bone and hemorrhagic regulation systems in women are attributed to it. As well as for the scalp and baldness. Walnuts, almonds, hazelnuts and chestnuts are nuts of great nutritional value as they provide with sufficient protein or calories compared to other fruits, as well as dietary fiber. Coffee is a fruit from whose drink mineral compounds and a mildly stimulating alkaloid, caffeine, are extracted, although it produces toxic physiological reactions. Palm Coconuts are nuts that grow retaining sweet milky liquid rich in protein as their white pulp that has a high content from which oil is extracted. Nances, loquats and olives are small Yellow Sweet fruits that are collected and eaten with a high of fatty acids. Finally, Oily fruits such as olives and sunflowers are presented, from which natural Oils of polyunsaturated and monosaturated quality are extracted, which are highly recommended for patients on a diet low in harmful trans and saturated fats, instead of palm Oils. this is in people with heart problems and obesity.

THE GRAINS

They are small and easy to prepare. They are in a great variety in all parts of the World. In the vegetable environment their nutritional value is only comparable to that of meats and they represent the greatest food source of all humanity throughout history.

They are also included among and in the grass family, thus the most consumed grains in their order of importance are rice, corn and Wheat. The grain of rice is the most popular in the diet of almost half of the planet's inhabitants. Studies carried out in the last decade show that the highest nutritional concentration of rice is found in its husk, which has proteins, complex vitamins B, E and K. On the Other hand, White grain contains 25% carbohydrates, and amounts minimal minerals such as iron and iodine, and protein. However, it is eaten cooked and white as a regular food. Estimating the value of rice bran like other cereals is very healthy.

Corn is native to America Indigenous cultures had already consumed it for centuries before the Spanish conquerors arrived and this was the basis of their diet. It was from the seventeenth Century that it began to cultivated in the north of Spain and then spread throughout Europe. Its edible part is the ear, which is the female flower at its base and the male at the tip. It grows amid Silky fibers such as hair or stigmas, and green leaves, with a variable number of seeds. Its nutritional value is based on its 13% protein and 7% fat, in addition to starch with few sugars. It is grown for feeding pigs, but it is also used in various ways for human consumption.

In North America the custom of eating it roasted in flakes is already known and, in Central America it is customary to crush it dry to cook it for the preparation of tortillas, as well as cream with milk, or ground cream already precooked to prepare tamales, which are made from its dough by filling of meat and seasoned spices that are rolled in vegetable banana leaves.

The oldest of these is Wheat, whose use dates back to the same prehistory in the Near East. Its uses in gastronomy are varied. They range from flours to make all kinds of pastries, and even pasta. Cereals are also made from this grain, whole grains with a high level of dietary fiber that improves the functioning of the large intestine and keeps the skin lean and firm. Likewise, Wheat has a high content of vitamins of the complex B, C, and minerals such as iron and zinc that are an obligatory part of a daily and balanced diet.

Other less popular cereals but of equal vitamin value are barley, oats and rye. The oat seed is rich in carbohydrates (64%), fiber (12%), proteins (12%) and fats (5%). It is attributed the property of helping to level the levels of fat in the as well as it is added in industrial such as ice cream, chocolates and peanut butters. Barley is consumed in some countries as food but in general it is marketed as a malt beverage and fermented for beer. It has a content of 67% of carbohydrates and 12% of proteins. And rye, a cereal that is Still used in temperate areas of northern to make bread and make malts used to make whiskey.

Peanuts, soybeans and peas: Legumes that do what Others cannot

These three seeds are the clearest example of legumes which are characterized by their fruit called legume, which is a pod that surrounds the seeds. They are distinguished by very rich in vitamins and proteins, a quality that is often visible due to their costs, more compared than other seeds. Peanuts are a dried fruit that is used in confectionery combined with raisins. It is very energetic and nutritious since it has 20 and 30% proteins and 40 and 50% fats and is a Source of B vitamins, which make it an ideal food to supplement the daily diet. Also called it is native to South America.

The use of soy, which is believed to be native to Southeast Asia, has spread due to its protein and Oil content. Beans, beans and chickpeas are other protein-rich legumes that supplement the daily demand for B-complex vitamins that both influence the metabolism and cellular functioning of the body. An acidic and somewhat sweet pulp that is also classified among these are the tamarinds that, when dissolved in drink, help regulate the intestine.

THE MEATS

If we look at the nutrition table, we can immediately realize that meats are the most complete food provided with the seven vitamin B complex nutrients and that they have another seven of the necessary minerals in the case of beef and amino acids. For Our subsistence this advantage is in doubt when addressing some negative of following a high protein diet from low quality or low-priced meat.

The main flaw is that high consumption of meat tends to raise the level of cholesterol in the which is an animal fat or steroid alcohol that influences cardiovascular function in people under 50 years of age. Although cholesterol is secreted by the sebaceous glands of the scalp and skin, in older than this age with diabetes and smoking problems; these diseases are added as risk factors for a cardiovascular event and suffering arteriosclerosis. In an order of higher nutritional value, we can classify meats into four types.

Firstly, would be those with red meat, which are those of beef or veal, rich in B vitamins and minerals, followed by White meats, which are poultry, such as chickens, eggs and turkeys with a little less B vitamins, vitamin D and minerals such as iron, phosphorus, and sulfur that interfere with the formation of hemoglobin, bones, and liver function. Bird eggs, which are the most consumed in the diets of many people around the World, are rich in three of the twenty amino acids derived for protein biosynthesis.

The lysine that participates in 7% in the composition of the proteins, the methionine that participates in 1.7% of the together with the functional group of the sulfur mineral and the tryptophan that intervenes in the formation of the vitamin amide B3 , known as nicotinamide that functions as a controller of oxidation reduction reactions. Iron is involved in this cellular respiration; contained in green leafy vegetables, cereals, meat and poultry, with the Copper contained in the water.

Then there would be shellfish, fish, octopus, oysters and canned tuna, which in addition to those found in and eggs, contain essential minerals such as phosphorus, sulfur, fluorine, iodine, selenium and zinc.

Finally, there is pork that only provides them with vitamin B1 and saturated Oils and fats that provide at least energy. It means a low cost to other meats and the need to always accompany them with enough grains, seeds or legumes. Another Source of protein is dairy derivatives that are extracted from the mammary glands of cows and other animals such as goat in lesser frequency. Milk is a liquid food rich in vitamins A and D that are directly related to the sensitivity of sunlight, both in the retina of the eye and the skin. It is vitamin D that is related to the formation of bones and the maintenance of the joints.

Among the minerals it also has are calcium, which is involved in muscle contraction, the transmission of nerve impulses and blood clotting, others are phosphorus, chlorine, sodium, and sulfur. This white liquid is pasteurized or heated to destroy bacteria that it could contain, damaging the health of those who consume it and pulverized under pressure, the reduction of its fat globules is obtained, which is homogenization. In childhood it is very for both nursing mothers and their babies, as well as for children in their growing stage. It is known that in the adult stage, the liver is responsible for storing the excesses of these vitamins to release them later when necessary, so it is not as to consume them daily as fruits with vitamins C, and seeds and meats of the complex B.

The sugars and fats in milk make it for its various stages and forms of fermentation to be processed into other products that Still maintain their nutritional content. Separating whole milk from half of its fat using a centrifuge, semi-skimmed milk is obtained. Butter is made from the globules of fat in the cream of the milk that is homogenized. Yogurt is a cream that is eaten natural, used as a diet dressing or combined with artificial flavors, to whole or semi-skimmed milk that is added two bacteria to ferment it. The acidification of the milk through the addition of the enzyme renin, which separates the curd from the Whey, gives the solid of cottage cheese or cheese.

There are a lot of cheeses on the market. There is the cream cheese, recommended in case of diets since it has half the calories of buffer. There are white cheeses, white pressed or semi-soft, hard and flavored. The most recommended are the semi- soft or pressed since the hard ones have a higher fat content so it is not recommended for with heart problems. Ice creams are other products made with dairy derivatives, but with a 70% of milk fats, which are mixed with sugar and milk, beating in metal containers immersed in ice and salt that produce their homogenization. They have and vitamin B2.

SPICES AND SEASONINGS

Spices are those aromatic plant substances that serve as seasoning, while seasonings are everything that serves to season food and give it flavor. But the delight that we give to the sense of palate and taste can damage Our body.

Let's start with the natural seasonings. Those green leafy vegetables or bulbs, roots, seeds and even citrus fruits that in a non- artificially way, can provide the palate with the same or better flavor and seasoning than some artificial products. We refer to celery, which, as we mentioned before, is a long, juicy, grooved stem that is used as a condiment in gastronomy; of course, washed and minced, it is used as a vegetable in salads, or as an accompaniment to meats and stews.

Chili are another vegetable that is used in the preparation of meats, legumes and sauces. Also called chilies or chillies, you can eat green or Yellow which have a sweet taste, but it should be used in maceration since its intake irritates the intestinal tract. The red pepper is hotter and is used for artificial hot sauces, and its jalapeño varieties, which can also be irritating to the large intestine of those who follow special diets due to diseases and treatments.

One of the most used bulbs is onion and garlic. The onion is attributed stimulating, rubefacient and as well as purifying the also improving the respiratory and renal systems. Garlic is known for its tonic, antiseptic, antiasthmatic, antidiabetic qualities, making it a good condiment for meat and legumes. These qualities that We Will analyze better in the next chapter of the book.

Some of the green leafy vegetables included here are watercress, spinach, coriander, chives, parsley, bay leaf, oregano, basil, mint. Many of these have vitamins A, E, K and C. They improve the digestion of food and with minerals such as folic acid and iron that regulate the formation of enzymes, proteins and hemoglobin they are ideal for cooking with vegetables and pasta.

Tomato is a favorite condiment for many and children. A variety of sauces are prepared from this vegetable, most of them artificial or with preservatives, which give many vegetable and meat dishes an exquisite flavor that we must know how to mix with diced onion or celery to amortize the corrosive effect that can affect the intestinal flora to have at the moment.

It has been always for seasoning sugar and salt. That they should be used in minimal amounts Without exceeding a teaspoon, since on the one hand they tend to alter liver function; and on the other hand the acid-base balance of the organism affecting the nervous and arterial systems in hot seasons. Molasses is another result of sugars that is used to sweeten in Central American countries.

Other condiments that are used only in and should also be consumed are ginger, which is a flavoring root that can be boiled for tea that benefits the throat and prevents dizziness and accompanied with bananas and milk is an excellent dessert digestive and for women a painkiller. Olives are oily fruits that, when preserved in water, are an additional to accompany rice, salads and even eat them alone since they have 40 to 60% unsaturated Oils, as well as their purified Oil, which is a good dressing against cholesterol.

The main one of the native spices of India is the pepper which is an alkaloid, which are nitrogen organic with a moderate toxic reaction. Its use should be macerate and always be consumed with root or green leafy vegetables. Seeds such as sesame or sesame, are seeds rich in dietary fibers that maintain the intestinal flora, preventing diarrhea and flatulence. Coloring seeds such as achiote are another condiment that is used to give a red and attractive color to different dishes such as meat and rice, it is grown in warm regions of America.

Similar to this one, but of a more appreciated economic value is saffron. It is a flavoring colorant that is extracted from the stigmas of the saffron flower that is grown in Spain and Other regions. Finally we find a citrus fruit, the lemon. Its ascorbic acid content makes it ideal for dressing salads and thus reducing the frequency of consumption of mayonnaise, which is made from Oil and egg yolk and therefore unhealthy for the adult individual.

The aromatic species are the hard parts such as the seeds and bark of trees and shrubs from Asia and Indonesia, which are used to enhance the palate of hot drinks and light desserts. Some are also grown in Europe and the Mediterranean. Anise, from which its of Star anise is known, is a seed with carminative properties, that is, it is an antiflatulent and stimulant. Its smell is very pleasant and warm for both cream and tea desserts. An antiseptic and anesthetic used among spices is cloves, which from Indonesia spread to tropical regions. It is used as a tea and flavoring.

Cinnamon segments are cut from the bark of the cinnamon tree, which is also ground to be used as a condiment for meats and cream sweets. It has stimulating properties of the digestive and cardiac functions as well as antispasmodic. An aromatic seed with a very pleasant aroma used as a companion for tea and desserts is nutmeg, which is sold dry.

The seed of the coffee plant has became the most popular beverage today. The most obvious reason is that it contains 1-5% caffeine, an alkaloid that stimulates the central nervous system, increases the activity of the lungs and heart and causes the formation of urine. It also potentiates the effect of some painkillers such as aspirin, but it can irritate the intestine. Another substance analogous to caffeine in tea is theine, which represents a concentration of 2.5 to Within desserts or pastries, there is a Wide variety of sweet toppings that are used to enhance the taste of cakes made from fruit and Wheat flour.

Vanilla is a liquid essence that is sold bottled to be added to artificial or natural soft drinks and cakes. Condensed milk is a milk dessert made with sugar that contains protein and calories.

A natural elixir of health and beauty, and widely used, is the honey extracted from the of the flowers that is ideal for sweetening. [t has moisturizing properties and a caloric value in its glucose and fructose, which reaches 3,307 calories kilogram, which makes it ideal for people who suffer from fatigue and weakness. An ingredient that is used as a condiment for dairy drinks and cakes is chocolate creams. It has proteins, fats, vitamins and minerals. [t is mixed many times with milk, peanut seeds, and tree nuts. The cacao from which it is made was, like corn, a food used by the Aztec Indians before the Spanish colonization. It was carried to other parts of Europe, almost a century later.

What is the type of seasonings that may be damaging Our health and which ones are not?

Salty and spicy kitchen dressings are another vitally important ingredient in our nutrition. Far from harmless, consuming much of many of them can undermine the gastrointestinal tract, as they are mixed into the various meals eaten throughout the day.

This represents a permanent ban for people who are sensitive to and even more those who suffer from liver, kidney and intestinal deficiencies. Vinegar is made from the fermentation of alcohol with sugar and a yeast. Its result is acetic acid- There are also vinegars made from Wine, barley malt, and apple liquid. Its use is recommended in moderation since excess acidity in the body is counterproductive. Another of the irritating condiments of the gastrointestinal tract are hot sauces which are made from red peppers and black or red seeds.

It is customary many times to exaggerate the spicy flavor of some dishes, so you should try to avoid them as much as otherwise, sooner or later deficiencies of the stomach, liver, kidneys or colon will appear. The seasoning sauces are not as harmful as the spicy ones, but always together with the condiments of artificially processed flavors, they should be moderate in their use to marinate meat and rice. Seasoning creams such as mayonnaise, mustard, butter and ketchup have become a youth favorite in recent years. It is essential that we remember that its uncontrolled consumption represents a threat to the maintenance of the smoothness and softness of the facial skin. People who have oily skin should avoid them in the case of getting to suffer from uncontrolled acne. People who suffer from colon irritation problems should know that refined flours and sugar used to make fine pastries and gourmet sandwiches are usually harmful When not with a diet high in dietary fiber of vegetables and cereals.

At the end we find green leafy and berry condiments such as basil and vanilla, both species are commonly used for their aromatic quality for meats in the case of basil and vanilla for desserts and pastries. This antihumoral property is beneficial for people who perspire or sweat excessively, producing an Odor similar to onion or garlic due to the consumption of vegetables, a situation that can improved with their use as condiments.

MEDICINAL PLANTS

The curative remedies used by primitive and indigenous peoples around history from the ends of the earth are still used today by science. It means those who have known how to preserve the magnificent tradition of trust in nature, of those who testify to it with their health and vitality. Today, doctors call these plant elements tocopherols, and they have various effects associated with their properties on the human .

The plants, flowers, stems and roots, although some of them are not very edible or attractive to the palate due to their Slight bitter or itchy taste, they contain active principles that, cared for and collected in advance, are capable of curing human diseases and animals diseases. And they have the excellent advantage of not producing the various irritating side effects of the liver like some medications or drugs that are prescribed in some diseases.

Likewise, the methods that are followed to apply the remedies that are used in different diseases are called in various ways as we present below.

INFUSION: heat water and add the necessary part of the plant in the first boil. Then it is removed from the heat, covered and left to rest for a few minutes. The infusion once made should not It is usually prepared with the Young parts of the plant, such as leaves, flowers and even seeds.

COOKING: It is a process by which the plant is boiled in water for a certain of time. This procedure is used for the hardest parts, such as bark, leathery leaves, roots, and Stern s. REDUCTION: if the is carried out for more than 20 minutes, the reduction occurs. It is used for active principles that resist heat and which require a higher concentration due to their low proportion.

MACERATION: consists of letting the plants rest in Cold water for a few hours. It is used to extract active ingredients that are unstable against heat but soluble in water.

TINCTURE OR MEDICINAL WINES: it is the maceration made in alcohol and normally takes one part of the plant for five alcohol. It is used if the active principles do not dissolve well in water or have an unpleasant taste, generally using a dry plant. The cinchona wines or the blackthorn brandy (pacharán) are well known.

SYRUPs: they are solutions of sugar in water to which the plant is added later. JUICE: the fresh and juicy fruits of plants are crushed directly and then the liquid is strained or sifted to be drunk.

MEDICINAL OILS: like alcohol, Oil is another of the most Widely used solvents. In fact, there are certain plants that transfer their active ingr&lients to the Oil better. They are the most used for external use (rubs, massages or spreads).

CATAPLASMS OR COMPRESSES: they are made by boiling the plant or it to the action of water. The boiled plants are wrapped in thin cloths that are placed on the area to treated. VAHOS: they are prepared with aromatic herbs, which are boiled in water. The vapor that emerges from the container once it is removed from the fire is what must inhaled. The one made for nasal congestion is placed on a table and the sick person sits with his head covered with a towel to receive the steam. Other fumes are made for hemorrhoids and intestinal problems and are made by flushing the already w arm water down the toilet, with the antiflatulent herbs and sitting while receiving the medicinal fumes. They are for who work a long time sitting down and do not have a diet high in dietary fiber from cereals.

What are the qualities or properties in which they are classified?

The healing qualities, internal and external, that medicinal plants have are classified by various nouns. Some of these herbs and foods appear with more than one medicinal They are the ones listed below.

APHRODISIAC: It is Said of the substance or medicine that has the property of stimulating the sexual appetite. Some of these are parsley, ginger, and cocoa or chocolate.

ANESTHETICS: It is Said of medicinal herbs or fruits that cause general or partial deprivation of bodily sensitivity and sleep. These are chamomile, nutmeg and jasmine. ANTIEMETICS: It is Said of the plants that serve to prevent vomiting and nausea. These are Basil, Fennel, Sage, and Mint. ANTISPASMODIC: It is said of the herbs that heal or relieve spasms or involuntary contractions of muscles and nervous reflexes. These are: Jasmine, Manzanilla, Mint and Calaguala. And a spice, cinamon.

ANTISEPTICS: It is Said of the herb that it prevents infectious diseases, destroying the microbes that it causes and producing scarring. Those are: Sarsaparilla, Watercress, Calendula, Plantain, Dill, Thyme and Aloe Vera.

ANTIHELMINTICS: It is said of the vermifuge plant that serves to eliminate or expel parasites from the interior of the body. These are: Rhubarb, Ipecacuana, Ginger and Garlic. ANTIFLATULENTS: They are carminative herbs that help the expulsion of gases. Those are Oregano, Sage, Boldo, Basil, Fennel, Mint, Valerian, and Melissa.

ANTIPYRETICS: They are febrifuge herbs that lower fever. They are Eucalyptus and Aloe Vera.

ANTIHYPERTENSIVE: They are plants that have the property of helping to control and regulate blood pressure in people. Those are Chamomile, Linden and Aloe Vera.

ANTI-INFLAMMATORY: It is said of the plant that prevents disorders of blood circulation, heat, redness or pain. These are Aloe Vera, Watercress and Plantain.

ANTICOAGULANT: It is said of medicinal plants that help improve blood circulation. This is the Ginkgo that should not be taken in combination with Other alternative medicine herbs or synthetic medications such as pain relievers.

ANTIRHEUMATIC: It is said from the plant that it prevents painful inflammations of the muscular and fibrous parts of the body. These are Celery, Ruda and Sarsaparilla-

ANTIBILIC: It is Said of the plant that it helps to avoid anger, irritation and anger. These are the Rhubarb, Lemon, Grape and Boldo.

ANTIBIOTICS: It is Said of herbs and plants capable of stopping the development of pathogenic organisms. This is Aloe Vera.

ANTI-CANCER: It is Said that plants help prevent the proliferation of cancer cells in the organs or blood. These are lemon, Aloe vera, cat's claw, and green leafy vegetables.

ANTIOXIDANTS: It is said of the herbs that improve the functioning of the oxidation-reduction reaction of cellular respiration that causes vitamin B3. These are Noni and Chocolate.

ANTIDIARRHEALS: It is said of the plants that prevent liquid and frequent bowel movements. These are Salt, Sage and Carrot.

ASTRINGENTS: [t is Said of the plant that contracts organic tissues. They are: Eucalyptus, Laurel, Sage, Comfrey and Blueberry.

ANALGESICS: It is Said of the plants that soothe some pains of the These are Rosemary and Aloe Vera.

SOOTHING: Narcotic plants are Said to reduce or disappear a pain or Other annoying symptom. These are Valerian, Claves, and Linden.

CARMINATIVES: It is said of medicinal herbs that promote the expulsion of gases developed in the digestive tract. These are oregano and rhubarb.

DEPURATIVES: It is Said of the medicine that purifies the humors and mainly the blocff These are Watercress, Horsetail, Cat's Claw, Sarsaparilla, Lemon, Grapes.

DIGESTIVES: It is Said of the plants that help to improve the digestion of food through the stomach and intestines. They are the Grape, the Cederrón, the Dill and the Sage.

DIURETICS: They are plants that have the of increasing the secretion and excretion of urine. These are Celery, Tansy, Thyme, Horsetail, Fennel, Cat´s Claw, Valerian-

ESTROGENIC: They are the plants that help women to with discomforts related to their menstrual cycle. These are the Cohoch and the Salvia.

EXPECTORANTS: It is said of the herb that it helps to start and throw phlegrn and secretions that are deposited in the pharynx, larynx, trachea and bronchi through the mouth. These are Fennel, Plantai n, Mallow and Valerian.

LAXANTS: It is Said of the plants that help loosen the belly and soften the evacuation. This is Aloe Vera (consumed alone), Castor Oil, Rhubarb.

RUBEFACIENTS: It is said of the plant that it flushes the color of the skin and the scalp, as well as invigorates good health. This is the Onion.

SWEATS: It is said of the plant that makes you sweat or evacuate water through the pares of the skin. They are Fennel and Rosemary.

TONICS: It is Said of the plants that help to give energy, regulate the heart rate. This is the Mastranzo (Horehound), Laurel or oleander, Ruda, lemon grass, Betel seed, Nopal or prickly pear, Aloe (precisely its substance calcium isocitrate).

Why is the use of medicinal plants recommended instead of traditional Coffees?

As mentioned in the previous chapter, the natural leaf of Tea, often green or Japanese tea, from which the popular hot drink is made, has been found to contain 2.5 to 4% theine; a caloric similar to caffeine.

Although coffee was drunk as a stimulating drink and tonic throughout in 1657, the introduction of tea from Asia occurred in England, with the later consolidated tradition of meeting for tea at five in the afternoon and eating sandwiches that has been always the most popular. However, natural herbs have many more medicinal properties than the stimulants in coffee that can increase blood pressure in with high pressure.

OBESITY AND CALORIES

To refine our recommended level of calories in Our diet, trainers and nutritionists have conducted their research in the all-important field of nutrition. This is how each of us has the opportunity, and of Course all the responsibility, to put all the food on their plate and in the quantities that they want, but knowing beforehand what their approximate balance is. To do this we have been provided with a simple Calorie Calculation formula, in which we only have to know two things. One is how tall we are, and the other is how much we weigh.

This formula is reliable and in the public domain for easy reference IX)th in brochures and on the Internet. with this information, it allows us to find out two very useful data for Our dietary planning and how many calories we should consume in our daily meals to stay within our healthy weight, thus knowing when we go overboard, in the case of obese people, or how much we still need to gain in the in the case of bulimics and anorexics, to maintain the optimal energy level; that is to say, always slim, and according to the activities we do every day.

Of course, spending every morning and night doing addition or subtraction, and weighing yourself on a scale to See how Your body is doing, is too tedious and unbearable. However, if we really care about Our appearance and health, we will learn little by Little how to control the calories that accumulate until we look our-self fat.

CALCULATE YOUR HEALTHY CALORIE LEVEL AND BODY MASS

There are two for calculating calories. The first helps you to know a minimum of Kilocalories, which is the term that defines the unit of thermal energy that the body requires for its and is equivalent to 1,00c) calories, adding 100, 2(X) or 400 extra calories to your diet for each level. activity higher than your calculated minimum. The second method is a bit more complicated, but more accurate since you don't have to add additional hundreds to the total obtained.

It is enough that you know your weight in kilos and height. Both methods use the numerical value of Your weight in kilos, not to convert from to kilos, divide Your weight in pounds by 2.21. Example:

If your weight is 128 pounds, you divide it like this: 128x2.21 – weight in kilos is 57.91.

CALCULATION FOR THE MINIMUM KILOCALORIES

Knowing this personal information is as simple as multiplying. Women have to multiply their weight in kilos by 21.6. And men multiply their weight in kilos by 24. The result is the minimum calories consumed in a day to remain at rest and do simple housework. More calories should level from the table below. Example:

Woman of 49 kilos X 21.6 1,058 is her minimum calorie.

72 kg man X 24 =1,728 is his minimum calorie.

Finally, if the Man of 72 kilos, in addition to working with little heavy efforts and also going to the gym on weekends, his total caloric plan will remain like this: 1,728 200 400 2,328.

In the other case, assuming that the 49-kilogram Woman lives in an apartment and decides to start a light routine to walk for an hour on Saturdays, the total caloric expenditure plan will be as follows; 1,058 100 200 - 1,358.

For people who want to lose weight, there are other calculation options where food servings are adjusted for the BMI, in addition to gender and weight, and are mentioned immediately in the next section of this chapter.

CALCULATION OF KILOCALORIES BY HEALTHY WEIGHT

If, in addition to your weight in kilos, you know your height in meters and centimeters; you can follow another formula that also works due to the level of activities that are carried out. It consists of two parts. The first is to calculate, according to sex, the recommended healthy weight according to height, and then it is obtained from that same result by the indicated (of three levels), the amount of kilocalories to consume daily is obtained to maintain that healthy weight recommended. The second part helps you discover the Body Mass Index that represents the indicator that you are at an inappropriate weight for health, considerably underweight, underweight, normal weight, overweight, obese or clinically obese. This data is used by a health specialist to detect the risk of heart disease, cancer, and others. A simple example is the following. To do this calculation you need to know three things.

First get your weight in kilos, height and the level of physical activities you do, according to your gender.

Follow these four Steps as an example: I. Multiply Your size twice:

1 .65 x 1.65 2.7225, which When rounded is

2.72. 2. This value should be multiplied by 21 for women, and 22 for men, like this: 2.72 x 21 57.12 This result represents Your healthy weight in kilos.

3. To know the amount of calories that should be included in the daily diet, use the number of the level of physical activity that you are used to. In the example below , it is light activity for women. 57.12 x 28 I , 599 This result represents the number of kilocalories needed for each day.

What follows is to choose individual servings of food from each of the five groups, which are.

KNOWING THE RIGHT PORTIONS OF FOOD

The portion of a regular diet of each food can represent about 200 calories, as seen in the image at the beginning of the chapter.

(Measure used is 1 Cup or 1 spoonful)

We can assume in a general way how much money to to Our grocery bag. But it is from the following table that you can have a more precise idea of the amount of food or portions that it represents to complete the daily caloric requirement or expenditure, according to the calculated kilocalories that Will be divided into the three meals; breakfast, lunch and dinner, and one or two snacks; morning and evening. Thus, each of sugars represents 1 or 2 tablespoons of sweets or a medium piece (in the case of ice cream). In Oils and fats (such as margarine, butter, and mayonnaise) a serving is I tsp. of the animal proteins, a serving is a unit of cheese, sausage, eg or two slices of ham or Other sausage, and half a cup of milk. In meats of any type, a portion is a piece of 30 grams. For vegetables and tubers, a serving is 2 cups of lettuce, spinach, beets, or celery, or I cup of mushrooms, broccoli, or Swiss chard- In fruits a serving 3 units of small fruit such as plums, I cup of medium or large fruits such as watermelon and melon, and in citrus a serving is two units. In grains and legumes, one serving represents half a cup. In minerals, a glass of regular water, at the rate of eight a day, and salt a teaspoon.

Calculation of the Body Mass Index

The calculation of the mass index (BMI) is achieved with the weight in kilos and is divided by the height, twice. This result allows us to know exactly where we are within one of the seven weight levels, ranging from low to normal with overweight or clinically obese. As follows:

Since the result was 21, the woman in this example is at her normal weight. To help you better understand this method of calculating BMI, body mass index, recommended healthy weight and total daily kilocalories for a diet, a table developed with broken down heights and weights is presented below.

DIET FLOW CHARTS

When we feel fully healthy and every system in our body is Willing to complete the complicated process of food metabolism Without suffering sudden physiological consequences, we can release a little of the restrictions.

Some examples of menus are opportune to know them to became familiar with them enough to with ease in the kitchen, When eating out is not the best option. For those who love culinary art or gastronomy, it Will be a matter of gathering the money and a small list to prepare the home pantry with the indicated foods in healthy nutrition.

We bring Five examples of basic diets by caloric expenditure by age for Children, Adolescents, Men, Women, and the Elderly can be described below.

CHILDREN'S DIET

Morning Menu - 275 cal. 1 plate of flavored cornstarch (150 cal.) 1 ham sandwich with cheese and tomato sauce (7 5 cal.) 1 fruit (Optional banana, apple, pear, mango) (50 cal.)

Evening Menu - 160 cal. two cups of chopped carrot, and celery broth (160 cal)

Afternoon snack - 175 cal. A cup of with a of butter (175 cal.)

Night menu - 510 cal. 1 cup of rice (60 cal.) 1 cup of kidney beans (120 cal.) 1 serving of beef (270 cal.) 1 / 4 cup ice cream (60 cal.)

Note: With this daily menu, the child is provided from the morning with enough energy provided by the cornstarch in the cornstarch, carbohydrates and minerals from the fruit and animal and dairy protein in the sandwich seasoned in an attractive way for those of this age. The rest of the day is supplemented with the same nutrients and vitamins in slightly more complete portions.

JUVENILE DIET

Morning Menu - 650 cal. 1 bowl of cereal with milk (160 cal.) 2 tortillas toasted in butter (400 cal.) 2 servings of fried chicken fillets or (70 cal.) 1 cup of citrus juice (30 cal.)

Evening Menu - 260 cal. two cups of mashed potatoes with coleslaw and carrot (260 cal)

Afternoon snack - 295 cal. 8 Units of crackers (120 cal.) 1 cup sour-sop smoothie (175 cal.)

Night menu - 450 cal. 1 cup saffron seasoned rice (60 cal.) 1 cup of stewed chickpeas (120 cal.) 1 serving of chicken meat (270 cal.)

JUVENILE FEMALE

Morning Menu - 390 cal. 1 bowl of cereal with milk (160 cal.) 1 sausage sandwich Without butter (200 cal.) 1 cup of citrus juice (3 0 cal.)

Evening Menu - 310 cal. 2 cups mashed bananas with salt and a of butter (260 cal) I cup of lettuce salad with tomato, watercress or spinach seasoned with vinegar or yogurt. (50 cal.)

Afternoon snack - 260 cal. 1 Units of granola cookies (200 cal.) 1 cup fruit drink shake (60 cal.)

Night menu - 510 cal. 1 cup saffron seasoned rice (120 cal.) 1 cup of stewed chickpeas (120 cal.) 1 serving of fried fish (270 cal.)

With this diet, which is intended for teenage girls and was made thinking about taking care of their beauty, they have a rich source of essential nutrients such as cereals, meats and vegetables that help sight and mental concentration, with minerals such as the match. It is also suggested to avoid excess fatty dressings such as butter and mayonnaise that tend to develop skin problems. Other snack options to replenish energy are proposed here following a diet of snacks instead of heavy meals. As for nighttime entertainment, alcohol consumption should be moderate with cocktails, since they tend to contain many more calories than is believed.

FEMALE DIET

Morning Menu - 540 cal. 1 regular bowl of cereal (120 cal.) 1 banana (50 cal.) 3 strawberries (50 cal.) 1/2 lemon (20 cal.) 2 medium yogurt (160 cal.) 1 toast with jam (140 cal.)

Evening Menu - 730 cal. 2 cups of seafood cream broth (260 cal) 1 roasted potato with a teaspoon of margarine (200 cal.) 1 grilled breast (270 cal.)

Afternoon snack - 180 cal. 1 Unit of celery (80 cal.) 1 carrot sprinkled with honey (100 cal.)

Night menu - 510 cal. 1 cup cooked brown rice (120 cal.) 1 cup of stewed lentils (120 cal.) 1 cup of mushroom, lettuce and tomato salad. (270 cal.)

The one who is a woman and a mother, and at the Same time a Wife and a worker, Well, she leads a busy and entrepreneurial life because she requires a more powerful reserve of nutrients but does not put her at the risk of becoming overweight, so she should avoid fast food from youth and get used to large amounts of red or green salads, with little starch from pasta and bakery. The meat portions of meat must be white, that is, fish fillet, chicken or turkey. Flaxseed in its various presentations is recommended to combat fat in the lower part of the female b co.

MALE DIET

Morning Menu - 720 cal. 1 skim milk shake with 1 banana and powdered chocolate (160 cal.) 3 grilled corn tortillas (300 caL) 1 egg cake with 1 slice of cream cheese 2 slices of ham (260 cal.)

Evening Menu - 840 cal. 2 cups of rice with beans (240 cal) 2 cup broccoli, bacon and salad seasoned with lemon juice and oregano. (210 cal.) 1 chicken thigh of 30 grams (120 cal.) 1 soft drink (320 cal.)

Afternoon snack - 320 cal. 1 yogurt (80 cal.) I cup unsalted peanuts (60 cal.) 1 walnut granule (180 cal.)

Night menu - 560 cal. 1 portion of liver stewed with onion and tomato (120 cal.) 2 cups cooked rice (240 cal.) 2 cups spiced noodles in toast crumbs (200 cal.)

Note: With this diet the adult person receives the average level of kilocalories, suitable for an intense work rate, without becoming overweight and allowing a light exercise routine of at least 20 minutes, 2 to 3 times a week. How to get used to at this stage of life. It is presented as an appropriate dietary option to keep cholesterol consumption at a low level and the importance of vitamins present in fruits and vegetables.

SENILE DIET

Morning menu (502 cal.) 1 cup of linden leaf tea (12 cal.) 8 units of crackers (120 cal.) 2 slices of White cheese (120 cal.) 2 slices of whole Wheat bread with fruit jam. (250 cal.)

Evening menu (480 cal.) 2 cups of rice with corn (240 cal) 1 cup of broccoli, chayote and cabbage salad seasoned with yogurt and oregano. (120 cal.) 1 chicken thigh of 30 grams (120 cal)

Afternoon snack (200 cal.) 2 cups of guava drink (80 cal.) 2 small unit of egg bread (210 cal.)

Night menu (420 cal.) 1 serving of grilled turkey with onion, watercress and tomato (120 cal.) 1 cup cooked vegetables (120 cal.) 1 cup garlic coriander noodle broth (180 cal.)

The elderly one should eat a diet low in Salt, fat and cholesterol, which is derived from animal meats, such as White meat such as chicken and turkey are the best and should be with just a teaspoon of unsaturated Oil such as sunflower and Olive oiL This diet presents a light option, not very high in protein, which gives energy, but abundant in cooked vegetables that protect the fragile teeth of the elderly, as well as fruits that can varied to suit each person. According to recent research, vitamin K helps delay the effects of aging and is contained in spinach and watercress.

THE DIGESTIVE SYSTEM

The digestive system has the mechanisms that transform into nutrients necessary to maintain Vital activity. For this reason, inadequate diets can trigger various alterations in the entire digestive process that will manifest themselves in modifications of the body and personal appearance. We can observe changes in the hair, skin and nails that lead us to the conclusion that external care provided to the the body is not enough if it is not accompanied by internal care. It is important to know the functioning of the digestive system, since the application of techniques that promote blood circulation, improve access and distribution of nutrients to the tissues and organs of the human body.

Digestion is the process by which food; too large particles are by physical and chemical treatments into simpler substances that the body can assimilate. Absorption is the passage of substances already assimilated, through the intestinal mucosa, to reach the blood circulation.

STRUCTURE of THE DIGESTIVE APPARATUS. The digestive tract is made up of the digestive tract, which is made up of a series of organs located after another through which food circulates in various States of waste from this process.

• Mouth: It is the entrance orifice of the Where the teeth chew and grind it together with the saliva.

• Pharynx: It is an organ with a double function, in the digestive system it facilitates the passage of food into the esophagus.

• Esophagus: It is the tube through which food descends to the stomach.

• Stomach: It is the organ Where food mixes with gastric juices to chemically transformed into increasingly simple substances.

• Large intestine: It is the final part of the digestive tract and Where mineral salts and vitamin K are absorbed.

The digestive glands in the mouth with the salivary glands which are distributed throughout the interior of the mouth, clean the teeth and facilitate the passage of the food mass towards the pharynx. Already located in the lower abdomen we find the liver, which is the largest gland in the body, it acts as a producer of bile, a yellow-green substance that helps both absorb nutrients and eliminate undesirable substances. Another digestive gland is the pancreas that makes hormones like insulin which regulates the level of glucose in the blood. In the process of functioning of the digestive system, we can observe the following stages:

• Mechanical grinding of food: The teeth together with salivation and the tongue carry out this process that forms the food bolus.

• Gastric digestion: The food bolus is transformed into chyme When it is received by the gastric juices of the stomach.

• Intestinal digestion: It is the phase that prepares the absorption stage, which is the main Stage of digestion. The bile of the gallbladder connected to the liver and the juices of the pancreas that regulate the acidity of the chyme to be received by the intestine.

• Defecation: The remains of food that have not been absorbed in the intestine, form feces together with gases and waste products of the fermentation of positive bacteria found in it.

The alterations most related to aesthetics are dental cavities, gastritis, ulcers, hepatitis, constipation and diarrhea. Chronic constipation can cause darkening of the skin due to the accumulation of toxic substances in the blood. The aesthetic professional can provide abdominal massages, stimulation currents to promote intestinal transit of these, fiber is recommended since it makes you chew more, and also removes a lot of water from the intestine at a nutritional level. The loss of fluids that When suffering from diarrhea can lead to or dry skin.

All types of hepatitis present with a manifestation of yellowish pigmentation of the skin known as jaundice.

SEX AND NUTRITION

From the aspect of nutrition, the property of stimulating the sexual through some substances, medicines or foods is what is indicated as aphrodisiac. Some of these substances are parsley, ginger, some shellfish and cocoa or chocolate, eggs and others. In a way, this ability to produce an enhancing effect on the sexual life of those who consume them is surrounded by a certain mysticism and disbelief. Although there are multiple biological factors such as hormones, sensory perception, in addition to the circumstantial factors that influence each individual from puberty to menopause in the case of women and andropause in question for men, to bring about a style satisfying sex life. The glands are part of the endocrine system of our body.

The female reproductive system is made up of the breasts, which are externally defined by the breasts, the areola, and the nipple. Internally to the breast, there are the mammary glands that are made up of fatty tissue that is ideal for the production of breast milk through progesterone.

Also in the lower abdomen area we find the vulva that is made up of the external parts that constitute the internal vagina, such as the labia majora, the labia minora, the hymen, and the clitoris. Internally it contains the vagina, which is a fibrous, membranous tube or duct that carries urine.

The labia are the folds that cover the entrance to the vagina, followed by the hymen, which is a membranous fold that reduces the external orifice of the vagina while preserving its integrity. The clitoris is a fleshy erectile body, which protrudes in the highest part of the vulva. In a vestibule located between the hymen and the labia minora, are the Bartholin glands that secrete mucus. Nearby is the cervix, which is a Structure located in the lower part of the uterus that occupies a third of this organ and constitutes a communication channel.

The cervix has a thinner and more flexible musculature than that of the uterine corpus. in women the secretion of cervical mucus in the neck is continuous and is not subject to cyclical changes as occurs in the body of the uterus. These secretions constitute a true mucous plug that acts as a barrier preventing the entry of germs into the uterus. Its consistency , fluidity and amount of cervical mucus does Vary throughout the female menstrual cycle and this characteristic is used in contraceptive methods to know the fertile days of a woman. The uterus is a hollow, flattened, pear-shaped organ located in the pelvis of the female and female of most mammals. It is the organ Where the fertilized ovum is implanted that begins gestation or reproduction.

The uterus is suspended in the and has a base or fundus, the neck or cervix that is slightly directed backward, and a mouth. When there is no pregnancy, the uterus is about 3 inches long by 2 inches Wide and I inch thick. The walls of the uterus are elastic and stretch during pregnancy to accommodate the growing fetus. The uterus is prone to infection. On each side of the uterus are the oviducts or fallopian tubes, which are two tubes that extend from the ovaries to the upper area of the uterus. Its name comes from its discoverer, an Italian anatomist named Gabriel Falopio. The woman's tubes are 2 centimeters thick and approximately 10-13 centimeters long.

Its function within the menstrual cycle is to lengthen the maturation period of the ovule that leaves the ovaries once a month and is propelled into the uterus by projections called cilia that are located on the inner surface of the tube. Infections at an early age must be taken care of since they are usually caused by obstructions in the fallopian egg duct that end up producing reproductive sterility in women.

The fimbriae are the edges of each fallopian tube that joins the ovary and also play an endocrine function through their hormonal production in the bloodstream. The ovaries are oval and flattened like an almond and are 3-8 centimeters long. The eggs or ovules consist of two parts: the outer or cortex and the inner or medulla. In the adult woman, the tissue of the ovarian cortex produces an enormous number of follicles of different sizes that contain ovules or female reproductive cells. It Will take a new cycle for each follicle to secrete a large amount of estrogens, which are the storoidal hormones involved in the development of secondary sexual characteristics in women, in the regulation of the menstrual cycle and in pregnancy. The ovary can suffer acute or chronic inflammation as a result of injuries suffered in childbirth, after operations or infections acquired through sexual intercourse.

The blood flow that from the uterine lining or endometrium of women of age is called menstruation. The development or female puberty begins between 10 and 16 years, and extends until 45 to 55 years, which is When the fertile age of women ceases. Menstruation is a natural process of the hormonal system that prepares a woman for pregnancy. When the lining of the vagina with blood flow has increased, it breaks and is eliminated for a period that covers between 3 and 7 days, which forces the adolescent to lose blood through the vagina and take care of herself with the use of feminine pads.

Female or development is a period in the life of every woman in which her hormonal maturation that is, of her own cells created by the immune system, and implies the ability to this maturation is manifested in women with their first menstruation, which indicates the beginning of their 28-day cycle. It involves the following physiological changes: It usually occurs between 11 and 14 years, they assume that it is earlier than in men. Puberty, which occurs at approximately 9 years of age, can be a cause of confusion in some adolescents, such as the myth of the suspicion of early sexual intercourse, however some physiological disorders in the secretions of the anterior lobe of the pituitary or adenohypophysis, together with the adrenal glands can another cause of a prominent development of the body in the adolescent.

The increase of the sexual organs is more evident in the breasts and the hips are Widened. The appearance of hair in the armpits, legs and is abundant forcing the use of razors to most and body creams.

In both sexes, the accelerated development of the sweat glands can cause acne on the face and back, forcing them to take care of some excess intake of saturated fat in their diet. Sometimes these changes can also alter behavior and mood, which forces the young adolescent to take some psychological assistance and counseling. The inclusion of sex education from any educational level is a matter of discussion yet to defined.

The menstrual cycle has some connotations for personal hygiene and family planning measures. The interval period one menstruation and the next marks the date from which each woman usually has her ovulation bleeding. This interval is 28 days, of which 12 days are the minimun or maximum fertility risk of obtaining an unwanted or unplanned pregnancy, between the ninth and the twentieth day, right in the middle of the 28-day cycle.

Therefore, it is affirmed by the practice of the contraceptive method or menstrual rhythm, that the 8 days before the menstrual effusion there can be no fertilization in the woman and the 8 days after the 12 days of risk there can be no fertilization because in those the egg has died in order to be fertilized. Only in these 16 days, which are added before and after, can there be sexual contact or vaginal intercourse between the couple with the security of avoiding an unwanted pregnancy.

A disorder that accompanies or precedes menstrual effusion is menstrual cramps or it is an acute abdominal pain that precedes the date of regular menstruation that may be due to the lack of acidity in the diet, but it is not limited only to this organ, but also to other diseases or neighboring organs. Colic can be difficult to locate for the patient so it should be verified if they are of intestinal origin, it is characterized by its contractions in the intestine that are preceded by the ingestion of irritating foods or infections.

These are confused with appendicitis and There are also renal colic in the bladder and bile ducts in the liver that are located by palpation of the abdomen and not the lower area. Its natural treatment includes the use of a tablespoon of natural or apple vinegar dissolved in a glass of water during the days that the discomfort lasts. If you take vinegar supplements you should drink a lot of water to avoid the sensation of burning in the stomach.

Persistent pelvic pain that is aggravated during menstruation is what is diagnosed as endometriosis. It has been accept that the immune response to eating meats and some cereals such as oats can trigger episodes of pain. The causes of this disease are not yet known and are Still the subject of debate among medical specialists.

In general, the most likely explanation is that during normal menstruation part of the endometrial tissue can flow retrograde or in the wrong direction towards the fallopian tube, and implant in the abdominal cavity, according to the regurgitation theory, in addition to evidence that later, the cells that line the abdominal cavity make metaplasia; which is the ability of certain tissues to mutate from one type to another, and form the obstruction. The cells then spread through the invasion of the blood vessels of the circulatory system that transports them to other parts of the body such as the lungs.

Other conditions associated with the menstrual cycle are amenorrhea, which is diagnosed by the absence of regular menstrual There are two of amenorrhea: primary amenorrhea is that which occurs in adolescent girls up to 16 years of age, who apparently healthy have not had any menstruation. This delay occurs due to some disorders of the sexual maturity of women, such as a genetic disorder known as Turner syndrome and other congenital processes with alterations in the development of the vagina or uterus that are associated with the consequence of female sterility. .

The second type is secondary amenorrhagia, which is the sudden disappearance of menstruation in an adult woman. This is when you are not pregnant, breastfeeding, or in menopause. Amenorrhea can have various causes such as:

- Excess medications such as birth control pills.
- Intense physical exercise in the pelvic area.
- Weight loss from severe diets or anorexia nervosa.
- Endocrine gland disorders such as pituitary tumors.
- And alterations in the function of the ovaries.

The case of resistant ovary syndrome is diagnosed when there is no physical cause, considering an inaccurate premature menopause, since many of the patients subsequently regain their normal ovarian function and menstruation. Another disorder that commonly occurs in the function of the ovaries is the polycystic ovary syndrome or Stein-Leventhal, which is characterized by a marked irregularity of menstrual cycles, with excessive growth of body hair and there may be an abnormal morphology of the ovaries with multiple small Cysts and some obesity. Its treatment is to restore fertility and regularize menstrual periods. The levels of male hormones in the female are reduced by anti-androgen hormone treatments such as cyproterone acetate and spironolactone. The contraceptive pill may be appropriate if you have irregular menstrual bleeding. Partial removal of the ovary may be helpful in this case.

Dysmenorrhea is the ailment that some women experience between the first and second day of menstrual effusion with severe menstrual cramps, which were to have a psychosomatic origin, recent research indicates that they are caused by chemical and hormonal changes in the female body that they are attributed to the absence of a diet very low in dietary fiber. Stress, mood swings, and nervousness are also associated with this picture of menstrual cycle symptoms. When the level or amount of blood flow shed by the womb during menstruation is excessive, it is called menorrhagia, and it is characterized by its extension in days, between 4 consecutive days and more.

If the stroke lasts for more than seven days in a row, it is called hyper menorrhagia. Its cause is considered to be associated with hyperthyroidism, which is an irregular increase in the function of the thyroid gland that is accompanied by excitability, tremor, tachycardia, and weight loss. Metrorrhagia is bleeding from the womb that outside of a woman's menstrual period, which is normally 28 days, interrupting its usual rhythm and originating from the cervix or cervix. Its causes are pathological such as the growth of tissue or accumulation of fluid that emerges from the mucous membrane as They grow from a narrow base or as a narrow Stern as a result of the accumulation of or malignant cells, pus, and degenerative tissue with malformations. Polyps can appear on almost all mucous membranes in the body, but are most common in the nose and small intestine.

A subject of repetitive interest in women is contraceptive that prevent the occurrence of unwanted pregnancies, which help to have a more adequate balance with respect to their own personal goals and family planning. Hormonal contraceptives are chemical substances, treated in laboratories, that work by altering a woman's normal hormonal pattern so that it does not produce ovulation.

These act on the uterine lining to prevent the implantation of the fertilized in the uterus, and the of the cervical mucus. To be administered to patients, they can select from various methods such as in its oral form by pill, by the injectable method or by implants. They do not offer protection against sexually transmitted diseases, but they are effective methods supported by social birth control programs because of their effectiveness. Oral contraceptives or contraceptive pills are combined, taken for 21 consecutive days, after which 7 days are rested, and contain estrogens and progestin; which is a synthetic form of progesterone.

They are 94 effective in preventing pregnancy. They also relieve menstrual pain, but do not prevent breakthrough bleeding, produce headaches, gain weight, and decrease sexual desire, among Other side effects. When the natural method is practical, but for some reason it falls into the of intercourse, the pill is an emergency contraceptive that can be taken up to 72 hours after sexual contact to avoid a pregnancy. Medroxyprogestorone contraceptive injection is the injectable drug of the synthetic form of progesterone, which is given every three months. Its side effects are depression, headache and abdominal pain, irregular bleeding and decreased sexual desire. In recent years it has been applied as a measure of birth control in homes with more than three children, it is surgical sterilization by tubal ligation in women which is 100 percent effective, so the mother should be aware that the Effects of the is not reversible. or general anesthesia is required in the tubal ligation surgical procedure.

It is carried out by cutting the tube and ligating the edges of the two ovules that carry the ovum from the ovary of the uterus. Other contraceptive methods provide a lower margin of effectiveness to avoid pregnancies, such as the one known among religious circles that prohibit contraceptive methods as Ogino-Knaus that was already explained in this chapter, and you get an 81 percent chance of not getting a pregnancy, and the method of coitus interruptus that consists of the withdrawal of the before ejaculation which has a 76 probability.

In contrast to male ejaculation, the woman experiences a climax or culmination of the sexual act with the pleasure of orgasm. Sexual frigidity is the abnormal absence of sexual desire or enjoyment.

Some of the aforementioned contraceptive methods also remain effective after a long period of use, so if it is intended together with the couple to obtain a pregnancy, it may take several months before having a child or baby is achieved. Pregnancy is the gestation of the woman within the human reproductive process.

In order for a pregnancy to begin after intercourse or sexual encounter, the female egg or ovum must be fertilized by a male Fertilization is the fusion of the ovum and the sperm that, like two nuclei of two gametes, give rise to the formation of a zygote or embryo. The first three months are the most critical in the growth of the fetus, which is When it develops its brain, internal organs, and the extremities of the arms and legs. Some eggs are implanted on the surface of the uterus Without fertilized, they are known as ectopic pregnancy, requiring a surgical removal. This first trimester, special care should be taken not to take medications of any kind, Without the prior advice of Your doctor. X- rays should avoided, in addition to avoiding tobacco use.

The alteration of the hormonal schemes in the manifests itself with some symptoms such as:

• Increased frequency of urination.

• Weight gain which is recommended not to exceed 24 punds at the end of pregnancy.

• Fickle cravings also eat in some women for cornstarch, ice, and chocolate banana ice cream.

• Tenderness in the breasts.

• Tiredness, nausea, and sudden mood swings.

• Sensitivity to odors.

• If abdominal pain and bleeding occur in the first weeks, you should See a doctor urgently.

It is Common for these symptoms to remit when the first three are fulfilled and Others appear such as breast enlargement and darkening of the nipples. If the pregnant mother is over 35 years of age, it is mandatory to perform an amniocentesis, which is a test that allows the early detection of genetic problems. In 9 5 percent of cases the fetus is normal. In the next Stage of pregnancy, between the fourth and eighth month of gestation, symptoms such as:

• Sudden weight gain due to edema, or soft swelling that is caused by serocity infiltrated in the cellular tissue, which is between 11 and 13 kilos in a month, of lost proteins in the urine test.

• Retention of liquids. These symptoms indicate the of a clinical picture of toxemia gravidarum, which is characterized by the presence of toxins or toxic materials in the blood, which can be bacterial, chemical or hormonal. When diagnosed, the baby is removed to protect him and the mother from contamination. The inability to conceive and give birth to a child is what is known as infertility or sterility. [t is considered that out of every 100 cases of infertile couples who fail to conceive after a year of sexual intercourse, 40 of the cases are due to problems in women and between 30 and 50 infertility is caused by male problems, the rest of the cases between 30 and 10 are caused by alterations in members of the couple that when interacting in produce infertility.

Possible causes of infertility are as follows:

• If it is due to malnutrition or the symptoms are reversible.

• Internal injuries caused by venereal diseases.

• The age of the couple is between 35 and 49 years, which represents the decrease in normal fertility in the sex glands.

• Hormonal or structural abnormalities of the reproductive system such as the absence of ovulation in the woman, in the uterus or obstruction of the tubes.

• Diseases of the male reproductive system such as insufficient production of volume.

• Excess alcohol consumption in any of the couple.

• infertility from excessive use of contraceptive

The treatments applied in female sterility initially focus on checking that there are no mechanical or chemical obstacles between the ovum and the sperm for fertilization to take place, if there is tissue obstruction it could be treated by surgical correction. Ovulation can be stimulated by hormones. If these conceptual methods fail in the woman and her partner, we proceed to artificial insemination methods. The possibilities are according to the condition of the

• In the event that the woman not produce eggs, she can ask her sister or close relative for an egg to be inseminated with her husband's. In the case of the woman, she has a uterus capable of supporting the pregnancy but does not produce eggs, the insemination is done in her own womb.

• If the woman does not have eggs or a womb capable of sustaining the pregnancy, then she can choose to rent a womb from another woman.

However, economic, legal and social factors can influence the decision making of those who assume to try these assisted reproduction techniques such as in Vitro fertilization which spreads rapidly, gamete implantation, zygote implantation or intracytoplasmic sperm injection. At 40 weeks gestation, the doctor estimates a delivery date that is counted from the patient's last menstruation. The normal duration of a for a new mother is 13 to 14 hours, and about 8 to 9 hours before she has given birth before. Labor begins with irregular contractions of the uterus every 20 to 30 minutes.

When complications during the delivery process such as bleeding in the parturient, lack of oxygen in the fetus, unusual of the fetus or difficulty in dilating the cervix for the passage of the placenta, a cesarean section is which is a consistent surgical intervention. In the extraction of the live fetus through an incision in the abdominal wall and the uterus. This name, according to tradition, comes from a of childbirth dating from the times of the Roman Empire in which the mothers who gave birth to the Caesars in this way would have already died, however the mother of Gaius Julius Caesar survived after that. The myth that a woman who has had a cesarean delivery cannot have a natural delivery again has long been disproved.

In the event that a pregnancy is interrupted before the fetus can develop its life independently of the mother, it is called abortion. This usually occurs before the sixth month of pregnancy. After the first 24 weeks there is talk of premature delivery, Where the fetus can be around 0.5 kilograms. There are two types of abortions on the situation in which they OCCLtr. abortion is one that for an unknown reason, and it is estimated that 25 of human pregnancies end in this way. If successive miscarriages occur in a woman, her chances of carrying a pregnancy to term are reduced and she is considered to have a predisposition. The causes of a miscarriage are not precise, but the following are estimated.

Some serious vitamin deficiencies are known to have resulted in abortions in laboratory animals. Folic acid and thiamine supplements are currently recommended. In 50 of cases it is because there is an alteration in the development of the embryo or in the placental tissue, which involves an alteration in the implantation of the fertilized ovum. Stress produced by the maternal environment such as extreme anxiety and other psychic disturbances.

Another percentage of cases are attributed to acute infections, systemic diseases such as nephritis, diabetes, or severe trauma. Loss of blood flow during the of pregnancy is harmless in half of the cases, however if vaginal bleeding is profuse and accompanied by intermittent pain it means a threat of abortion and it is recommended to carry the pregnancy with bed rest, plus even When it is a recurrent situation in women.

The concept of deferred abortion is When the fertilized embryo does not exceed the first three months that are key in its development for some reason and dies but is not expelled from the cavity because the mother did not know that she was pregnant, or if she did, she did not she knew it could be a twin pregnancy, obstructing the exit. Doctors recommend surgical excision of all embryonic or placental remains and ensure the possibility of infection or irritation of the mucous.

The deliberate interruption of pregnancy by consent of the mother herself, is the case of induced abortion. The method used for infanticide is applied depending on the gestation in which it is carried out. Among the clandestine or clinical interventions that are carried out are the following six:

• Curettage: an old metal instrument with a Sharp, spoon-shaped edge, with which the surface of the uterus is separated and the entire fetus is left in its placenta to die in the open.

• Chinese technique or aspiration: It was introduced in China in 1958. It consists of the use of successive dilators that help to gain access to the uterine cavity through the cervix or cervix, a flexible connected to a vacuum pump called cannula to remove the fetus. The method can be used up to the twelfth week and lasts ten minutes and does not require a hospital stay.

• RU-486 pill: It is a substance that blocks the progesterone hormone in women and is effective in the first 50 days of pregnancy. Its use is legal since 1988 in France.

• DC - Dilation and curettage: Sometimes combined with forces, the patient must remain hospitalized because the technique can cause bleeding and discomfort after the intervention and combines the two previous techniques.

• Saline infusion: Starting at week 15, the method used as a birth control measure, health recommendation for diseases and others, is the needle or fine with which a small amount of amniotic fluid is extracted from the uterus through the abdominal Wall. This is slowly replaced by a 20 saline solution. Uterine contractions occur between 24 and 48 hours, culminating in the expulsion of the fetus from the uterus.

• Hysterotomy. In cases of late abortions, a major surgical intervention is applied, similar to cesarean section, but which is through a smaller incision in the lower part of the woman's abdomen.

Regarding world abortion legislation in various parts of the World, opinions are diverse regarding the freedom of women to exercise their free will over the fate of their embryo. Considered a punishable offense or a recommended health measure in some exceptions, abortion must be marked within family planning and the right to life, which poses a challenge to us due to the reproductive difficulties of some couples who cannot have a Child before whom they do not assume timely contraceptive methods.

Gradually the pregnant woman reaches 289 days of gestation, although sometimes women give birth before the scheduled date which gives rise to a premature child of 37 weeks. If the pregnancy lasts more than 42 weeks, the delivery is called delivery. There are some home remedies in botany that help the woman in labor to up her birthing process.

Natural childbirth is the process by which the baby is from the uterus through the vagina, Without the intervention of any invasive medical or botanical method. One that some women choose is the reduction of labor discomfort with the use of anesthesia in the pelvic region at the end of the procedure. Until the last century, due to the development of science, those women who attended deliveries in the homes of women in labor were called midwives, at a time when plagues proliferated amid poor sanitary measures that maintained a high number of stillbirths. [28 81, or did not survive the first 28 days after delivery. Currently, the changes experienced in the field of obstetrics allow us to affirm a notable decrease in infant mortality that has been improved through increasing attention to nutrition together with an improvement in the techniques of specialized doctors.

The three in which a delivery is divided are the following:

• Dilation: This period is from the onset of pain or contractions until the cervix has fully dilated or expanded. It begins with irregular contractions of the uterus every 20 to 30 minutes that more frequent until the water breaks.

• Expulsion: This period begins when the fetus begins to exit through the cervical canal, once it has yielded, and ends When the fetus has already emerged and its umbilical cord is cut.

• Delivery: When the umbilical cord is cut, the placenta remains inside with part of the amniotic fluid and the membranes inside, so it mu St be completely removed. It is then When, after delivery and the normalization of the woman, the called the puerperium is located. It lasts approximately 5 to 6 weeks, Where the week immediately after delivery is the most delicate. The most Common disorders are regularly:

• Discomfort of the perineum, or area between the vagina and the anus.

• Breast discomfort such as adaptation to the simple act of breastfeeding the newborn.

• Postpartum hemorrhages, which can endanger the mothers Postpartum incontinence is when small amounts of urine can leak from the mothers bladder due to increased pressure in the abdominal cavity during times of laughter, coughing, and even certain sports activities.

Postpartum depression, also known as or postnatal depression, usually lasts for two weeks and is characterized by frequent crying, distinguished as sadness and excessive worry for the baby. It is even described in early Greek medicine. It is associated with genetic problems, the emotional temperament of the baby and economic problems and family dysfunction. In extreme cases of psychosis there may be rejection of the baby and even wishes to harm him that must be attended to by a psychiatrist.

In the situation of a mature woman who has had repeated deliveries throughout her fife, we of uterine prolapse, which is a pathological protrusion, or herniation of the adjacent womb and Structure through the vaginal canal, in such a way that it pushes the cervix through the introitus or external lips. In its most serious degree, the entire uterus protrudes through the vagina, inverted and is unfavorable due to the congenital weakness of the tissues. It produces pain, a feeling of pelvic heaviness, ulcers and bleeding in herniated structures. It is recommended to attend a permanent diet that on the care of organic and muscular tissues.

Continuing with the different stages of the functions of the female sexual organs, we find motherhood and lactation, which refers to the Stage of caring for and breastfeeding the baby. The mammary glands are wow the surface of the skin and form several small nodules on the areola. There are between fifteen and twenty milk ducts that extend through the different lobes or subdivisions of the breast and reach the nipple, where they The secretory parts of the glands produce milk after childbirth, during a of time known as lactation. Mastitis is the name given to inflammation of the breasts. Some more complex of discomfort in breast care are mentioned below as cancer prevention.

Recommendations while breastfeeding the baby:

• Breast milk is the only food for the baby during the first five months of life, so the mother must take care of her own nutrition. By tradition, it is believed that there are varied options for nursing mothers to choose in place of the well-known "cravings" that are caused by the lack of glucose that lead them to mistakenly prefer sweet foods or desserts. Breastfeed your baby for six months to a year if possible.

• Remember that formula milk is a second feeding priority and there are ones for newborns and when they reach three months.

• Clean your nipples with natural solutions such as olive oil or aloe vera to avoid the cracks that often cause discomfort when breastfeeding your baby.

• In this case, it is recommended to ingest infusions of the stimulating of breast milk such as anise, whole milk and dairy products together with malt cereals, shakes or barley drinks that have a high protein content.

• Changing height can sometimes affect normal circulation. Choose loose clothing, mainly in the belly area- Also choose gowns or dresses that make breastfeeding easier.

• The two months after Your baby is born are for the to return to its normal size. Take walks, do not lead a sedentary life where the immobility of Your limbs emphasizes the sufferings or of pregnancy.

• Avoid alcoholic beverages in excess, your baby Will thank you in the future.

• After 6 months of breast milk feeding, the baby should a diet that complements with a greater amount of iron, calcium, vitamins and energy for optimal growth. In addition, as recommendations for the guide next to this table for feeding the baby, it is suggested:

• Box cereals should not be used to thicken formula milk, but to give consistency to liquid baby

• If the child refuses a food, continue to insist on Other days.

• Children should eat with their own utensils such as a plate and spoon for exclusive use.

• You should not add salt or sugar to the vegetable or fruit porridge, you should get used to the natural flavors of the food.

• As long as the baby does not reach his eighth month, the baby should not be given Wheat or bread crackers, or barley, or rye.

• For the care of baby's milk teeth, artificial sugary drinks, coffee or soft drinks should not given.

• When Your child is 1 year Old, you can drink whole milk and formula for Older children.

• By the time the child reaches its first year, it can already fed with food made from honey, doing so earlier runs the risk of poisoning the baby.

Galactorrhea is a milk secretion outside pregnancy due to excess prolactin in women that is associated with hormonal alterations produced by the pituitary adenoma, which is usually excretory. Continuing with the diseases of the female reproductive system, the inflammation of the cervix or cervix, known as cervicitis, is mentioned. The one that is derived as a symptom of alterations of the menstrual cycle, birth trauma or oral contraceptives are ectopias of the endometrial mucosa. Its cause is venereal diseases and there are two mucopurulent cervicitis and the most serious one, ulcerative. Mucopurulent is characterized by a purulent and exudate discharge that can caused by Chamydia, gonorrhea and, less frequently, other such as Ureaplasma urealyticum. In the ulcerative it has as a consequence of contagion with genital and syphilis, while in developing countries it occurs together with symptoms of chancroid, lymphogranuloma and donovanosis. In its treatment, antibiotics are administered to the patient and their sexual contracts. Bacterial inflammation that occurs in the vagina is known as vaginitis. It can from contact with a woman's dirty hands and is not exactly caused by sexual contact.

When there is a controlled increase in the number of cells in an organ or tissue in some parts of the body, it is called so. In physiological hyperplasia, it in the glandular epithelium of the Young adolescent breast When it receives hormonal stimuli at puberty due to the production of estrogens. In pregnancy this is produced by progestogens that affect the inner lining mucosa accompanied by hypertrophy in the smooth muscle of the myometrium, which is the muscle layer.

In those cases in which the bacterial infection of the female genital tract affects the uterus, fallopian tubes and ovaries, it is called pelvic inflammatory disease or PID. Its symptoms that begin a few days into the menstrual period, are fever, chills, vaginal discharge or and abdominal pain that is often confused with appendicitis. It is often caused by gonorrhea or chlamydia bacteria. Its diagnosis is made by physical examination that demonstrates tenderness in the uterus, ovaries, and fallopian tubes. In severe cases, an abscess may form in the pelvis, and it carries a risk of topical pregnancy and is a cause of infertility. When presented with liver problems, it can lead to death. The accumulation of pathological or foreign material to the organism in a liquid or semisolid state that forms inside as the form of a membranous bladder that can sometimes be and attached to the surface of the vagina, it is what is called ovarian cyst. The rupture or torsion of an ovarian Cysts can be mistaken for an of inflammatory disease which requires a lampaoscope examination.

Among the circulatory problems of women we find varicose veins, which are frequent in the veins of the legs that become prominent or visible with their bluish color. They can lead to ankle swelling or skin ulcerations. They are treated by applying pressure with an elastic stocking along their path, covering them with a solution or excising them aesthetically with laser treatments, verifying that neighboring veins work well since the blood they contain is diverted towards the next.

Among the aesthetic ailments of general interest We can mention cellulite, which is a French term-There is no consensus regarding its cause, but it is known that among the of bacteria that cause human diseases is the bacteriurn Vibrio aeromonas hydrophila that can be found in underwear and this effect on the skin due to sweating and toxins of the itself. However, most doctors consider it an accumulation of fat around the hips and thighs, more Common in women.

The lymphatic system is responsible for the purification of waste prcm1Cts or toxins from the tissues, if for any reason the lymphatic circulation does not work toxins accumulate in this area that breaks the chains in the adipose tissue. Avoiding this situation depends on muscle contractions, so lack of exercise, tight clothing, altered high heels and even the fact of crossing the legs is responsible for lymphatic circulation. It means the retention of water through proteoglycans and a greater number of water-binding molecules. Repeated dietary regimens can cause a loss of skin elasticity and contribute to the development of cellulite.

Consumption of harmful toxins such as alcohol and coffee should be lower than the nutrients in dietary fiber. Local massages and the application of can help its treatment, together with herbal Oils with astringent properties and earthy creams or ash, which, applied regularly, improve their effects on the of the skin. Continuing with the aesthetic issues in women due to the effect of age are wrinkles or skin folds. Wrinkles are due to various nutritional, expressive and environmental factors. For example, it is common to observe in some elderly women the dryness of the skin obtained throughout maturity, which is marked mainly in the well- known "crows feet" or the contour of the eyes, eyelids and dark circles, in addition to expression lines around the lips and cheeks.

A daily water intake of at least 8 glasses is recommended, between meals to improve moisture and skin elasticity with an intake of beta-carotene and carotene from orange vegetables and leafy greens, as well as collagen from the eggs and pulps crystallize from Aloe Vera. For skin care, an ideal natural cosmetic mask for sun protection, wrinkles, blemishes and Other skin problems is to mix the following ingredients :

- A medium branch of aloe vera,
- Three of honey.
- 1 egg White.

Mix all the ingredients in a container, place on the face and neck leaving it to act for 20 minutes and remove with warm water and a clean towel. You can keep the leftover in the refrigerator for another application for up to 24 hours.

The accumulation of tissue in areas of the woman as she undergoes pregnancy, intense work, and family life can bring a problem of overweight and obesity that is accentuated being more difficult to reduce or lose weight. A slimming process applied to habits and a change in lifestyle can improve appearance, self-confidence, the dynamic ability to perform various activities at the same time, such as and study, and above all to improve. a longer and more satisfying sex life.

In women with a thin complexion, there may be a low intake of known as exogenous, that is, a lack of certain or endogenous or secondary due to organic diseases, and fasts of psychological motivation. Symptoms of malabsorption due to poor functioning of the small intestine are characteristic. Also pregnancy, lactation, hormonal alterations due to hyperthyroidism, surgeries and convalescence are causes of loss of muscle mass that Vary with age. However, statistics show that the majority of the is obese and requires urgent implementation of social awareness measures through social campaigns and in the media that seek to eradicate the high rates of preventable deaths with a healthier lifestyle.

Voluntary weight loss plans should not be taken lightly, but through well-controlled diets, balanced by the inclusion of sources of nutrients and supplements, in addition to physical exercise. The risk of selective malnutrition is present in those tables of popular diets such as tea, pineapple that are accompanied by self-destructive fasting, and Others that are not related to current nutrition standards should be avoided. Anorexic drugs such as amphetamines carry a high risk of addiction in some patients who must take care of the symptoms that, as side effects, lead to Other little beneficial conditions in the medium and long term.

The female reproductive system can be affected by various forms of tumors, some of them with malignant development. Cervical tumor or cervical cancer or cervical cancer; it represents the leading cause of death in women according to study rates worldwide, and is followed by breast cancer. [t is characterized by the formation of tissue on both sides, at the end of the vaginal canal and between the entrance to the uterus. Fibroids and tumors of the ovaries usually have a more favorable prognosis. The Pap smear should performed in women aged 25-64 years. The earlier the diagnosis is, the greater the chances of improvement with therapeutic measures, such as radiation therapy or chemotherapy. Cancer can be asymptomatic until advanced stages of the disease. If suspicious cells are found, a biopsy should performed in which a larger tissue sample is analyzed to confirm or rule out the existence of cancer.

Finally, to complete this analysis of the most frequent ailments in the last stage of women, we the climacteric, which is the period of a woman's life in which she loses her reproductive capacity, and is the preamble to her menopause. It can begin with an absence of menstruation or with a definitive absence from the first moment.

As a consequence of the cessation of ovulation that takes place at the of the climacteric, there is a decrease in the production of progesterone, which is released in the corpus luteum after ovulation, and a relative increase in estrogens due to anovulatory cycles that also decline the levels of these others. To be considered menopausal arrival, there must be a definite lack of menstrual bleeding that lasts for a variable minimum of at least nine months to one year. In almost all women this decrease in estrogen occurs between the ages of 45 and 50.

Osteoporosis, or deterioration of the bone Structure of the spine, is a sign of the onset of menopause, with hot flashes and sweating, accompanied in some cases by vaginal dryness, burning and pain during intercourse. Surgical ablation or disabling of the ovaries from other causes can induce early menopause at any age in women. These disorders can be treated by prescribing hormone replacement therapy, which has unfortunately been associated with an increased risk of endometrial cancer. Before it was believed that depression and emotional disorders accompanied the onset of menopause in women, however their achievement is questioned in most cases.

The most drastic surgical treatment performed on the female system is hysterectomy. This is the surgical removal of the uterus, and one of the most common surgical procedures. Sometimes only the cervix and corpus are removed; in other cases, what is called a total hysterectomy is done, in which the uterus, neck, fallopian tubes, and ovaries are removed. Hysterectomy is indicated in a large of cases, ranging from life-threatening situations such as cancers, fibrous tumors, excessive bleeding and uncontrollable bleeding, recurrent inflammatory conditions, or serious infections. with the application of this the woman regularly older than 40 years, will not present menstruation nor will be able to conceive a child.

HEALTHY RECIPES

The detoxifying diet is a therapy proposed by natural or alternative medicine through medicinal plants and fruits for having unique regenerative properties among all the elements of the plant and animal kingdom.

Those who have ever heard of its immediate effects have thought it a matter of native ancestral magic, witchcraft or the illusory fascination of some group of But many testimonies around the world attest to its infallible healing power from Peru, through the Amazon rainforest of Brazil, to China, India and the Mediterranean. This knowledge was first collected in Parkinson's Theatrum Botanicum in 1640. We must then recognize that botany, as a plant science, has contributed to traditional science many non-synthetic drugs that are extracted directly from plants, leaves, stems and roots that are harvested and packed for conservation When climate changes affect their production. The quality of purifying the toxins produced by the catabolism of the cells, which is the stage of purifying the waste of the body and mainly the blood, is one of the most important that known medicinal plants have, which stimulate and produce beneficial effects on the body. man. If toxins are not eliminated, over time they accumulate and precipitate towards deficiencies in the functioning of organs such as the stomach, liver and intestines, and then in serious diseases that affect the immune system with irregular inflammations and overload the spleen work.

The so-called botanical cures are Common of alternative medicine that use natural drinks that are taken in the morning and on an empty stomach, one to three times a day, Without eating anything so that their effect is more effective. They should always be done after a long of illness, sedentary life, consumption of alcoholic beverages, smoking or consumption of artificial anabolics and medications. They should not accompanied by taking medications as in some cases there may be interactions due to side effects contrary to the cure. The consumption of alcoholic beverages should be avoided. Some of these are harmful for with large intestine problems and pregnant women, such as grape cure and rue tea, which are tonic cures of the natural alternatives for the cure there are the most Common ones such as grape, watercress and lemon. The grape, which is the round and juicy berry of the vine, is a natural cleanser of the digestive tract, which stimulates the secretion of gastric and pancreatic juices, influences the secretion of bile by activating the liver, as well as having a laxative function by decrease intestinal fermentations. It also increases urine production and regulates the presence of uric acid. All this influences, toning the heart nucleus and stimulates the appetite, reducing fatigue. This affects the health of with diseases such as anemia, arteriosclerosis, arthritis, gout, hemorrhoids, hypertension, liver diseases, nervous problems, obesity, psoriasis and rheumatism.

Watercress, which is an aquatic plant with a temperate climate, is collected before flowering and its leaf is used as a condiment for salads in food. As a green leafy vegetable, it has a lot of vitamin A and C, and blood cleansing acids. It is used in cures of people who suffer from the habit of smoking or drinking, helping to eliminate the desire to do so. It also helps in others such as cough, fever, thinness or low weight, as well as heart problems and heart rhythm and nerves.

Lemon is an excellent citrus fruit to purify the skin of varicose veins and facial blemishes. Its content is ascorbic acid, it prevents oral bleeding, relieves rheumatism and arthritis, and stimulates the healing of the skin of the lips and wounds as it regulates the pH or acidity in the discomfort of women. Lesser known are the roots of sarsaparilla and horsetail, and also the stem of the cats claw plant. Sarsaparilla is a plant from which the root is extracted to make the infusion of its tea that is used for arthritis, rheumatism and gout for people with joint problems and inflammation. Horsetail, due to its plant name, is used for respiratory, stomach and menstrual bleeding ailments, as well as liver and kidney problems. Another infusion is extracted from the stem of the herb called Cat's Claw that is believed to have regenerative properties of the immune system as in primary cancer under treatment and even use in patients suffering from the immunodeficiency syndrome, AIDS. As well as women's diseases such as varicose veins, menstrual complications and fibroids, and kidney deficiencies.

For the urgent treatment of food poisoning When the patient has symptoms such as heartburn, vomiting, heart palpitations and skin rashes after eating or harmful substances, a natural antidote is recommended that prevents the absorption of the into the body and consists of mixing bread burned and have the intoxicated patient swallowed together with milk of magnesia dissolved in a cup of strong tea.

IMMUNE SHAKE

METABOLIC EFFECTS: The amino acids, such as acemannan, contained in aloe vera leaves are effective in treating many diseases of the immune system such as colds and flu, leukemia, arteriosclerosis and AIDS.

INGREDIENTS : 1 liter of malt 3 tablespoons brown sugar 3 of flower or / ounces of honey 1/2 carrot, 2 half leaves of aloe vera or aloe drink 1 lemon 1 Sprig of chopped celery, 2 capsules of vitamin B complex (in separate bottle)

PROCESS : On a cutting board, the carrot, aloe vera leaves and celery are cut into slices. They are put into a blender along with the malt, the or honey and the sugar. A strainer is placed on top of the jug and the lemon juice is squeezed out. The strainer is removed, covered and liquefied. They are drunk, along with a daily tablet of complex B, with two or three cups of the drink daily for 3 to 14 days, on the improvement.

FRUIT SHAKE

METABOLIC EFFECTS: The high vitamin content of green leafy vegetables and lower in Other elements such as nitrogen and alkaloids, together with the Vitamin A contained in yogurt, activate the body's lymph, regenerating our white cells.

INGREDIENTS : 2 medium yogurt of preferred flavor I lemon, I Fruit of preference (banana, apple, kiwi) 20 grams of the heart of a White cabbage, 3 of sugar 1 pinch of salt I cup of ice water Cup of semi-skim milk of oat flakes to taste

PROCEDURE: The cabbage is cut into strips or julienne strips on a chopping board and placed in the blender with the milk, water and yogurts. The oats, the pinch of Salt, and the sugar. A strainer is placed over the blender and the lemon juice is squeezed out. The strainer is removed and liquefied. two cups are drunk daily for one (1) day.

DIURETIC SHAKE

METABOLIC EFFECTS: The nutritional components of carbohydrates contained in apple and lettuce combine to create a tonic that together with salts, minerals and sugars stimulate and regulate digestive, gallbladder and liver function.

INGREDIENTS :

1 medium fresh lettuce 1 red apple 3 cups semi skim milk 4 tablespoons honey or brown sugar 1 pinch of salt or baking soda

PROCESS : On a chopping board, cut the lettuce and apple into pieces, preferably with the peel. Add with milk, honey or sugar and a pinch of Salt. Blend for I to 2 minutes. Drink Cold as a refreshment after

ANTIOXIDANT SHAKE

METABOLIC EFFECTS: The of carrots are excellent, since the carotene contained in its Orange fiber contains vitamin A and fat and is of great for the health of eyes, skin and intestinal tract. The fiber or starch in fruits serves to regulate intestinal functions and prevent diarrhea. The antioxidants and vitamin C of the Orange complete a drink with many nutrients required in large quantities.

INGREDIENTS : 1 tablespoon of Turmeric 1/2 carrot, chopped 3 or anges 2 tablespoons sugar or honey 1 pinch of salt 2 cups of water

PROCESS : Blend all the ingredients with the juice strained from the oranges. Take as a drink with meals.

ENERGIZING SHAKE

METABOLIC EFFECTS: Beets contain a lot of calories and sugars, as well as vitamin A and C, some protein and fat. The Same ones that help to have energy and increase muscle m ass.

INGREDIENTS : 2 sliced beets I Orange or banana 3 brown sugar or honey I pinch of salt 2 cups of water I Cup of barley pre-baked or microwave 1 tablespoon of peanuts

PROCESS : Chop the beets and squeeze the Orange juice or banana (preferably). Add the water, sugar, Salt, and precooked barley and beat in the blender. two cups are drunk daily between meals.

TONING SHAKE

METABOLIC EFFECTS: Ice cream is a rich dairy fat treat that is ideal to to any palate, but mixed food is usually healthier. The healthy fats in nuts are sometimes hard and difficult to eat whole, so smoothies are used to give a flavor to fruit salads and are mixed to create an appetizer with carbohydrates and sugars ideal for any time of the day. day.

INGREDIENTS : 2 cups of ice cream of the flavor of preference 1/2 Cup of bananas or bananas 1/2 cup pineapple 1 / 2 cup berries or kiwis 1/ 2 cup of dried fruits (almond, walnuts and pistachio)

PROCESS: All the fruits are washed and chopped and chopped into pieces. In a blender, combine all the fruits with the ice cream and that's it. They can be served with whole grain cookies.

SLIMMING SHAKE

METABOLIC EFFECTS: Cereals are a rich Source of B vitamins, which must be consumed daily, as well as fiber to avoid many diseases.

INGREDIENTS : 1 tablespoon chia 1 tablespoon flax 1 1/2 cups whole grain cereal 1 1/2 cups low-fat milk 1 tablespoon sugar, Raisins to taste

PROCESS: Blend all the ingredients in the blender and refrigerate to serve.

PEANUT AND RAISIN COOKIES

DESSERTS RECIPES WELD: 18 to 24 regular cookies.

METABOLIC EFFECTS: The peanut seed along with the raisins make a powerful combination rich in energy and unsaturated fat.

INGREDIENTS // 4 cups of Wheat flour (I pound) 1 1/2 cups of sugar 2 and 1/2 bars of light margarine 3 eggs 1 cup peanuts 2 cups of raisins I of baking or baking 2 vanillas

PROCESS // 1 - Preheat the oven to 3502 F. Melt the light margarine in the microwave or a saucepan.

2- In the blender the raisins are crushed at medium and set

3 - In a deep container or bowl they sift; or pass through a sieve, one by one, all the powdered ingredients: flour and baking powder to break up lumps.

4- In the bowl of the mixer, beat the butter, eggs, vanilla and sugar, until they are well combined. On the Same container, add the sifted flour and the crushed raisins, until a hard and compact mixture for cookies is formed.

5 - Grease, with the remaining half Stick of margarine, a sheet or with sunflower or soybean Oil.

6- with a spoon, place on the tray, one by one, of the biscuit mixture in balls until the Spaces are filled. Immediately take the peanuts and place the seeds to taste, one by one on each cookie. 7- Put the tray in the preheated oven and let it bake for 10 to 12 minutes. 8- Remove from the oven and let the tray cool before taking them off. Repeat 5, 6 and 7 with the rest of the mixture.

CINNAMON COOKIES

YIELD. 12 to 20 regular cookies.

METABOLIC EFFECTS: Cinnamon is a natural stimulant for the digestive and muscular system. The apple is a fruit rich in phosphorus that is attributed with properties to fight anemia, neutralize cholesterol and prevent

INGREDIENTS // 4 cups of Wheat flour (I pound) 1 cup of brown sugar 2 and 1/2 bars of light or low fat margarine 2 eggs, 1 and 1/2 tablespoons of powdered milk 2 tablespoons ground cinnamon 2 red apples, chopped into pieces with their skin 1 of baking 2 vanilla

PROCESS/ 1. Preheat the oven to 3509 F. Melt the light margarine in the microwave or m a saucepan.

2- In the blender, crush the apple peels and set aside. The peeled apples are into Small pieces.

3- In a deep container or bowl they sift; or pass through a sieve, one by one, all the powdered ingredients: flour, baking powder and cinnamon to break up any lumps.

4- In the bowl of the mixer, beat the butter, eggs, vanilla and sugar, until they are well combined. On the same container, add the sifted flour and the crushed peels with the chopped apples, beating until a hard and compact mixture for cookies is formed.

5 - Grease a cookie Sheet or spray Oil with the remaining half Stick of margarine.

6- with a place on the tray, one by one, portions of the biscuit mixture in balls until the spaces are filled.

7- Put the tray in the preheated oven and let it bake for 10 to 12 minutes.

8- Remove the tray from the oven with a flat utensil and let the tray cool down before taking them off. Repeat procedures 5, 6 and 7 with the rest of the mixture.

GINGER COOKIES

YIELD: 12 to 20 regular cookies.

METABOLIC EFFECTS: Ginger is a tuber that gives a light and peculiar spicy flavor to Stimulates the female respiratory, immune, digestive and reproductive Systems.

INGREDIENTS 4 cups of Wheat flour (I pound) 1 1/2 cups of sugar or 2 cups of honey or grated scrape 2 and 1/2 bars of light or low fat margarine 3 eggs 4 tablespoon s grated ginger 2 tablespoon ground ginger 5 tablespoons of powdered milk 1 tablespoon of baking powder 2 tablespoons vanilla

PROCESS // 1 - Preheat the oven to 350e F. Melt the light margarine in the microwave or m a saucepan.

2- with a ray, the ginger root is crumbled until obtaining 4 tablespoons.

3- In a deep container or they sift; or pass through a sieve, one by one, all the powdered ingredients: flour, baking and cinnamon to break up any lumps.

4- In the bowl of the mixer, the butter, eggs, vanilla and sugar, until they are well combined. The sifted flour and the ginger zest are added to the Same container, until a hard and compact mixture for cookies is formed.

5- Grease a cookie Sheet or spray Oil with the remaining half Stick of margarine.

6- with a spoon, place on the tray, one by one, of the biscuit mixture in balls until the spaces are filled.

7- Put the tray in the preheated oven and let it bake for 10 to 12 minutes.

8- Remove from the oven and let the tray cool before taking them off. Repeat 5 , 6 and 7 with the rest of the mixture.

DRY FRUIT STRUDEL

METABOLIC EFFECTS: Nuts are necessary fruits for a balanced diet. Its flavor is special and its nutritional value in carbohydrates and proteins make it ideal to combine with desserts, as well as being combined with an antioxidant such as chocolate produced from cocoa.

INGREDIENTS FOR THE PASTA / / 2 cups flour 1/2 of salt I of White sugar 1 1/4 cups low-fat butter 1/4 cup low-fat milk fruit juice of half a lemon FOR THE FILLING // 2 Pounds of Fruit (Noni) fruits 1/2 cup brown sugar 1/2 cup of almonds 1/2 cup of grapes or pine nuts 1/2 cup raisins 5 of powdered chocolate, 1 teaspoon cinnamon, 1/2 cup crumbled cookies 2 of cooking rum FOR THE DECK // 2 tablespoon of flour 1/2 quart of butter 1 of jam 1 yolk

PROCESS // 1 - Start the pasta by mixing the flour, Salt, sugar, buffer, lemon juice and eggs. The milk is added little by little until it reaches the hardness and firmness of the paste.

2- Peel the nonis, remove the core and cut them into very thin or transparent slices. Mix them together with the grapes, raisins, powdered, cinnamon, sugar, crumbled cookies and liquor.

3- Flour a napkin and place the pasta on top. Roll it out to a thickness of 3 to 4 millimeters. Spread the melted butter over the pasta with a teaspoon or brush and then the jam.

4- Put the filling little by little on half of the pasta. Wrap the pasta with the filling inside, curing its funnel (take it by the napkin so that the pasta does not break).

5- with the help of the napkin, place the strudel in a greased mold sprinkled with flour. Paint the surface with the egg yolk and the melted margarine that is left. 6- Bake at medium level for 40 to 45 minutes, until the surface is golden brown and remove the mold.

MANGO AND PINEAPPLE CRUMBLE

YIELD•. 8 servings.

METABOLIC EFFECTS: Ripe mango is a delicious fruit rich in acids, but accompanying it with pineapple helps it digest Without digestive discomfort as they sometimes prcxiuce, making them another balanced dessert option.

INGREDIENTS FOR THE STUFFING // 1 and 1/2 pounds of ripe mango I and 1/2 pound pineapple I/ 3 cup White sugar 2 ground cinnamon I lemon juice FOR THE DECK // I cup of flour I cup of brown sugar I pinch of salt 1 Stick of low-fat margarine, melted

PROCESS // 1 - Preheat the oven to 37 F. / 2- Peel the mangoes and pineapple and mix them in a flat glass bowl with the sugar, cinnamon and lemon juice. 3 - In another bowl mix the flour, brown sugar and Salt. Mix them with the fruits and add the butter and join the ingredients with a stick, until it is lumpy. 4- Bake for 45 minutes and leave until golden. 5 - Remove and let COOL It can be served immediately with vanilla Ice cream

CORN AND CHEESE CAKE

YIELD: 12 servings.

METABOLIC EFFECTS // Corn is a grain rich in carbohydrates and proteins that help build muscle mass. Accompanied with cream cheese, they complement it with vitamin A and unsaturated milk fats.

INGREDIENTS FOR THE BASE // 3 and 1/2 cups of Wheat flour 4 cups whole corn precooked 1/4 cup vegetable or sunflower Oil 1 1/2 cups brown sugar 1/2 of salt I and 1/2 of baking powder 6 eggs 1/2 cup of water 1/2 Stick of margarine, Oil or grease spray

FOR THE DECK //

2 regular jars of cream cheese (3 ounces each) 1 pound creamy Yellow cheese or mozzarella, whole and unsliced (1/2 pound of each may be optional) 1/2 cup milk 1 egg 3 tablespoons cornstarch cornstarch 1/2 of salt

PROCESS // 1- Preheat the oven to 3 502 F.

2- In a deep container or they sift; or pass through a sieve, one by one, all the ingredients: flour, baking and salt to break up lumps.

3- The precooked whole corn is beaten in the blender with half a cup of water.

4- In the bowl of the mixer, beat the Oil, eggs, and sugar, until they are well combined. The beaten cooked corn and the mixed flour are added to the Same container, until a thick and compact mixture is formed for the sweet.

5- Beat the cream cheese with the egg, cornstarch, milk and salt for the cover.

6- with a grating, the pound of cheese is crumbled (without slicing).

7- Grease, with the remaining half Stick of margarine, a glass pyrex (9 inches in diameter) or with cooking spray.

8- The corn base is emptied over the pyrex, after placing it carefully so that all the cheese does not go to the bottom. Then the cream cheese topping is added.

9- Put the tray in the preheated oven and let it bake for 40 to 45 minutes.

10- Remove from the oven and let the container cool before serving. Garnish with almonds, a sprig of parsley and about two tablespoons of melted margarine, as an option.

GRANOLA BARS

METABOLIC EFFECTS: Grains and cereals are foods rich in B vitamins, which When mixed with eggs and peanuts make a complete triplet of energy, nutrients and unsaturated fats for the balance of the functions.

INGREDIENTS : 1 cups of Wheat flour I bar of butter 1 cup of brown sugar 2 egg yolks I cup chocolate 1/2 cup oat flakes 1/2 cup flaked barley 1/2 cup of rice cereal 1/2 cup corn cereal 1/2 cup of ch 1/2 cup of Wheat bran 1/2 cup of chopped walnuts or almonds I cup of whole grain cereal 1 cup of raisins 1/2 cup of honey (to varnish) 1 cup of strawberry jam or flavor of preference

PROCESS : 1- Mix the flour with the melted butter, the egg yolks and the sugar, beating well.

2- Add the remaining ingredients starting with the rice cream and the corn cream, beat until it melts.

3 - Work with Your hand to form the lumps and now continue with the Wheat bran, the chocolate, the flakes, the walnuts or almonds , the peanuts and the raisins.

4- Cover a refractory mold with wax and press the mixture until the entire mixture in the mold is covered.

5- Bake at 3502 F for 15 minutes.

6- Remove and let stand for 30 minutes. In a dry blender, blend the whole grain cereal. Add a layer of honey and then the strawberry jam Spread cereal over base to coat.

7- Bake now at 225e F to brown.

8- Remove, unmold and refrigerate for a few hours. 9- Already cold, cut into long bars and serve.

NUTRITION BLOG ARTICLES

"WHY DO YOU NEED TO TAKE CARE of YOUR NUTRITION?

"It is vital that you take care of Your nutrition. Your food Will be like the fountain of the elixir of eternal youth. Is trying to get sick less, to live longer and better We resumed this blog in 2014 to share health and wellness information for all of you. The nutrition boom is reaching its climax. Lees just watch the media for an hour. For example, the written press and magazines are always presenting us with articles and interviews of all kinds in which updated and recent information on thousands of topics is expanded- They have only one in common: Our culture, Our lifestyle. This to take hold as a capitalist more than 30 years ago When a diversity of products were introduced to the international commercial World that try to improve Our make us more attractive and last but not least; younger.

Aesthetic values are making our lives what they want, sometimes placing them above intellectual and spiritual values. They are always the essential, the first impression. The fight is really against aging, which means a fair impact on our habits, equal to the natural degeneration of every human being, without distinction of age, sex or social class. To start worrying to horror, let's just remember the most interesting headlines of recent months: Increase in in the World Detection of cancer cases in humans and animals, Climate changes that harm crops in many countries, Cycle decontrol of nitrogen and selenium in soils in nature and Discovery of new epidemic diseases worldwide: AHI NI.

What should be known and put into practice "Only the strong survive" dictates a maxim from the past. And if imitating is one of the statements of aesthetics, which is one of the most accepted by the majority, as a bran ch of Aristotelian philosophy, then we have no doubt that we are, from time to time and in one way or another, victims of these trends. Food is one of the vital values as is clothing and housing. In order not to go so far, it is Worth remembering the French philosopher Henri Bersong who defined this science as "the use of intelligence to create a system of that describes reality even though the real world falsifies it."

"MYTHS AND TRUTHS of GAINING AND LOSING WEIGHT

"After my personal experience with oral anabolics, of those caloric shakes with artificial steroids sold in supplement stores, I can testify beyond What I previously wrote about this controversial topic.

We continue with this criticism and positive complaint on the subject of our health and And it is that according to other web writers comment, this issue is no longer being paid for by millionaire research laboratories for its better study. Rather, only its risks are warned. To know it you don't have to be a doctor, just be a regular reader or observer, that's enough. For those who have made the decision to follow the advice described in the first article of this series, it is now necessary to know much more about what happens after they have started to follow it. of course, the side effects in the long run are somewhat negative for our health.

Virtually all medications have them, and whichever does not believe it, just take the medicine boxes they take and take a careful look at what is said, on the Internet or in pharmacology directories, who with honest clarity from the laboratories themselves producers, capsules, syrups and another medicines that you frequent, warn you. Everything thus seems to have a good side, but another bad. The nitrogen balance When I replaced my usual childhood vitamins with anabolic steroids, fueled by their promise to help me gain muscle vitality and weight, I couldn't even imagine the effects of not writing down the burly salesman's quick recommendations. It may sound comical now, but it wasn't. In one of the links that we can search on the net, this comment appears:

"The anabolic effects of nandrolone decanoate are reflected in a positive nitrogen balance. Nitrogen is part of the protein, Deca Durabolin causes the muscle cell to Store more nitrogen than it releases, as a result a nitrogen balance is achieved. A positive nitrogen balance is synonymous with muscle growth because the muscle cell, in this phase, assimilates a larger amount of protein than When 1 used them, 1 did not know that the CONTINUED USE of these contained in the shakes had a limit period of 8 to 9 weeks, that is, two and a half months. I took them for a of more than 4 months and then I left them, because as they themselves warn, it happened to me that I no longer felt the effect of before.

The worst of all is that I never gained enough muscle mass, because I simply reduced the recommended dose When I noticed that sometimes its consumption unleashed a strange state of palpitations and tachycardia, which I do not know if they are always normal. or they are another of the effects to my food allergy. On the same page, the following is noted: "The moment you notice that progress slows down to the of being irrelevant, you should stop taking it and rest for a few months.

Unfortunately, the rush to obtain spectacular results and the unawareness that some show off lead to situations that we could classify as and absurd at the very least. Nothing can replace hard training, proper nutrition, rest, motivation and "To summarize, we must know that even these new and surprising physical bodybuilding treatments, whether or need a balanced diet; that is to say with ALL the food groups. In my case, the nitrogen cycle manifested itself with the same past blog post episode of chronic fatigue, signs of overweight, stress, drowsiness, and then a lack of But this did not mean the beginning of hepatitis, but a notable absence of this nutrient along with other minerals such as selenium and silica in the foods of my regular meals. For those who want to write them down, just add a lot of green leaves to the super cart in salads such as cabbage, spinach, artichoke and garlic; as well as tea, such as green tea and horsetail, available at alternative medicine stores or pharmacies.

"WHEN WE DEMAND MORE FROM OUR BODY"

"The Slight bodily symptoms that we suffer daily and they appear recurrently in our life in a short or long term, they are undoubtedly signs. Pain is defined as the distressing and annoying sensation of a part of the due to internal or external causes. They are the nerve endings or receptors that are found from the skin until they are distributed throughout the body, with varying degrees of sensitivity, which warn us. Let's remember the very first effect that we some of the many times When we feel pain. Whether due to an external or internal cause, it has always been a mechanical stimulus that through nerve fibers reached our brain to indicate that our back; for example, he no longer had the strength to continue working. Although it is also that pains are to other parts of the for example from the back to the thorax after a pericxl of reflection that affected the spleen, with a feeling of anguish. It could even be that a virus already inside our mouth made us think about the need to get an analgesic. The first thing we do when the cause of that shock or shock is internal, is to ignore it, however, it is not until the pain or discomfort persists that we make any precise decision to solve it. Going to the doctor is the most common, and we know that they are undoubtedly the best option.

But what When we do not, could it known in advance which organs are located in the area in which we pain ? Each pain is a different disease. Perhaps those of us who have not had a direct relationship with the area of science do not yet know the importance of the immune system in our what its function is and how we should enhance its ability to protect ourselves from the diseases that swarm around By destroying the pathogens found in the it defends us against autoimmune diseases such as allergies, others that are hereditary or congenital and benign, but Others such as cancer and AIDS are deadly and are Still being studied. Vitamins, along with proteins, fats, carbohydrates and minerals, are the natural anabolics that, through our diet, supply us with essential nutrients to maintain health and have normal development.

The natural Source to obtain vitamins is to have a balanced and complete diet, that is to say that it includes all the food groups of the pyramid, according to their meats and derivatives; fruits and vegetables; grains and cereals; and minerals.

But you should know that in the cases of people who do not have an optimal diet, either because they cannot include any food due to allergic causes, whose health status fluctuates constantly, those who have come out of surgery, or who simply use to skip the meals due to lack of appetite or other reason, they eat too many processed foods, those who make diets to lose weight, those who have the habit of smoking or drinking and even the elderly; they may be requiring the use of vitamin supplements. It is also important to note that throughout our lives, our body requires different levels of intake of certain nutrients.

For example, babies and children who are constantly growing need a nutrition high in calcium and vitamins A and D. In adolescence, it is sometimes used to neglect regular feeding for junk food because it is more appetizing which it can also bring nutritional deficiencies.

From maturity Our eating habits fluctuate for different reasons, and in Old age, Our begins to lose the ability to absorb certain nutrients. Recently, international organizations such as the World Health Organization and the FAO have evaluated the established maximum levels (or ULS) for iron, vitamin A and B12 and folates, due to the risk factors associated with their high intake. This is done in order to establish internationally regulated intake levels. This seeks to go beyond the "recommended daily intake" (RD], in its English acronym). And such is the importance that has been given to them, that it is suggested to consider them already food instead of drugs. Knowing more about the functions of each of the vitamins can help us to reduce, to a certain extent, our frequent visits to the doctor, by identifying, by our own symptoms, what vitamin deficiency we are having.

When diseases appear In the event that we suffer from leg cramps or experience heart problems, it could be that we have a lack of vitamin BI in Our diet. Alterations of the nervous system, dizziness and depression, reflect a lack of B2. Tooth bleeding and loss have been shown to depend on the consumption of vitamin C, not its consumption to prevent colds. Vitamin D deficiency manifests itself in rickets. And iron deficiency causes anemia, in women. For these reasons we must know that to include green and Yellow leafy vegetables, fruits, as well as liver, and cereals; they are the foods richest in these vitamins. If you are one of those who frequently neglect the nutritional value of what you put in Your mouth, you should consider talking to Your doctor including vitamin supplements in Your healthylife.

THOUSAND AND ONE DIETS

We hear them from everywhere, we read them from books and magazines, or at work, or Our friend tells us about them. But there is much that is ignored the expression: "This diet worked for me, I recommend it. " And it is that despite the fact that their origin is uncertain, we never hesitate to try them, unaware that many of these weight loss proposals do not follow the minimum guidelines of a balanced diet and are done Without medical Even in the worst of cases they can the trigger to fall into diseases as serious as bulimia and anorexia. Diets are voluntary weight loss They come in all colors, flavors and duration. There is no doubt that over the years they continue to be a necessary practice for many individuals who See in them a hope to regain their normal weight. We have surely heard of of their flashy names, such as the Atkins diet, the Scardale diet or the Montignac diet and the Barry Sears diet. All of them famous nutritionists who in recent years have revolutionized the eating habits of many in the World, including well-known celebrities.

There is also the office diet, that of artichokes, and so the list goes on until we find others as unlikely as the diet, based on the influence of the star on the liquids we ingest. The bad thing about diets While some allow some foods to be eaten, others prohibit Others that should not be eaten together. Some emphasize carbohydrate consumption; like greens, vegetables and fruits. Among these, the tomato soup diet, due to its few calories, with which you can lose up to seven kilos in a allowing you to eat brown rice and coffee. The Montignac diet against all carbohydrates such as rice, bread and Just as it prohibits eating fruits after meals. Other diets, such as the anti-diet, is one of the least recommended since avoiding the consumption of carbohydrates increases the level of uric acid and cholesterol.

On the contrary, others include the consumption of pure carbohydrates, such as honey, sugar and jams that provide us with calories that give us enough energy as in the sportsman's and psychological diets. In the case of fats, the only ones that are allowed is uncertain, we never hesitate to try them, unaware that many of these weight loss proposals do not follow the minimum guidelines of a balanced diet and are done without medical even in the worst of cases they can the trigger to fall into diseases as serious as bulimia and anorexia. Diets are voluntary weight loss They come in all colors, flavors and duration. There is no doubt that over the years they continue to be a necessary practice for many individuals who See in them a hope to regain their normal weight.

We have surely heard of of their flashy names, such as the Atkins diet, the Scardale diet or the Montignac diet and the Barry Sears diet. All of them famous nutritionists who in recent years have revolutionized the eating habits of many in the World, including well-known celebrities. There is also the office diet, that of artichokes, and so the list goes on until we find others as unlikely as the diet, based on the influence of the star on the liquids we ingest. The bad thing about diets While some allow some foods to be eaten, others prohibit others that should not be eaten together. Some emphasize carbohydrate consumption; like greens, vegetables and fruits. Among these, the tomato soup diet, due to its few calories, with which you can lose up to seven kilos in a allowing you to eat brown rice and coffee.

The Montignac diet is against all carbohydrates such as rice, bread and just as it prohibits eating fruits after meals. Other diets, such as the anti-diet, is one of the least recommended since avoiding the consumption of carbohydrates increases the level of uric acid and cholesterol. On the contrary, others include the consumption of pure carbohydrates, such as honey, sugar and jams that provide us with calories that give us enough energy as in the sportsman's and there are even psychological diets. In the case of fats, the only ones that are allowed to act on the or Vice versa; from body to mind.

On the Other hand, is a condition characterized by a great sensitivity of the nervous system with habitual sadness and constant and distressing concern for health. Bath descriptions bring us closer to what is known as biological medicine and chiropractic. Peelings, personality, and pain The flow of blood through the superficial capillaries of the skin is the most obvious reflection that emotions give us away.

The blush that forms on the face and neck is an effect of anxiety as the blood is driven to the skin or, suffering from high blood pressure is the aggravating State of this reaction When it is accompanied by physical and mental Stress. The case is paling, as the blood is propelled into the muscles. Insecurity or fear can leave us in evidence in many moments of life. Poor circulation in the hands can also cause the nerve spasms of the so called "Cold hands and feet." For this, recommend unmasking yourself by saying what you are really trying to hide, for example in a meeting or before a love date, then just take a deep breath and relax.

In the case of low back pain, the lower back is Said to be caused by living an overloaded life by trying to be too responsible. Balancing activities in a rational way and taking a break from a diet high in calcium and iron can solve this. Speeding up in what is Said and thought brings contradictions to Taking a break and listening is the way to prevent Your tongue, probably badly washed, from choking. Finally we can find a urological condition, which is related to safety during sexual intercourse with the partner. According to the tension experienced causes a to acquire infection on the vaginal tissue in women and in the urethra in m en.

"GREAT NUTRITIONISTS of YESTERDAY AND TODAY "

They are men and women from the area of medicine and science who have discovered and tested theories valuable for the betterment of human life through scheduled consumption of each nutrient group We could find a list of hundreds of nutritionists from all over the World who bring their knowledge and conclusions in the field of human nutrition to the public light. However, few names are collected from the various currents and trends that have saturated the media, the comments and the critics with their spirited and durable international diffusion.

In my vast experience as a reader and follower of these books and articles published from various sources; which, although at times they may seem to some like "cheap lies", can now be more than by professional medical teams and in the field through the incredible rejuvenated faces of those who practice them. They warn and we must know each of us can Our own judges when it comes to eating. Facing the risks and combining the new discoveries of World science with a conscientious responsibility to control ourselves could add or take years from our own life expectancy. In this article we have chosen three of the most popular diet proposals of the last 45 years to highlight the good and not so good news they brought us.

1970: Atkins LOW Carb' Concept Appears

After on the television show "Tonight Show and subsequently in the women's magazine "Vouge," the diet regimen of New York-based cardiologist Robert Atkins began to welcome famous. Inspired by his own episode of already overcome by medical advice with the elimination of sugars from his diet, the doctor started a revolution in American nutrition. His successes at that time were to control with his suggested food menus, the amount of carbohydrates in the diet of the with this, it eliminated many fruits and vegetables, which had the disadvantage of eliminating according to its critics. The Worst of Atkins' advice, and which was discovered much later by doctors, is that the intake of saturated fat was ignored, which years later came to endanger the health of the nutritionist himself. with the diagnosis of heart problems and subsequent strikes overcome, a blow on a Winter ice walk took his life at the age of 72.

1995: Staying in the Sears Zone Some time later, a Young and academically prepared competitor to patent blood tests that showed that his patients were staying within the recommended level coming from that wave of products that characterized a "new age lifestyle in those decades, biochemist Barry Sears created his "The Zone" diet which to achieve healthy sugar levels, hormonal balance, lower inflammation and maintain a range of good health. But, as he confessed, ghosts around Barry would inspire him to devise this diet to overcome his fear of dying Young like most of his family [n its time this diet was very famous among entertainment stars in the United States. Among the nutrients Sears has set out to promote are Omega 3 Oil capsules and low-cholesterol lipids from foods.

2012: A coach suggesting their OMG to teens In recent years you can Still hear a new initiative originated in the UK by a trainer with experience in Young people, who recommends an intense 6-week plan. Her pseudonym is Venice Fulton. Its acronym comes from the English phrase "Oh, my God" , and it is number one as a reference work since after the self-publication of the e-book "6 weeks to Oh, my God, you get to be the slimmest of Your friends! " unseat a diet they called Dukan, which we will talk about another time. The good thing is that the plan is ordered to achieve weight loss in that period of time, after that the patients Will already be hungry enough not to fall ill. It is based on fasting with physical exercise routines that can be strenuous, eliminates some vegetables that have antioxidants from its list and recommends eating Others. And curiously, he urges you to bathe with Cold water, to keep Your temperature metabolically stable such fasts.

2013 : An American actress in nutrition and a arrives on television While science and technology continue to evolve, a charismatic doctor bursts in from hospitals with a television that brought the simple talk from the office to the patient to a mass audience Where the use of dynamics and experiments has clarified some of the most doubts. Common to specific diseases. His name is Dr. Oz and his program transmitted from a North American television network has led him to translated into Other languages and reach a huge audience. Another of the stars of the media is the American comedy actress Cameron Diaz who, together with her team of collaborators, has published two books, "The Body Book" and "The longevity book" in which it exposes its secrets to its readers to preserve their health, their beauty and to be successful on the cinema screen through an entertaining essay. What you liked best about the they may be that it does not a time frame to achieve the goals of the plan. According to the book's preface, it was written strictly to share her formula for becoming a happier, healthier, and stronger woman with a guide with embarrassing answers for girls, based on science and inspired by her own personal experience. which became number one in sales among the New York Times

CHAPTER 8 PROTOCOL & LABEL

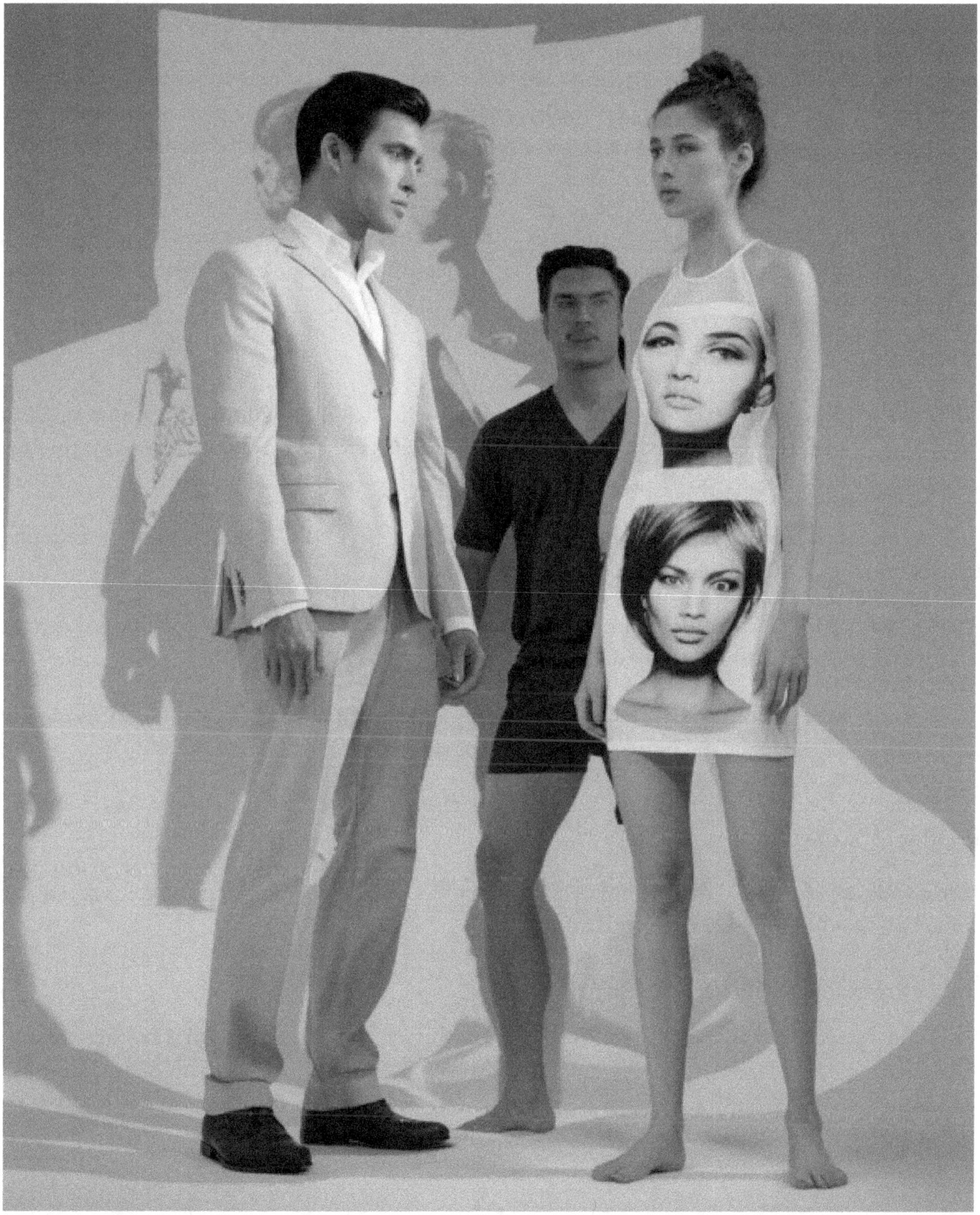

CRACKING THE PERSONAL IMAGE CODE

Personal image is the hallmark that defines us to the world, a combination of physical, tangible, and intangible elements that reflect our personality, lifestyle, and values. It is the perception others have of us, based on what they see, hear, and perceive from our verbal and nonverbal communication.

In the world of modeling, personal image plays a crucial role. Physical beauty is undoubtedly an important factor, but it is not the only one. A successful model must possess a comprehensive image that combines harmonious physical attributes with a captivating personality, self-confidence, and a positive attitude.

Building a Solid Personal Image

Building a solid personal image does not happen overnight. It is an ongoing process that requires dedication, effort, and a constant search for self-knowledge. Below, I share some key tips for cultivating an attractive personal image that's consistent with your professional goals:

* Get to know your body and face thoroughly:** Discover your best angles, your most flattering features, and the clothes that highlight your figure.

* Define your personal style:** Experiment with different looks and trends until you find a style that makes you feel comfortable and confident.

* Take care of your health and well-being:** A balanced diet, regular exercise, and plenty of rest are essential to looking radiant and projecting an image of vitality.

* Cultivate an attractive personality:** Develop social skills, such as effective communication, empathy, and active listening.

* Boost your self-esteem:** Trust in your abilities, strengths, and skills. Accepting and valuing yourself is essential to projecting a confident and positive image.

Professional Projection: Your Passport to Success

Professional projection is the ability to effectively communicate your skills, experience, and values to potential clients, employers, or collaborators. It's how you present yourself to the professional world and leave a memorable impression.

In the competitive world of modeling, social media, and entertainment, professional exposure is essential to opening doors to new opportunities and achieving the success you desire. Below, I share some key tips for developing an effective professional exposure:

* Define your professional goals:** Set clear and precise goals about what you want to achieve in your career.

* Develop your professional skills:** Take courses, workshops, or participate in activities that allow you to strengthen your skills in the areas that interest you.

* Create a solid portfolio:** Gather your best work, photographs, or projects in a portfolio that reflects your talent and experience.

* Build a network of contacts:** Attend events, join professional groups, or use online platforms to connect with relevant people in your industry.

* Develop a personal brand:** Create a coherent professional image on your social media, website, and presentation materials.

* Take care of your verbal and nonverbal communication:** Project confidence, enthusiasm, and professionalism in your interactions with others.

Personal Image and Professional Projection: A Winning Combination

The combination of an attractive personal image and effective professional projection is the formula for success in modeling, social communication, and entertainment. Remember that your personal image is a reflection of your inner self, so cultivating an image consistent with your values and professional goals will allow you to achieve your goals in an authentic and memorable way.

Dare to shine with your own light! Cultivate a solid personal image, develop effective professional projection, and achieve your dreams in the exciting world of modeling, social communication, and entertainment.

SELF-CONFIDENCE IN PERSONAL SUCCESS

** Self-Confidence: The Fundamental Pillar of Personal and Professional Success

In the intricate world of psychology and motivation, **self-confidence** emerges as a beacon that guides people toward achieving their goals and personal fulfillment. More than just an attitude, self-confidence is defined as the belief in one's own abilities and skills to face life's challenges. It is the cornerstone upon which strong relationships are built, sound decisions are made, and success is pursued with determination.

Why is self-confidence so important?

Self-confidence plays a fundamental role in various aspects of life, from personal to professional. Below, we explore some of the reasons why it is so crucial:

1. Impact on Decision-Making:

People with high self-confidence are able to make decisions with greater confidence and assertiveness. They trust their judgment and don't let fear of failure or uncertainty paralyze them. This allows them to explore new opportunities, take calculated risks, and pursue their goals with determination.

2. Improved Performance:

Self-confidence has a direct impact on **performance** in various fields. In academia, students with high self-confidence tend to perform better, as they are not intimidated by challenges and believe in their ability to learn and overcome obstacles. In the workplace, employees with high self-confidence are more likely to take initiative, assume responsibilities, and excel at their tasks.

3. Strong Interpersonal Relationships:**

Self-confidence also plays a crucial role in building **strong interpersonal relationships**. People with high self-confidence express themselves clearly, defend their ideas respectfully, and set healthy boundaries. Additionally, they are more likely to be empathetic, understanding, and supportive of others. **4. Emotional Well-being:**

Self-confidence is closely linked to **emotional well-being**. People with high self-confidence experience less anxiety, stress, and depression. They feel self-assured and are less susceptible to external criticism. This allows them to face life's challenges with greater resilience and optimism.

5. Goal Achievement:**

Without a doubt, self-confidence is an **essential ingredient for goal achievement**. People who believe in themselves are more likely to set ambitious goals, develop action plans, and persevere in the face of difficulties. Their belief in their abilities allows them to overcome obstacles and achieve their dreams.

How to develop and strengthen self-confidence?**

Although self-confidence can be influenced by genetic factors and early experiences, it is possible to develop and strengthen it throughout life. Below are some strategies to achieve this:

1. Recognize Past Achievements:

Making a list of past accomplishments, no matter how small they may seem, can be a powerful exercise in strengthening self-confidence. Recalling experiences where you have triumphed, even in the face of challenges, can reinforce your belief in your own abilities.

2. Set Realistic Goals:

Setting achievable goals and consistently working toward them is an effective way to build self-confidence. Gradual success in achieving goals reinforces belief in your own abilities and motivates you to keep going.

3. Accept and Learn from Failures:**

Mistakes are an inevitable part of learning and personal growth. Instead of avoiding or denying them, it is important to **accept them as opportunities to learn and improve**. The ability to face failures with resilience and learn from them strengthens long-term self-confidence.

4. Mind Your Inner Language:**

Internal dialogue plays a fundamental role in building self-confidence. It is important to maintain a **positive and constructive dialogue**. Avoiding excessive self-criticism and focusing on the positive aspects of oneself fosters a more favorable self-image.

5. Practice Self-Expression:**

Speaking clearly and assertively is a way to express self-confidence. Defending ideas and opinions respectfully, even in the face of dissent, strengthens self-confidence and the ability to relate to others effectively.

6. Accept New Challenges:**

Getting out of your comfort zone and **accepting new challenges** is a way to test and strengthen your self-confidence. Overcoming obstacles and achieving goals in new areas reinforces your belief in your productive abilities and increases your motivation to respond to criticism from others and your self-esteem.

SELF-ESTEEM DYSMORPHIC DISORDERS

Facing Body Image Distortion

In the complex framework of mental health, body dysmorphic disorders (BDD) emerge as a condition that distorts the perception of one's body image, generating profound emotional and behavioral discomfort. Unlike eating disorders, where the concern centers on body weight or shape, BDD focuses on perceived defects, often minimal or nonexistent, which generate intense self-criticism and social isolation.

** Delving into Perceptual Distortion

Individuals with BDD experience an obsession with their physical appearance, convinced they have defects that make them unattractive or even deformed. This self-image distortion can manifest itself in various ways:

* Excessive concern with specific details:** A mole, facial asymmetry, a scar, or even the texture of their skin can become the focus of their attention, generating constant mental rumination about their appearance.

* Degeneration of minor defects:** A slightly asymmetrical facial feature, a temporary pimple, or a small skin blemish may be perceived as significant deformities, generating intense distress.

* Constant comparisons:** The person tirelessly compares themselves with others, seeking to reaffirm their negative self-perception, intensifying their emotional distress.

* Compulsive behaviors:** To avoid social exposure or camouflage their perceived defects, they may resort to behaviors such as:

* Avoiding mirrors or photos:** Confronting their reflected image can generate anxiety and discomfort.

* Excessive use of makeup or baggy clothing:** They attempt to hide perceived defects, affecting their personal style and comfort.

* Seeking unnecessary cosmetic procedures:** They seek to modify their physical appearance to fit their distorted image, without obtaining lasting satisfaction.

* Social isolation:** They avoid social events or gatherings for fear of being judged on their appearance.

** Emotional and Behavioral Consequences

ADD has a devastating impact on the lives of those who suffer from it, significantly affecting their emotional and behavioral well-being:

* Low Self-Esteem:** Constant self-criticism and negative self-perception significantly deteriorate their self-esteem, generating feelings of shame, humiliation, and inferiority.

* Anxiety and Depression:** Constant concern about one's physical appearance and fear of social rejection can trigger anxiety and depression, affecting their quality of life.

* Eating Disorders:** In some cases, an obsession with body image can lead to eating disorders such as anorexia or bulimia, as a mechanism to control their appearance.

* Social Isolation:** Fear of judgment and shame lead them to avoid social situations, limiting their interpersonal relationships and opportunities for personal development.

* Suicidal Ideation:** In severe cases, profound desolation and feelings of unworthiness can lead to suicidal ideation.

** Finding the Path to Recovery

Despite the challenges, ADHD is manageable with the right treatment. Psychotherapy, particularly cognitive-behavioral therapy (CBT), has been shown to be an effective tool in helping people with ADHD:

* Identify and challenge cognitive distortions:** Learn to recognize and question negative and distorted thoughts about their appearance.

* Develop a more realistic body image:** Work on accepting and appreciating their body, recognizing its beauty and intrinsic value.

* Reduce anxiety and improve mood:** Implement relaxation techniques and strategies to cope with anxiety and improve their emotional state.

* Develop social skills:** Increase their interpersonal confidence and improve their skills in relating to others.

* Promote a healthy lifestyle:** Adopt healthy habits such as a balanced diet, regular exercise, and adequate rest.

In some cases, medication can be a useful complement to therapy, especially to manage symptoms of anxiety or depression. Family and social support also play a crucial role in the recovery process, providing understanding, empathy, and encouragement.

** A Message of Hope

If you or someone you know is experiencing the symptoms of ADHD, it is important to remember that you are not alone. With the right professional help and the support of loved ones, it is possible to overcome these difficulties and build a full and meaningful life.

* Beauty lies in diversity and individuality.

GESTURE LANGUAGE AND HUMAN RELATIONS

Key to deciphering human relationships and personal motivation

Beyond words, there is a universe of nonverbal communication that shapes our interactions and defines much of our human experience. Body language, that silent dance of gestures, facial expressions, and body postures, plays a fundamental role in psychology and personal motivation, revealing hidden aspects of our emotions, intentions, and motivations.

Decoding Emotions Through Gestures:

Gestures are windows to the soul, revealing emotions that words sometimes fail to express. A furtive wink can indicate attraction, while crossed arms can reflect distrust or discomfort. Science has extensively studied body language, identifying patterns that allow us to decipher the emotions of others.

* Microexpressions:** Small, fleeting facial movements that last less than a second, revealing emotions such as happiness, sadness, anger, or fear.

* Macroexpressions:** Longer-lasting and recognizable facial expressions, such as a

A genuine smile or a frown.

* **Body Postures:** The way we sit, stand, or walk also conveys information about our emotional state. A slouched posture can indicate shyness or discouragement, while an upright posture with shoulders back reflects confidence and security.

The Influence of Body Language on Human Relationships:

Body language not only allows us to understand the emotions of others, but also influences how they perceive us and the dynamics of our relationships. A study from the University of Glasgow revealed that people who use more open and expansive gestures are perceived as more outgoing, pleasant, and trustworthy.

* Empathy and Rapport:** The ability to interpret and respond to the body language of others allows us to establish a deeper emotional connection, generating empathy and rapport.

* Negotiation and Persuasion:** The effective use of body language can be a powerful tool in negotiation and persuasion. A firm handshake conveys confidence, while direct eye contact demonstrates interest and attention.

* Attraction and Flirting:** Body language also plays a crucial role in attraction and flirting. A light touch on the arm or a flirtatious smile can spark the other person's interest.

Body Language as a Personal Motivation Tool:

Beyond deciphering emotions and relationships, body language can also be a powerful tool for personal motivation. Studies have shown that adopting power poses, such as standing with your shoulders back and hands on your hips, can increase testosterone levels and feelings of confidence.

* Fake It Till You Make It:** The idea of "fake it till you make it" has a scientific basis in body language. Adopting postures and facial expressions associated with confidence and determination can influence our own self-perception, prompting us to act with greater confidence and determination.

* Visualization and Self-Affirmation:** Visualization and self-affirmation, popular techniques for improving motivation, are based on the power of body language. By imagining and verbalizing our goals with congruent gestures and facial expressions, we increase the likelihood of achieving them.

In Conclusion: Body language is an essential component of human communication, revealing emotions, intentions, and motivations that words sometimes fail to express. Understanding and using body language effectively allows us to improve our interpersonal relationships, increase our self-confidence, and achieve our goals with greater motivation. By deciphering the body language of others and consciously using our own gestures, we can open up a world of possibilities in the fields of psychology and personal motivation.

PROTOCOL AND CEREMONIAL

Problems of this nature affected the European Courts until they were resolved in the Congress of Vienna (1815), the Congress of Aachen (1818) and, in more recent times, in the meetings that took place in Vienna to draft a Convention Diplomatic Relations in 1961. As a result of these meetings, diplomats were divided into three classes:

- Ambassadors, legates and papal nuncios who are accredited to the heads of state;

- Envoys , ministers and other persons accredited to the heads of Attachés accredited to the ministers of foreign affairs.

Precedence among foreign representatives in a capital is currently governed by age. The oldest person in the diplomatic corps is dean, who as a rule represents the entire diplomatic corps in ceremonies and in matters of diplomatic privileges and immunities. The most concise summary of diplomatic protocols is the Vienna Convention on Diplomatic Relations, which consists of 5 3 articles drafted under the auspices of the ONU.

ORIGIN OF THE SOCIAL LABEL

It is a term that arose as the thinking man was leaving his barbaric attitudes to assume through the centuries the civilized culture that left the battles in cold blood, to assume customs in the manners to be used, hunting activities and clothing appropriately when everybody is stirring on you. Etiquette can be exercised as a social instrument. The external adoption of the superficial gestures of a group in which, for the sake of general social advancement a concern for others, is considered by many a form of snobbery, lacking in virtue.

The earliest indications of what would later become a label date from the 3rd century BC. when Ptahhotep wrote his famous Maxims, which were precepts that enhanced civil virtues such as truthfulness, self-control and goodness, where he taught that greed is the basis of all evil and the search for justice was emphasized. In China it was Confucius who, with his works, introduced personal and governmental morality with his philosophy.

The Renaissance was an immense cultural flowering. The textile industry was strongly linked to the bourgeoisie, so, from that moment there was an exclusive fashion for the middle classes. The handkerchief was the object that delimited the social classes of the time. The only sector that could use it by law was the nobility. It was from the 16th to the 20th centuries that some norms or criterion of conduct converged from various parts of Europe that delimited the expectations so that social behavior within each group remains within the conventions regularly accepted within a society, class or group.

Fashion began to acquire greater importance, and became a concern of the wealthy bourgeoisie. The garments began to be seen as an investment, some time was devoted to their maintenance and repair. The use of shirt, doublet and jerkin, by men, and the use of dresses or skirts, by women, a constant until the seventeenth century. Fashion began at this time as clothing loses its universal character and each nation wanted to differentiate itself from the rest, so unique and different details were devised, at the same time that clothing the symbol of wealth and The clothes of this era can characterized under the influence of countries such as France, Italy, Spain and England. It is what is known as a label, which is a term of English Origin that dates back to the fact that across its it was assumed and modified in France with the meaning of "label" and from there it was probably transmitted to the rest of Europe Louis XIV (1638-1718) transformed a royal hunting house in Versailles, a town 25 km southwest of the capital, into one of the largest palaces in the world, officially moving his court and government in 1682. It was in this imposing context in which Luis tamed the nobility and foreign dignitaries impressed, with entertainment, ceremony and a highly codified system of etiquette, affirming his supremacy.

Centuries later in the age of the Enlightenment with the formation of Cavalry Clubs, gentlemen seeking to be identified as middle class in the midst of the bourgeoisie adopted artistic preferences and standards of behavior. It was in this century when the strictest standards of modesty were established among women, such as when to show emotion, maintain posture, and how to act courteously.

Other philosophers such as Lord Shaftesbury encouraged the use of courtesy as the art of being pleasant in Company. Thus, the "etiquette" model was formed from concepts, such as courtesy, civility, manners, and education, which were openly manifested in good social customs such as clubs, meeting for conversation, tea, and level assemblies. of government.

It was Philip Stanhope, 4th Earl of Chesterfield who first used the word "etiquette" in its modern sense, from letters to his Son in the art of becoming a man of the world and a gentleman. This work made up of more than 400 letters written from 173 7 or 1738 and continuing until the death of his son in 1768, mostly they were instructive letters on various subjects. The letters were first published by his son's widow Eugenia Stanhope in 17 74. Chesterfield tried to disassociate the subject of mores from conventional morality, arguing that mastery of etiquette was an important weapon for social progress. The letters were full of wisdom and elegant perceptual observation and deduction. Chesterfield personified the restraint of 18th century good society, writing, for example, in 1748:

While the Victorian era began in England in 1837 when a revolution finally consolidated disputed economic, social and religious dilemmas; in France one of the most important economic movements in history flourished with its "Belle Epoque" that would later influence European modernism. This marked the beginning of many precepts that we adopted in America more than a century later that included the refined customs of civilized culture that Still persist in postmodernism today. In Victorian times, etiquette had become an exceptionally complicated system of rules that governs everything, such as the proper method of writing letters and using silverware; the closely regulated interactions between different classes and gender.

Among the authors who have studied this period in depth, we Can mention the book The Process of Civilization by Norbert Elias, who argued that manners arose as a product of group life and persist as a way of maintaining social harder. He theorized that manners proliferated beginning in the Renaissance in response to the development of the "absolute state" the progression from a small group living to the centralization of power by the state. Elijah believes that the rituals with manners in the Court Society of England were closely linked to social status. For him, manners demonstrate an individual's position within a social network and act as a means by which the individual can negotiate that position.

This is how according to Curtis, three categories of manners are Specifically denoted; hygiene, courtesy, and cultural norms, each of which help explain the multifaceted role manners play in society. These categories are based on outcome rather than motivation, On individualized manners and behaviors and can fit into 2 or more categories.

• Hygiene manners: these are manners that affect the transmission of diseases. They are likely to be taught at an early age, primarily through parental discipline, adherence to positive around continence with bodily fluids (such as toilet training), and avoiding or eliminating the elements. that pose a risk of illness to children. It is expected that, in adulthood, hygiene manners are so ingrained with one's own behavior; they second nature. Violations are prone to elicit upset responses.

• Polite manners: demonstrate the ability to put the interests Of Others before Your own. They help maximize the benefits Of group life by regulating social interaction. The conduct of avoiding illness can sometimes be compromised in the observance of courtesy manners. They can be taught in the same way as hygiene customs, but they are likely also learned With direct (that is, observing the interactions of others), indirect (that is, through the functions of the brain The learning of manners of courtesy can take place at an older age than hygiene manners, since individuals must have at least some means of communication and some self-awareness and social positioning, violation of polite customs most often leads to social disapproval.

• Manners of cultural norms: usually demonstrate identity within a socio-cultural group. Adherence to cultural norm customs allows the demarcation of sociocultural identities and the creation of borders that inform that it is trustworthy or that it Will be considered as others. The manners of cultural norms are learned through the daily life and routinization of the "family and through exposure to others. Cultural norms, by their very nature, have a high level of variability groups, but are likely to common to all who identify with a group identity.

SOCIAL AND BUSINESS LABEL

In trying to recognize current trends in the use of rules of etiquette for the workplace and social events, there is to some a set of rules, which, although they are not definitive or the same in all parts of the world, have marked a milestone in World and emerged from the end of the last century, and remain during the nineteenth century.

Many of these norms are already known to us because we have adapted to the customs considered and we have molded ourselves within a standard been modified by clothing accessories that we cannot assure that they change or imitate the fundamentals of style when dressing that is used. has or is obliged to be used by all of us to establish a link of group membership.

For the purposes of study in this aesthetics manual, have consider clothing, clothing, footwear, folkloric or ethnic dresses and other clothing accessories as part of the etiquette of a social group. sociology, which is the science that studies development and social function, leaves the study of human beings in charge of anthropology from a biological, and humanistic perspective. It is divided into two broad fields: physical anthropology, which deals with the biological evolution and physiological adaptation of human beings, and social or cultural anthropology, which deals with the ways in which people live in society, that is, the forms of evolution of their language, culture and customs. That is why anthropology is fundamentally multicultural.

Leaving the natural and aromatic dyes of some primitive and indigenous cultures, which from New Zealand to ancient Egypt used to decorate the body, has been attributed magical Powers against the enemy, or protecting themselves from high temperatures, are the first historical indications of the use of makeup in the actuality. The cultures of the Mediterranean adopted them from the Hebrew culture, which passed to the Roman one and spread throughout the European colonies.

More recently, in full modernism we find two pioneering women in cosmetology and fashion design. One of them is Arden, who was born in 1884, and was a renowned American beautician and cosmetic manufacturer of Canadian origin, Her deep interest in chemistry and her nursing knowledge her to bring a scientific approach to the cosmetics industry. One of his maxims was: "Beauty must combine nature and science " She was a brilliant salesperson who knew how to create her own feminine makeup products and improve those already on the market, adding more Pleasant fragrances. In 1910 he opened his own beauty salon on New York's prestigious Fifth Avenue, the painted front door of which would became a famous Company hallmark. A short time later, he opened his second salon in Washington, DC. Between 1915 and 1920, he brought more cosmetic formulas to the market than any other manufacturer. By 1929 his company, which already had salons in London and Paris, was making a gross profit of $ 40 million a year, through direct sales or by mail order.

He created the notion of "color harmony" by suggesting that women could choose makeup according to what they were wearing rather than according to the color of their skin. In the 1930s he opened the first nursing homes dedicated to beauty and health, and extended his industry to the perfumery sector. His first fragrance was called Blue Grass.

The other of the forerunners of the great international fashion houses is Coco Chanel. She was a French designer who died in 1971 and was turned into a myth thanks to her distant and enigmatic personality. He knew how to impose a timeless Style regardless of all fashions. The famous suit that bears his name remains a symbol of elegance.

In the immediate aftermath of the war, Chanel gradually began to Create one of the most important couture houses of the time. Her male relationships often provide her with inspiration, thus creating, for example, costumes with Slavic motifs during the time that she frequented Grand Duke Dimitri, cousin of the last Russian Tsar. Later, he adopts elements of the clothing of the Duke of Westminster, a man reputed to be the richest in England, such as the Wool sweater, the fur coat, the sailor beret or the tweed vest to adapt them to female clothing, giving them a modern and dynamic touch, combining comfort and elegance. Chanel became one of the first Women to launch the fashion for short hair, resolutely opposing the Sophistication advocated by the couturier Paul Poiret who accused her of wanting to transform women into "undernourished Little telegraphers".

It encourages a carefully studied simplicity with practical suits, such as the first trousers, the short pleated skirt, the jacket suit with pockets and the famous black short dress (color until then reserved exclusively for mourning): a fitted garment, without collar, with sleeves long and without cuffs, in Crepe de chine according to the masculine style to use. Called "a Ford signed Chanel" by Vogue magazine, this suit was copied countless times and would Soon became a women's fashion classic.

Rejecting the qualification of poor gender, with which her creations were often Chanel knew how to distinguish sobriety from poverty: women's clothing must be simple but, in return, it must be accompanied by the appropriate accessories. For this she resorts, for example, to costume jewelery, mixing semiprecious stones, rhinestones and fake pearls, bracelets with the motif of the Maltese cross, Byzantine inspired or animal, floral or shell motifs. The creation of these accessories was directed by Étienne de Beaumont, Paul Iribe and above all, 1929 and 1937, by Fulco di Verdura, who knew how to bring an identity of his own to Chanel jewelry.

DRESSING: FROM THE INFORMAL TO THE FORMAL

In the business world, the customs of good dress are more demanding, the etiquette within a company is the set of written and unwritten rules of conduct that make social interactions work sticking to foreign etiquette is an important complement to culture shock, providing an interesting market for company manuals. Other resources include business and diplomacy institutions, which are only available in some countries such as the UK. As for the job search stage, these rules often resonated throughout an industry or economy. For example, 49% of recruiters surveyed in 2005 by the American National Association of Colleges and Recruiters observed that nontraditional attire would a major influence in considering a potential candidate for the position. The particular office etiquette applies to a working group of interaction, excluding interactions with external contacts, such as Customers and suppliers. When conducting group meetings in the United States, the assembly could follow Roberts Rules of Order, if there are no Other Company policies for the control of a meeting. In 2011 a group of etiquette and an international business group formed a nonprofit organization lead to help the human resources (HR) of multinationals in the to measure the etiquette skills of potential employees, it was done during the process through image standardization and label examination, similar to what ISO does for industrial process measurements.

The rules of labor, social and daily etiquette when it comes to dressing apply in a similar way for both ladies and gentlemen, however to distinguish the informal, semi-informal Style and the completely formal Style, its scope of use in events, colors of most accepted use according to complexion, Shapes according to body height and when to wear accessories or not; are compiled below exclusively.

• Informal Style: It is the way that each of us have to express our personal taste through the meticulous selection of each garment, it means comfort and freedom, but it also has its limits in terms of the texture of the fabrics colors and cove e. of the extremities.

That is, we can group "informality" as a style that does not keep the rules of decency, seriousness and punctuality such as sport style, clothes to be at home, and summer. When dressing to attend events, vacation or beach walks, only in this style white, cream and colors so striking even neon are allowed examples of types of casual clothing in women are sleeveless blouses, T -Shirts, miniskirts, shorts and dresses with a simple cut at the that are accompanied by slippers or flipflops, sneakers or tennis Shoes with always low soles, sandals and hats or summer hats. In the case of men's casual clothing, we mention t shirts, shorts, sports or mid-calf pants for camping or outdoor activities, these outfits can be accompanied by hats, glasses and slippers or flip-flops, sneakers or tennis shoes. Here the very tight and loose converge to convey comfort when dressing. Full swimsuits, men or women's thongs are also considered informal. Wearing tattoos uncovered, the use of piercings, earrings and woven Or leather bracelets are also considered informal that denote artistic expression of ones own personality and should be covered by makeup or clothes with long sleeves and long hems in case of dressing more formally.

• Casual or Semi-formal Style: It is a Style that moves away from the breakdown of the informal and approaches a little to the moderation of formality without going to the extreme, which as a general rule assumes the use of jackets, vests, bodices , jerkins and jacos. Clothing that is too baggy and tight should avoided, as is the Case with the formal Style. a system for manufacturing and selling fashion made in series, with vario us stipulated sizes. It is a French expression that means "ready to wear', often used in opposition to the classic haut couture or haute couture fashion system, where each garment was custom-sewn in the workshop itself. In fact, ready-to-wear meant the full incorporation of industrial design into the world of fashion, where it introduced or reinforced concepts such as the economy of production, functionality or consumption. The term had its origin in the textile industry of Great Britain and the United States (where the English equivalent ready to wear was used), but it was in France, around 19 5 0, where the concept was incorporated, in the postwar period, to the culture quality fashion.

Also, depending on the Weather season and severity of the event; clothing accessories are added such as the use of hats with a short or medium brim, berets, only those in bright or warm colors, or pastel tones and printed motifs, but never white. Without even including the rigor of top type hats, high heels or complex feminine hairstyles.

In men, this character describes the use of long sleeved shirts without pastel colored designs, fumes, trench coats, leather jackets and vests combined with classic style shoes without laces or brown ankle boots, socks in the color of the pants that can be caky, gray or black with some pleats at the hip. The types of pants that mark the semi formality are the long ones, or shorts to the mid-calf or at the knee, they can be jeans of any color or of the folded type of fabric. On the other hand, women who dress in a casual or semi- formal Style wear blouses with half sleeves or long ones buttoned at the wrist or free.

The color options are broader for the female sex, always applying a rule of contrast between warm tones with another ocher or dark color, never combine two striking tones, or two types of prints. As for footwear, sandals and medium heeled shoes are allowed, never low soled, open or with bare toes. Flannel or coats are regularly paired with semiformal shirts. There is no definitive rule regarding accessories such as handbags, scarves, jewelry or watches since certain freedom of combinations is allowed, a situation that does not occur with formal etiquette_ The ethnic, typical or folkloric dresses of each country can also be included in this group, taking into account the solemnity of the events or celebrations that are commemorated annually and are specific to each culture.

• Formal or dress Style: Although we are not supporters of capitalist doctrines, we must recognize the rigor of quality and Price in the selection of formal clothes to wear formally when attending events of great social lineage that is limited to urbanized areas. As jackets and pants, the type of linen, and silk fabrics are distinguished from synthetic fabric garments that, although they may be cheaper, are also more uncomfortable. Navy blue Or dark gray suits or suits are recommended, which are formal tones that translate into formality.

The black tuxedo must be impeccable without fabric lint from wear or fading, it is not recommended to use coffee as it is considered to transmit. The cut is generally always straight, classic type, without pleats. The shirt is generally white with long as it is considered that it gives more light to the whole and transmits neatness, with the exception of the vertical stripes. The tie should always be chosen from tones, avoiding the informality of combining them with elaborate figures Or scribbles denote a complicated and untidy personality, while logos or cartoons in an area that does not correspond or is unrelated to the event should be avoided to some degree of habit- The color code On ties exists and Can summarized as follows: Formal shades are blue, gray or Silver and pastel Shades. of the pastel shades, Pink and lilac or violet are the least popular for projecting naivety and exaggerated candor. Red projects action or aggressiveness so it tends to be very striking. While gold transmits monetary interest Vertical lines are recommended for people of short stature, while checkered patterns or horizontal lines are recommended for thin people as a general rule.

Finally, in the gentlemen who dress formal, accessories or accessories are added such as leather briefcases that are accepted in the executive field where it is recommended to maintain order and neatness in the presentation of documents such as the resume. The capes or raincoats are a winter complement in countries with temperate climates together with high boots that are also used by women, as well as gloves. Women's suits should be "haute couture", or haut Couture encompassing clothing from exclusive collections, made by individual designers for a Small and wealthy clientele, such as clothing from international brand Stores. The main fashion houses in Paris are Dior and Chanel. Spain Balenciaga, Paco Rabanne, Adolfo Domínguez and Vittorio & Lucchino, among others. In Britain the most important haute couture houses are Norman Hartnell, Hardy Amies and Belville Sassoon, all famous for dressing the royal family.

In Italy, Giorgio Armani, Gianni Versace and Romeo Gigli stand out. Other famous companies distribute high quality lingerie and perfumery to large stores. Evening or gala dresses are the ideal pattern for the woman who dresses formal where the fit of the figure and the length to the ankles, as well as the neckline with or without sleeves are the Style established in the current era without extreme changes that have accepted. Delicate and high-gloss fabrics such as Organza, satin and others are exclusively for women at all levels of formality. High-heeled shoes and elaborate, carefully styled headdresses are the other characteristics of this style. This is the appropriate dress style to keep the level of solemnity high, such as weddings, government events, corporate job rank such as partnerships, corporations and senior management. Perfumes are also another of the aesthetic senses that are capable of creating a good impression in our social relationships, which is why, due to their high commercial value, good hygiene practices are considered part, although it is suggested to use it moderately since exaggerating gives the impression that something is being hidden.

In business environments, male or female formal dress uniforms are the characteristic clothing of members of commercial, government, military and other services that distinguish them from civilians and other groups. Although soldiers, nurses and doctors have always worn specific clothing, including protective armor, the military uniform did not begin to evolve into the form in which it is known today until the second half of the 17th century. In the past, Some military units, notably palace guards and royal personal escorts, wore uniformly patterned clothing, although most soldiers fought in a motley assortment of civilian garb. Other professions that use them a Iot are in the tourist field such as waiters, hostesses, aviation. In recent years we See how the private services of sea or marine vessels have also adopted their own dress in contrast to those belonging to government offices. There are cases where the amount of clothing is almost Zero, such as dancers in nightclubs or table dancers, etc.

Business etiquette can vary considerably depending on the country, which is invariably related to its culture. For example: A notable difference China and the West in business etiquette is the avoidance of conflicts between partners. Chinese companies prefer to look to the management of relationships to avoid conflicts, while the West leaves the resolution of conflicts to the interpretation of the law through contracts and lawyers.

CUSTOMS AT CULTURAL LEVEL

On this side of the planet we are governed by the Christian or Western tradition that was conceived in past centuries until it was preserved, expanded and by subtle differences between each region or country but from the same Latin root. However, in other ancient cultures the rituals of ceremony and even the simple act of having dinner or receiving the New Year, entail rules of behavior that must be applied even being foreigners in an unknown Land, in order to keep and values strict social fundamentals. Other times the traditions of other nearby cultures mix with those of the East, resulting in later events. For example, lees compare the different rites and social events of religious intimacy that are practiced in different continents, such as births, baptisms, weddings and funerals where folk or ethnic dresses are used and not Western dress, among other characteristics. Some of these continents Or regions are: Asia, the Middle East, Oceania and Europe.

Luck and future destiny have always been a constant concern in the mind of man throughout history, to the point of causing fear in the face of the expectation about the future in terms of prosperity and health, always produced by the trend. to believe in God or before the threat of the supreme gods who control the forces of nature, the time of harvests, droughts, the sky, diseases, the afterlife and death itself. Superstitious beliefs and practices are common in situations involving high risk, chance, or uncertainty, as well as in times of personal and social stress or crisis, when events seem ta escape human control. However, defining "What is it" or what is not superstitious is a relative matter One person's beliefs may be superstitions for another. All religious and practices Can be branded as superstitions by non-believers, while religious leaders frequently Condemn certain unorthodox folk practices, calling them superstitious parodies of the true faith.

Among the rites of passage, as the Belgian anthropologist Arnold vann Gennep called them, it begins with the initiation rites, which go from the gestation period and culminate with the public presentation and the choice of name for the neophyte. The circumcision of males eight days after their birth is an initiation ceremony in the Jewish religion. Islam also requires male children to be circumcised before marriage. The water baptism ceremony is an example of a religious ritual of birth practiced by Jews and Christians throughout his-tow, which involves the admission of the neophyte into the religious Community.

Meanwhile, in Western tradition weddings there is a tradition from Eastern weddings and that of throwing grains of rice at the joining couple. Other things that are thrown from the bride is her bridal bouquet to the single public or sometimes it is her lingerie.

Finally, we find burials, which is a funerary practice that consists of depositing the corpse in a grave or grave underground. Other burial Systems are: the deep-sea funeral throwing the Corpse into the water over the side of a ship, the exposure of the body to the atmospheric elements, a custom practiced by the Inuit people or cremation. These practices are usually preceded and accompanied by different funeral rites, such as embalming. In the years following the fall of the Han dynasty in 220, the arrival of foreigners and political instability affected the idiosyncrasies of Chinese art. Buddhism, introduced in the first century, brought new Styles of architecture, sculpture, and painting from India. Furthermore, with the Buddhist doctrine, which introduces the concept of reincarnation, the custom of opulent burials declined. Sometimes mourners, who are not relatives of the deceased, are hired to cry and mourn.

Also the times and places Where family members must show their sadness can be defined by traditional rules. Some anthropologists have observed that, despite the great variation in burial practices, there are always four main symbolic elements. The first symbolism is color. Although the association of the color black with death is not universal, the use of black clothing to represent death is Widespread. A second element is the hair of the relatives, which can be shaved or, conversely, long and messy as a sign of sadness. A third element is noisy activities with beats of the drum or any other instrument. Finally, and as a fourth element, there is the use of some worldly practices in the procession with the corpse. The classical interpretation regards the ceremonies surrounding death as well as those accompanying birth, initiation to and marriage as rites of passage.

In social terms, the symbolic meaning of death is seen more clearly at the funerals of the rulers. Cremation is practiced in some cultures with the intention of releasing the spirit of the dead. Outdoor exposure is Common in Arctic regions and among Parsis followers of an ancient Persian religion, Zoroastrianism, where it also has religious significance. Less Common practices are throwing the corpse into the water after a boat transfer and cannibalism in India.

In cultures Where the tribe or the nation is personified in the ruler, these funerals become a drama in which the entire country participates. The pyramids of Egypt, for example, became a symbol and a test of royal authority. Since the pharaohs embodied social permanence and spiritual and temporal authority, their death endangered all of these elements. The participation of his in funeral rituals provided a sense of continuity. In Thailand, after the monarch's cremation, the new king and members of the royal family traditionally searched the ashes for bone fragments. These relics became objects of worship that indirectly signified the continuity of the presence and authority of the deceased monarch.

In pre-Columbian societies in America, death was a highly ritualized event, which required ceremonies of all kinds, accompanied by offerings, food and accompanying objects and very useful gifts during the long journey that began after death. Among the Mayans, burial was differentiated according to the class and category of the dead. Ordinary people were buried under the floor of the house, but nobles were often cremated and funeral temples were erected on their graves. The Aztecs, who believed in the existence of paradises and hells, prepared the deceased for a long road full of obstacles. They had to fight to be able to reach the end and offer gifts and presents to the lord of the dead, who decided their final destiny.

In diversification societies as England, 18th-century France, and the Shilluk in the Sudan, the funeral rituals of monarchs were related to cultural ideas about the nature of the monarchy, the political order, and the transfer of authority. The burial of a ruler is not just a religious event, it is an event of considerable political and cosmological con sequences.

• China: A watch should never be given as a gift as it is considered bad luck. However, When the Chinese New Year celebration is held, which is based on the lunar calendar and is celebrated between January 21 and February 19, donuts or boiled eggs dyed red are given as a of prosperity. It is the most important event of the Chinese year and traditionally the festivities last two weeks with each year being assigned the character of one of the 12 typical animals in China. During this cities and towns are adorned with colorful lanterns, flowers and brightly colored banners that wave congratulations. In Chinese communities in Great Britain, Hong Kong, and anywhere in the World outside of China, the usual Cantonese grating is Kung hay fat choy, in which prosperity .

• Scandinavia: In northern Europe, as the group of countries consisting of Denmark, Norway and Sweden was formerly known, the tradition of receiving luck was adopted. When in the prairies characteristic of their relief it is customary to find some clovers among their four-leaf clover and Scandinavian mythology included dwarves, goblins, and the gnomes, who distributed lots among mortal s.

• Turkey: Turkish men greet each other by kissing their cheeks. This is a normal custom in Turkey. A Turkish man kisses men, women and a Turkish woman kisses men and women on cheeks. Turks have a habit of removing their shoes before entering the house. When a is born and circumcised, relatives and friends give them a gold coin with a red bow. The most religious women do not kiss men. There is a ritual when a younger person greets an older person from the same family or a friend where the younger person kisses the Older hand and brings their hand up to their forehead, as a sign of Turkish families love to offer something to their guests. It can be lunch, dinner, or tea, so if you have an invitation to Visit a Turkish family, you leave on an empty stomach. Usually the Wife of the family cooks delicious dishes throughout the day and hosts a feast. Savor a little of everything because if you reject something, they Will be disappointed.

• Middle East: In Muslim culture menopause; which is the natural cessation of menstruation, it is a gradual process of changes in the woman's that includes two of the three phases of a rite of passage: the loss by the person of their previous status and the acquisition of one new. In some Mediterranean societies women in menopause dyed their clothes black and covered their heads. These signs indicated that the men could not flirt or converse with them and that the woman had changed her role. It was considered that according to Muslim law the absence of adornments is symbolized in the use of black as the traditional "burqa", however their women are allowed to dress in any color that does not incite lasciviousness.

• Africa: We can observe some Common aspects such as the important role of dance as a vehicle for expression or social or spiritual communication. In Africa the dancer is more than a the dancer is also a teacher, a historian, a social a priest, a spiritual medium, a healer and a storyteller. In some of these the woman, who gives birth to a girl is immediately deflowered at birth without the right to maintain her virginity.

LABEL ON THE TABLE

Table behavior when eating food has been a social norm among cultures from East to West for centuries. For example, in rigid hierarchical cultures like Korea and Japan, alcohol helps break down the strict social barrier between classes. Allow a touch of informality. It is traditional for host and guest to take turns filling each Other's glasses and stimulate each other to gulp. For someone who does not consume alcohol, except for religious reasons, it can be difficult to escape the ritual of social drinking. In Hausa culture, standing while eating can be seen as offensive and ominous behavior, even insulting the host shows a lack of for food shortages, it is known as "eating with the devil" or "committing santi In China, a person who takes the last item of from a Common plate or bowl without first offering it to others at the table can be seen as a glutton who is insulting the host's generosity. Traditionally, if customers do not have food scraps in front of them at the end of a meal, it is to the disgrace of the host. In the United States of America, a guest is expected to eat all the that is given to them, as a complement to the quality of the cuisine. However, it is still considered polite to offer food from a Common plate or bowl to Others at the table.

Traveling from East to West, we observe that the cutlery, which are the utensils used to serve food, is different as we See the oriental chopsticks that are held between the thumb and index finger, and the forks and spoons for each occasion of West. The appearance in England of the Sheffield plate method in 1743, Whereby cutlery was with a thin layer of copper, lowered the Price and made possible the enormous proliferation of styles and designs that has continued to this day.

Designs for the included a family crest or seal. The handles of and forks gradually became curved for easier use, and in England the pistol-grip knife handle became popular. In France, the terrible shortage Of silver led to an increase in the use of fine porcelain for utensil handles. At the Same time, many other cutlery items appeared, such as saucepans, tea strainers, grape scissors, fish serving utensils and sugar tongs. In addition, many variants from the three basic instruments emerged, teaspoons, coffee, tureens and Salt; dessert knives, fruit, butter, fish and carvers, as well as salad, dessert and fish cutlery.

ARTISTIC PROJECTION

In the broad entertainment industry, a high standard of artistic and is also required that combines many or almost all the frameworks of aesthetics and the expression of artistic concepts. For many, this ideal of professional realization entails many years of improvement in academies of various artistic expressions such as modeling, singing, acting, the artistic direction of theater, radio, film and television, and even in the management of public relations and beauty pageants.

Each artist has their own Style, and that is why we always see diverse artistic movements or expressions in the midst of society that seek to highlight ideas, values, concepts and abstract metaphors that can be interpreted to be admired or rejected by a demanding and capitalist society of the that Our opinion is also part.

Making the decision to become an artist means starting a process of learning the appropriate techniques to Shape the talent (s) required to be considered by the long-awaited "talent scouts", juries or investment partners. The degree of disappointment is high among the great majority of dreamers that swarm in global society, with whom we can by throwing ourselves or simply "trying our luck", while we do not assume either the great commitment of work, deprivation of society and risk involved in signing the various contracts that require compliance with a promotional agenda.

On the Other hand, qualities are inherent and inherited. In the past it was considered that every son of an artist should be an artist too, or that the son of a baker should learn to make bread, the son of a blacksmith grow up welding iron and so on. The intelligence of a child is considered to be the ability to learn and understand and emphasizes the skills and abilities to handle specific situations, through sensory experience. Create experimental conditions, reveal the potential that can be measured in quantitative terms that give it a level of qualification above its making it stand out for demonstrating its capabilities Without much effort and naturally in the midst of its actions in daily life.

We cannot assure that courses, study, or class hours Will guarantee us success in Our artistic career if we do not meticulously follow the Steps to achieve it Artistic are always influenced by physical limitations, which is what is called the social rank of artists. The scrial rank of artists has been changing in the West over the centuries. In classical times and in the Middle Ages, and writers, using only intellectual capacity for their works, were considered creators of a higher rank than actors, dancers, musicians, painters and sculptors, who used manual or physical skill. But today the occurs, where singers, actors and dancers turn out to attract a Wider consumer audience than writers and painters as in other decades.

For Your better understanding, we address them separately with the purpose of listing some recommendations as well as defining their social functions.

• The voice: In the music industry, the media and international entertainment stand out the handling of the voice through the locution, the song, the petic declamation and the dubbing of voices. It refers to the handling of the voice as a sung without accompaniment, with rhythms and melodic contours closely related to the rhythms of speech with the pertinent inflections of the text. The locution is more related to the field of broadcasting, both and digital, television and the journalistic field already involves maintaining a medium tone of voice, with the help of the sound amplification of the microphones, a command of fluent and correct language without the use of babbling and idioms. In recent years, poetic recitals have made their way into cities, restaurants, Parks and Other cultural events with a renewed presence of representing the most varied literary trends. Finally, in relation to the use of the voice, we can mention that among the musical genres that have impacted the evolution of current cultural expressions, the most are Still African-American hip hop, electronic music, pop, classic romantic ballads, reggae. and national folklore.

• Movement: The performing arts such as theater and dance in contemporary society, dances provide young people with occasions to meet, express conceptual figures of everyday life and the rhythms or genres that emerge in urban areas and suburban, to convey something without using words but with their own dress Style. It is also feasible to work on concepts aided by dance.

Rhythmic movements are capable of making work faster and more efficient, as in the Japanese dances performed in rice plantations. In some cultures, such as the Latin one, dance is an art form, and in the 20th Century some dances that were originally religious rites or Court entertainment have been adapted to the theater. Thus, according to the classicist models, it differs from that of its in a greater formal care in the plots and verses. In his Works, vices are always condemned, in the manner of a happy and exemplary ending, against the pattern of the new comedies of the Spanish Lope de Vega, Tirso de Molina, Guillén de Castro, Francisco Rojas Zorrilla, among Others, who used draw exemplary consequences from situations Where Christian values border on ambiguous and even dangerous limits. It is not until the middle of the 20th century that Latin American theater has acquired a certain personality, by treating its own themes, taking as a starting point the reality of the spectator to whom it is intended. When attending a model scouting call or acting casting, some recommendations are kept for those wishing to embark on an artistic career. Looking for a representation agency can be exciting and stressful at the same time, but in any case, it is to know that not all agencies are the Same or seek the Same characteristics of models.

• During Your search, make an to apply according to the preferences of each agency. Doing Otherwise than impact Will send Your application to the trash.

• When casting calls are it is especially crucial to follow the rules to side with the seeking agency. Remember that part of being a good role model is having the ability to follow directions. If you are unable to qualify for an open call and attend, this makes a bad first impression and may imply to the agency's scouting staff that you are not following directions well.

• Casting calls: When you are looking for a model scouting Call, you should know that not all agencies make open calls for availability. The best way to find Chis information is by visiting the modeling agency's website. Any details about the casting call Will be indicated if it is offered or the agency can establish that they do not organize open casting calls. If they don't mention them; that's that they don't use it.

• Know your agency well and follow it: Never miss a casting Call. Always check the information on the modeling agency's site to find out how they handle their database, When they at what time, and estimate What wardrobe you should wear. Following the instructions you leave the simplest things to the agency. Hundreds of hopeful models show up for casting and only a few, properly prepared, will spend some time working with the agency team

• Prepare Your photo booking: A professional photographer is the ideal to help you create a "booking" which is an English term that designates a portfolio of previous modeling work that you have done as a model. If you are a beginner model, you must also have a booking of at least one photo session that includes versatile Styles, both classic, modern and eccentric or ethnic cuts, since you never know in which of these the agency directors can you- consider, depending on the concept design of each marketing campaign.

• Before the casting appointment: Each modeling agency establishes its call days, it can be from one to two days a week, once a month or even less such as once a year. The duration of a casting is approximately two hours, so if you apply to more than one agency you must be very organized and keep a meticulous agenda. Remember that you are not the only one to attend it is preferable to arrive before the stipulated time and be patient to Start, even if the line of people is already there.

• Bring Company to Your casting: If you are a minor then Your guardian or authorized relative must attend with you when attending the casting. Without exceptions, only one parent should be brought, babies or small children should not be carried. For over 18 years of age and Older, they can go alone although it is customary to attend with a image assistant who should not go the dressing room area since their job should only consist of providing help with makeup and wardrobe . You should never enter the casting Studio.

• Dress wisely: Attending a casting call is your chance for the agency to know who you are. The purpose is for them to get to know you briefly and assess Your It not mean that you attend to demonstrate the best pieces of wardrobe Couture, but to demonstrate versatility of Your character. Some agencies give them suggestions of the type of clothes they should wear on the day of the casting, if there are no detailed ones then a certain degree of informality is allowed, such as clean sneakers, jeans and preferably solid colored t-shirts. If the casting is in the Summer season, it is recommended to include a two-piece swimsuit. Hair must be dry and manageable for each Style to styled.

• Avoid distractions: If you are attending school or college, avoid distractions such as talking on the cell phone, playing games or doing homework. You must show that the casting has Your full attention. Not doing it like that would show that you have better things to do than attend the casting. It has happened in some castings that the models are so distracted with their cell phones that the team ignores them and lets the Others pass, so we recommend that you Stay alert to the call to be evaluated or evaluated.

• Enjoy Your moment of glamour: The most inescapable advice for modeling, or for any other place is to relax, feel fulfilled and be yourself to show the team an extroverted and genuine personality. Also, don't overdo it by using many flattering phrases like: "wow, how wonderful the agency and its models are." The casting call is for you to shine, so listen to the agency, answer their questions to the best of your ability, and smile.

• If Your qualities go far beyond the handling of Your in a photographic studio and outdoors, having a good memory for dialogues, you master Your emotions and feelings to a striking personality before the cameras, Your dream may be to work as an actor or actress. Maybe for a long time you have been saying "do it", you have waiting for the phone to ring but there have been no return calls yet.

Well, it is said that what separates the true professionals from the is not inspiration, but preparation and execution. Take control of Your hearing with these ten helpful tips to improve your skills.

• Confidence: This sounds simple but it takes a lot of practice. Walk through the door with Your head up, be careful When moving your steps. If you don't get sympathy hooks and you're nervous, you're not feeling well, or you had a bad day. Leave it behind the door. You are being characterized from the second you Step inside, so practice good and language before entering. And do not forget to smile that is the only impression that you Will want to leave.

• Personality. Let it shine throughout. Don't give one-word answers When you have a conversation with the casting director, ask yourself. The industry is looking for bold and curious actors.

• Connection: Make one with the reader, memorize the material or familiar enough with it to maintain a of view. Knowing the dialogue is but making an emotional connection with the character is what Will make the scene look natural and believable.

• Character: Know Your character well. Read the entire script beforehand to any essay, as many times as We know a character answering the following: - What does he or she say themselves? - What Other characters say about him or her? - What does the script or writer say about him or her?

• Objective: Go and unravel the dialogue. What does he or she look for from the other characters?

• Obstacles: What is in the characters way to get what he or she wants? Acting is defined as what to you as you try to achieve Your goal, despite obstacles?

• Crying is not the only Way to show hatred or anger. Sometimes being as Still as you can aim is a powerful display of emotion. Playing opposite sides is a more interesting selection than being obvious.

• Love; Find love in the scene. Even offensive and ruthless characters need to played to a certain level of liking. As an antagonist you must also find a moment of love in the scene.

• Acting: Acting means doing, not talking. Find Your actions and interpret them, some acting books can useful here.

• Miscellaneous: Feel the levels and dynamics. Interact, don't play with just one emotion. If the character is angry and inflexible, find out when the character can show some vulnerability.

CHAPTER 9: BIOSECURITY

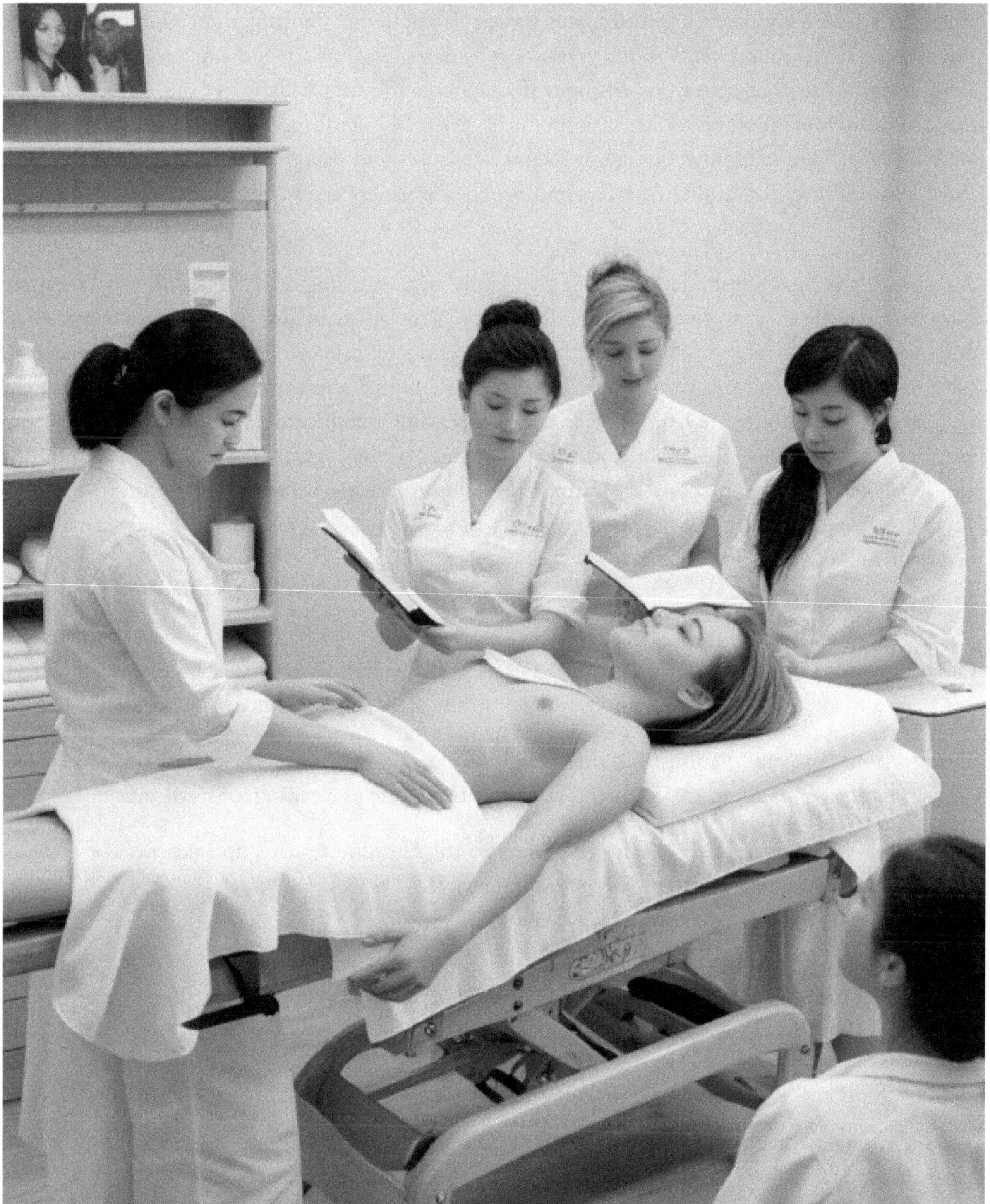

Biosafety is a set of standards, measures, and protocols applied to multiple procedures carried out in scientific research, businesses, public areas, and teaching work, with the aim of contributing to the prevention of risks or infections arising from exposure to potentially infectious agents or those with significant biological, physical, and chemical risks. Biosafety measures not only encompass laboratories that handle highly contagious strains of viruses and bacteria, but also natural habitats, especially agriculture, contaminated rivers and beaches, business activities, mass events, and public places.

Its terminology is a neologism derived from the Greek "bio," meaning life, and "securitatis," meaning safe or risk-free. In cases of risk when handling toxic substances or during global epidemics and pandemics, it usually refers to blocking the proliferation of microorganisms or living materials capable of causing respiratory or toxic infections in people, animals, or the environment. Government biosecurity policies proliferate from time to time, depending on citizens' health circumstances, and are subject to controversy. The goal is to ensure the control of biological agents that threaten public health by activating safety protocols that must be followed during a quarantine period or a period of forty days, weeks, or years of preventive isolation to which the population is subjected to verify clinical statistics of spreading diseases.

Biosecurity encompasses three main concepts:

- Contamination: The introduction of some type of substance or energy that harms living beings, causing almost irreversible damage. This may occur in the environment, water, or a product.

- Disinfection: The elimination of germs that infect or can cause infection in a body or place. Disinfection of a wound is an environmental organization's role in cleaning, or sterilization.

- Cleanliness and sterilization: Cleanliness refers to the cleanliness, care, and neatness of a thing, place, object, or surface, free of stains—in short, habitable.

Universal biosafety precautions

This set of precautions should be applied to all types of patients. For practical purposes, every person should be considered a carrier of communicable diseases.

- Handwashing: Use antiseptic soap before and after each contact.

- Use of personal protective equipment: Such as gloves, face masks, goggles or eye protectors, and impermeable aprons.

- Take extreme precautions to avoid injuries. All necessary precautions should be taken to minimize risk.

- Avoid mouth-to-mouth resuscitation as much as possible.

- Avoid performing procedures on patients with exposed wounds. Pregnancy does not increase the risk, but precautions should be taken.

Microorganisms and infections are living organisms smaller than 1 mm, so they are only visible with the aid of a microscope. The conditions for the development of microorganisms allow them to proliferate quickly, preventing others from growing, even destroying their habitat. These conditions are where they find nutrients such as carbon, nitrogen, and mineral salts. Water: if an environment lacks water, it is very difficult for a microorganism to develop. Regarding oxygen, there are microorganisms that live both in the absence of oxygen and in the presence of air. pH, or a measure of the acidity level in the environment, ranges from alkaline to acidic. Finally, we find temperature, where there are three types: those that grow in cold, moderate, and warm climates.

Infections are the effect that occurs after microbes enter and grow in another specific organism, causing damage that did not previously exist. The alteration or damage caused is called an infectious disease. When this infectious disease can be transmitted to other people, it is called a contagious disease.

Microorganisms are classified into four groups: bacteria, fungi, protozoa, and viruses. Bacteria are unicellular microorganisms, formed by a single cell, and can form spores. The most common skin infections are caused by bacteria. These include folliculitis, pustules, dermatitis, and acne.

Fungi are microorganisms that can be unicellular, like yeast, or form filaments by successive unions of cells. Among the diseases caused by fungi are mycosis of the feet and nails. Viruses are another type of microorganism that are considered particles, not cells, capable of reproducing and living as parasites of other cells. These include hepatitis and AIDS, and they are transmitted through many routes.

IMPORTANCE OF A DERMATOLOGICAL CONSULTATION

If you experience any symptoms of a skin condition, it is crucial to consult a dermatologist for an accurate diagnosis and appropriate treatment. The dermatologist will perform a complete physical exam, review your medical history, and, in some cases, may order additional tests such as biopsies or blood tests.

Treatment for skin conditions will depend on the specific cause and severity of the condition. Treatment options may include topical or oral medications, light therapy, surgical procedures, and even lifestyle changes.

ACNE

In Facial Aesthetics, we may encounter patients suffering from acne, which in dermatology refers to the inflammatory disease of the pilosebaceous unit. It is one of the most common dermatological pathologies, affecting almost 80% of adolescents between the ages of 13 and 18. Its appearance in the outermost layer of the skin has shown that in comedones, this microorganism secretes chemotactic factors and possesses chemotactic activity. This attracts polymorphonuclear leukocytes, which, upon entering the follicle, can phagocytize P. acnes and trigger the release of hydrolytic enzymes.

As we see in our following graph, these can be grade I, also called comedones and papules, and grade II, which present papules and pustules like deep acne. Here, acne is mild or moderate, where the patient may have oily skin and pimples, which appear as whiteheads or blackheads on the face, back, or chest. Most pimples will not cause any other symptoms.

In grades III and IV, pimples that have become inflamed or infected, such as pustules, nodules, and cysts, can cause pain. Lesions can be grade III (pustules and nodules) or grade IV (nodules and cysts). These are deeper lesions, develop much more slowly, and leave significant scarring when they disappear.

Acne is an inflammatory disease caused by multiple factors that affects the sebum-producing glands located on the face, back, chest, shoulders, and even the upper arms.

Comedonal acne is a type of acne in which the predominant lesions are open comedones (blackheads) and closed comedones (pimples). Inflammatory acne presents with redder, more painful "bumps," which are known as papules or nodules if they are deeper.

There are several etiological factors linked to the appearance of acne, ranging from genetic and hereditary factors, a healthy diet, psychological and emotional states, significant hormonal changes such as those that occur during pregnancy and menstruation, certain medications, and the improper use of some cosmetics.

If there is excess sebum and too many dead skin cells, the pores become clogged. Bacteria (especially those of the Propionibacterium acnes species) can then become trapped inside the pores and reproduce, causing the skin to swell and redden: the beginning of acne.

Depending on the degree of skin severity, the main acne lesions are:

Ø Papules: red, swollen lesions due to inflammation.

Ø Pustules: lesions filled with purulent material, containing whitish or yellowish pus.

Ø Nodules: more advanced lesions, larger in size, and located deeper in the dermis.

Another factor that can influence the appearance of acne is the foods that cause acne due to their composition. Foods that cause pimples are mainly foods rich in sugar and fat, such as chocolate, dressings, fatty meats, fried foods, sausages, fast foods, frozen ready meals, and excessive consumption of bread, cookies, sweets, junk food, milk, and yellow cheeses.

To treat these pimples and eliminate facial acne, you should follow some tips, such as:

Ø Change your pillowcase regularly.

Ø Avoid excessively greasy foods; avoid doing so once a week.

Ø Wash your face twice a day (no more) with warm water and a mild soap made specifically for people with acne.

Ø Do not pop pimples while they are ripening or drying.

Ø Avoid touching your face with your hands or resting it on objects that tend to accumulate sebum and skin residue, such as the telephone receiver.

For medication, consult a dermatologist, who will prescribe antibiotics that can help relieve the effects of acne:

Ø Oral antibiotics (taken by mouth) such as tetracycline, doxycycline, minocycline, erythromycin, trimethoprim, sulfamethoxazole, and amoxicillin.

Ø Topical antibiotics (applied to the skin) such as clindamycin, erythromycin, or dapsone.

Its terminology is of a neologism from the Greek "bio" which means life, and "securitatis" which means safe or risk-free. In case of risk when handling toxic substances or global epidemics and pandemics, it usually refers to blocking the proliferation of or living materials capable of causing respiratory or toxic infections in people, animals or the environment.

Government biosafety policies proliferate from time to time, according to the health circumstances of citizens and are the subject of controversy. The intention is to guarantee the control of biological agents that threaten public health by activating security protocols that must be complied with during a of quarantine or a of forty days, weeks, years, of preventive isolation to which they are subjects the to verify clinical statistics of proliferating diseases.

In biosafety, three main concepts are handled: • Pollution: It is the introduction of some type of substances or energy that threatens beings causing almost irreversible damage. Either in the environment, in the water or some product.

• Disinfection: Elimination of germs that infect or can cause an infection in a or place. The disinfection of a wound, an environmental organization in cleaning or sterilization.

• Cleaning and sterilization: Clean refers to the condition of cleanliness, care and neatness free of stains that may show a thing, place, Object or surface, habitable in a few words.

Universal biosafety precautions

This set of precautions should applied in all of patients. For practical purposes, every person should be considered a carrier of communicable diseases:

• Hand washing: Using antiseptic soap and after each contact.

• Use of personal protection elements: Such as gloves, face masks, glasses or eye protectors, waterproof aprons

• Take extreme precautions to avoid injuries, all necessary precautions must be taken to minimize the risk.

• Avoid as much as possible the practice of mouth-to-mouth resuscitation.

• Avoid performing procedures on patients with exposed

• Pregnancy does not increase the risk, but precautions should be taken.

Microorganisms and infections are living beings with dimensions less than 1 mm, so they are only visible with the help of a microscope. The conditions for the development of allow them to proliferate in a short time, preventing others from growing, even producing the destruction of where they are housed. These conditions are where they find nutrients like carbon, nitrogen, and mineral salts water, if an environment lacks water it is very difficult for a microorganism to develop. As for oxygen, there are microorganisms that live in the absence of oxygen and ventilated. The ph. o measure of the level of acidity in the environment ranges from alkaline levels to acids.

Finally we find the temperature where there are three types, those that grow in cold, medium and warm climates. Infections are the effect that occurs after the entry and growth of microbes in another specific organism, causing damage that did not exist. The alteration or damage caused is called infectious disease.

When this infectious disease can be transmitted to other people it is called a contagious diseases are classified into four groups: bacteria, fungi, protozoa, and viruses, Bacteria are unicellular microorganisms, made up of a single cell, and can form spores, the most common skin infections are caused by bacteria, dermatitis and acne.

Fungi are microorganisms that can be unicellular like yeasts, or form filaments by successive cell unions. Among the diseases caused by fungi is mycosis, of the feet and nails. Viruses are another type of microorganism that are considered particles, not cells, capable of reproducing and living as parasites of other cells. Among these we find hepatitis and AIDS and they are transmitted by many ways to the human being such as respiratory, sexual, or digestive.

SCIENTIFIC BASES OF BIOSECURITY

The word hygiene has two closely related meanings within aesthetics and cosmetology, on the one hand it means cleaning and on the other, it is a method or system dedicated to the prevention of diseases of any kind.

Microbial decontamination is the elimination of from a utensil, product or the environment in general. In aesthetic and beauty stores there are cleaning and disinfection standards that must be extreme in cases of suspected skin infections in a client. so it Will be essential to check if there are wounds or infections on the skin in all professional.

There are different levels within this concept. Decontamination systems or methods differ in their field of action and their effects.

• Disinfection: It is the method applied to objects and utensils facilities to destroy microbes, except and viruses. Ammonia, chlorines or bleach and derivatives of iodine are used.

• Fumigation: It is the system used to eliminate visible vermin and insects such as ants, rats, lice, worms and fleas so that they from the environment. Insecticides and rodenticides are used to exterminate

• Antisepsis: It is used in the case of injuries to and animals to avoid the effect of bacteria and fungi. Hydrogen tincture of iodine, antiseptic soap are used.

• Sterilization: It acts on microorganisms and parasites in cloches, utensils, containers and products. Temperature is used in furnaces, boilers, radiation.

In aesthetics, the most used removal methods are disinfection and sterilization and are broken down as follows:

• Moist heat with steam sterilizers at 200 0 C. There are devices Where the material to be sterilized is introduced, it is a quick and comfortable method.

• Use of 2% glutaraldehyde. For disinfection by glutaraldehyde we must prepare the 2% solution in water. This compound has great antimicrobial and can be sterilizing. If the material is kept submerged for 10 minutes, it acts as a disinfectant.

BIOSAFETY PRINCIPLES

Assume that all patients are infected as well as their own fluids and the objects used in their care.

a) Universality. Everyone must take precautions to prevent the skin from the mucous membranes that can give rise to accidents, Whether or not contact with blood is foreseen.

b) Use of barriers: Avoid direct exposure to and Other organic fluids.

c). Means of of contaminated material or material without risk.

CONDITIONS FOR HAND WASHING

• During care work.

• DO not wear rings on the fingers, or bracelets or watches.

• DO not use nail keep them clean and short.

HAND WASHING TECHNIQUES.

Hand washing is the simplest, most economical and most important for the prevention of infections.

HAND WASHING- Hand washing is an important procedure to prevent and control infection, minimize the transmission of microorganisms and the of contamination. And it is as follows:

• Wet your hands.

• Apply the antimicrobial soap and spread it all over the surfaces of the hands.

• Clean your nails with the brush

• Rub each finger in a circular motion.

• Rub the Spaces between Your fingers.

• Rub the wrists in their circular contour.

• Rinse with plenty of water, towel dry. Repeat if necessary.

Hand washing processing is also known as removal, there are two types of removal.

• Manual or mechanized removal: It refers to hand washing with liquid soap, leaving the in suspension, thus allowing them to be removed. It is done before any aesthetic, facial and ornamental procedure such as manicure, hairstyle, waxing or massage. Also between each client at the end of their care.

• Chemical Removal: Refers to deep washing with antiseptic solutions, managing to inhibit or destroy the growth of It is indicated in routine non-invasive procedures such as massages, facials and makeup.

SAFETY RULES

There are two fundamental aspects to consider regarding safety in our professional work are, on the one hand, those related to the accidents that may occur, both to the worker and the client, and the other related to the professional diseases that arise from the development of our work.

First of all, we can apply the most important measures such as prevention. Avoiding accidents and diseases entails developing preventive measures in the work area as well as in its organization and cleaning, including work material.

If an accident occurs or a situation arises that requires prompt and effective attention from the professional, it is necessary for the professional to know how to provide first aid before transferring the affected person to the medical center.

Accidents are injuries suffered by clients and workers due to non-compliance with basic safety regulations. The factors that regularly cause them are long nails and hands washed by the professional, improper use of different chemical products or deficiencies in the facilities.

Among the security measures that should be taken into account are mentioned:

• Risk reduction with sanitary training, the use of gloves and glasses, as well as the protection of the client with a blanket, in addition there should be a first-aid kit with hypoallergens, anti-inflammatory, anti-burn ointments and analgesics.

• Control of cosmetic doses and possible injurious agents, flammable as well as the temperature of the place and the use of devices.

• Maintain order of shelves and general order within the premises, such as the location of electrical cables and slippery floors.

TOXICOALLERGIC REACTIONS

90% of the accidents produced in aesthetics are caused by the cosmetics used. Allergic reactions to and color dyes stand out above all. However, reactions to facial treatment creams on the face, eczema around the nails due to the application of acrylates, and contact eczema to lipstick are also mentioned.

The main guidelines that must be followed to avoid any related problems are:

• Follow the instructions written on the cosmetic manufacturer's package insert.

• Consult if you suffer from allergic processes of any kind, to cosmetic, if so, we must see the convenience of applying the cosmetic.

• In the event of signs of irritation or in the client after applying the product, remove with water and refer to a

ASSESSMENT AND MEASUREMENT OF SKIN PARAMETERS

** Navigating the Cutaneous Microcosm: Techniques for Assessing and Measuring Skin Parameters in the Aesthetics Industry

In the dynamic world of aesthetics, the skin stands as the canvas upon which techniques and treatments seeking to enhance natural beauty are deployed. To optimize these procedures and ensure the best results,

For satisfactory results, it is crucial to master the techniques for assessing and measuring skin parameters. These tools allow practitioners to delve into the skin's microcosm, obtaining accurate information about its current condition and specific needs.

Diving into the Skin Microcosm: Assessment Techniques

1. **Visual Assessment:** Careful observation of the skin, under adequate lighting, is the first essential step. Texture, coloration, pigmentation, and the presence of wrinkles, fine lines, enlarged pores, vascular lesions, or blemishes are analyzed.

2. **Palpation:** Through gentle touch, the skin's elasticity, turgor, hydration, and tone are assessed, detecting possible areas of sagging or dehydration.

3. **Photographs:** Capturing high-quality images, under standardized lighting, allows for documentation of the skin's initial condition and monitoring of progress during treatment.

4. **Dermoscopy:** The use of dermatoscopes, devices that magnify the skin's image, facilitates the detection of early lesions, atypical moles, and other signs of dermatological problems.

Quantifying Beauty: Measurement Techniques

1. **Hydration Measurement:** There are various methods for measuring skin hydration, such as:

* **Hydrometer:** A portable device that measures the amount of water on the skin's surface.

* **Electrical Impedance:** A technique that evaluates the skin's electrical conductivity, an indirect indicator of its hydration.

* **Optical Techniques:** These use light to measure water absorption in different layers of the skin.

2. **Elasticity Assessment:** Techniques such as **cutaneous extensibility** and **elastometry** measure the skin's ability to stretch and return to its original state.

3. **Pigmentation Analysis:** Devices such as a **melanometer** are used to measure the amount of melanin in the skin, helping to detect hyperpigmentation or areas of lack of pigmentation.

4. **Roughness Assessment:** Techniques such as **profilemetry** and **skin topography** measure skin texture, allowing for the detection of wrinkles, fine lines, and other irregularities.

Applications in the Aesthetic Industry

1. **Treatment Selection:** The information obtained through the assessment and measurement of skin parameters allows the professional to select the most appropriate treatment for each patient, considering their specific needs and skin type.

2. **Procedure Personalization:** Quantifying parameters such as hydration or elasticity allows for personalized treatments, adjusting their intensity and duration to individual skin characteristics.

3. **Effectiveness Assessment:** By measuring skin parameters before and after treatment, the effectiveness of the treatment can be objectively assessed, allowing adjustments to be made and results to be optimized.

4. **Communication with the Patient:** The information obtained facilitates communication with the patient, giving them a clear understanding of their skin condition and the available treatment options.

Skin parameter assessment and measurement techniques have become indispensable tools in the aesthetics industry. By delving into the skin's microcosm and quantifying its characteristics, practitioners can provide personalized treatments, optimize results, and establish effective communication with their patients. Mastering these techniques allows them to accurately navigate the complex world of skin, ensuring the satisfaction and well-being of those seeking to enhance their natural beauty.

PROFESSIONAL ETHICS OF THE BEAUTICIAN

It is the set of principles, values and standards of action by which aesthetics must be governed in the development of their functions, with values thus maintaining a code of excellence. The appropriate conduct that the professional must have with patients, related professionals, in general and the environment.

The Code of Ethics to the trust that society has placed in the suitability of aesthetic professionals. The objective of aesthetic medicine is to prevent, improve and treat totally or partially the unsightly of the patient to their quality of life. The esthetician Will not discriminate against her patients for reasons of religion, ideology, race, sex, nationality or social extraction.

In his article I he tells us "The esthetician owes loyalty to the patient in the first and Will foster mutual trust." Regarding its preparation, the article tells us "The beautician must have academic and institutional This must be reliable and prestigious " Regarding the facilities, the article refers to "offering quality treatments, making the most appropriate products, equipment and facilities available to patients and clinical practice guidelines".

The modern legislation of each nation has established regulatory norms for cosmetry or cosmetology centers, training centers as well as non-formal education centers, and the like of the obligation to abide by current laws and certify accreditation, diplomas, and technicians as considering health requirements and regulations for cosmetics. It may grounds for the closure to incur irregularities, by the State educational or health authority, duly assigned for this purpose. No one may advertise, practice or as a cosmetologist, or open a beauty, cosmetology or aesthetic center to the public, without having completed a high school cycle and a Course with a program of at least 500 theoretical and practical hours.

The exercise of aesthetics and cosmetry will be governed by humanistic principles, health and personal image, which is why it must be developed in centers authorized for that purpose. The esthetician or cosmetologist may not perform any practice or act resewed for doctors or health professionals but only for techniques limited to cosmetic.

The procedures reserved for the cosmetologist are facial cleansing, facial and massages, waxing, lymphatic drainage and, in general, those invasive procedures that do not require surgical intervention and other medical health operations.

THE 10 PRECEPTS OF THE ESTHETICIST

The professional exercise of the cosmetic discipline indicates that it should be governed by the following

- The beauty center must present an impeccable, healthy and hygienic dress.

- You Will obtain the or authorization of the authorities of the same address where the cosmetic commercial activities will be offered and taught.

- Sterilized and disposable biosafety implements; biotechnology equipment and other instruments Will be provided.

- Will promptly and efficiently assist the user in the provision of aesthetic services.

- You will apply his knowledge and skills in a and conscious way and if he observes doubts regarding the diagnosis of the service user, you will refer them to a dermatologist.

- It will only apply to users the treatments with the protocols authorized by the state entities assigned to their country or region.

- You must refrain from serving minors without the person authorization of their parents or legal representatives.

- The cosmetologist will not expose his clients and regular users to any unjustified risk, and will have to make the previous warnings or contraindications of the treatments that will be applied and due

- The cosmetologist must attend events related to their occupation or specific area of the branch, as well as collaborate with the media.

- In the event that there is one, it Will attend to the possible modifications of the laws and decrees of public health issued by the organisms , offices and other entities of interest to public health.

These will be authorized to impose sanctions on Commerce that range from private and public reprimands, fines, temporary suspension of activities, to the closure or cancellation of the operating permit.

CHAPTER 10: RELAXATION THERAPIES

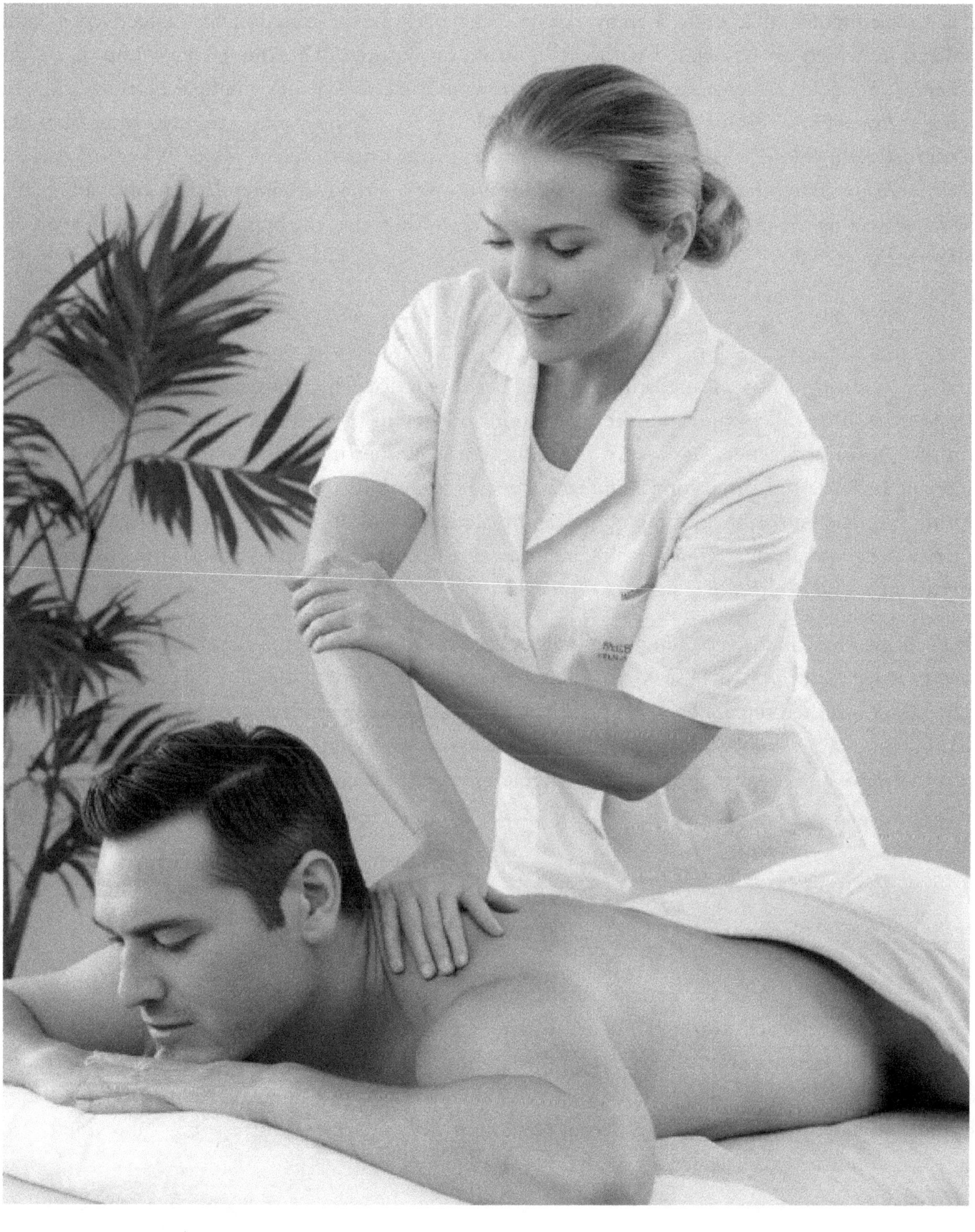

It is to distinguish that each therapy has its own precepts of functionality, effectiveness and application, which are associated with each culture or country. We cannot try to impose on an audience, or attract as constant a clientele as we would like, since they might feel an aversion to seeing themselves in certain situations, such as lodotherapy, Wine therapy or any Other of those mentioned here below. It is the responsibility of the staff of the different places Where relaxation services are given, to offer a package of services appropriate to the recommendations of their clients, always protecting the integrity of the client and the reputation that the brand or franchise relaxation and esthetic.

CHIROPRACTIC

Literally meaning "manual medicine," it has been practiced by physicians since the time of Hippocrates. Modern chiropractic medicine was introduced in 1895; today, it is the most widespread non-drug medical practice. Essentially, the treatment is neither medical nor surgical. Chiropractic medicine focuses on the prevention and treatment of conditions through psychological counseling, healing, hygiene, nutrition, and manipulation of the spine and other joints. The foundation of the practice is, in essence, that established regimens restore normal function to the body's joints, helping the patient regain health.

Osteopathic medicine is very similar to chiropractic medicine, and both have developed from the same practice. Chiropractors use X-rays more frequently than osteopaths and are generally believed to be better qualified to cure back pain and restore health. In general terms, osteopathy involves the manipulation of the body, and more specifically, the spine, with rhythmic movements and massage in areas that can cause constriction of nerves and blood vessels. Osteopaths also claim to cure numerous diseases.

COSMETIC BIOTECHNOLOGY

In this chapter we mention cosmetic is a branch of biotechnology to industry, mainly to the aesthetic care of manipulating cells through biochemical, toxicological and electromechanical processes. Also known as Aesthetic Apparatus, it refers to any medical, operational and functional device that brings together electrical, electronic, mechanical, hydraulic systems, including their computer programs that are intended to be used in aesthetic clinics and dermatological offices. It is subdivided into reductive appliances such as cavitation and vaccinia therapy.

HYDROTHERAPY

As its name indicates, Hydrotherapy, in alternative medicine, is the use of water in the treatment of diseases. Hydrotherapy was used by the doctors of Ancient Greece. The German Vincenz Priessnitz, the use of spas in Germany and other areas of Europe where it is still popular. There is little evidence that mineral Waters offer any specific effect that normal hot water or physical therapy Hydrotherapy has many applications. Hot water relaxes contractures; For this reason, hydrotherapy has been very useful in the treatment of disorders such as muscle strains and stretches, muscle fatigue and back pain. Heat is often used in conjunction with massage or other manipulative or stimulating treatments, such as baths. Sitz baths (sitting in hot water) are effective in treating painful and inflamed hemorrhoids. Water is also useful in physiotherapy since patients who carry out the exercises in a floating medium can mobilize the weakened areas of their body Without having to overcome the force of gravity.

CUPPING

Cupping therapy is also known by its spanish name, "Ventosas", which comes from "cup", which means "cup" in English- Cupping Therapy is a very old and universal therapy and consists of making a vacuum effect in which the suction cup sticks to the sucks the skin and part of the muscle, opens the pores and moves the blood and lymphatic circulation. In primitive shamanic practices, cupping was already applied in order to suck the disease-causing spirit from the body. In the glass suction cups the vacuum is generated in several ways, all of them with the use of fire.

The technique consists of consuming the oxygen inside the suction cup and immediately applying it to the skin before more oxygen enters again. In this way the vacuum is made.

The application of the suction cups consists of making a vacuum effect in which the suction cup sticks to the body, sucks the skin and part of the muscle, opens the pares and moves the blood and lymphatic circulation. In the glass suction cups the vacuum is in several ways, all of them with the use of fire. The technique consists of consuming the oxygen inside the suction cup and immediately applying it to the skin before more oxygen enters again. In this way the vacuum is made.

The plastic suction cups come with a suction pump that allows you to control the amount of air that is extracted from inside the suction cup. Another model of suction cups are the plastic ones with a rubber bulb that extracts the air. Suction cups can be used in Several ways:

• In massage: In this case, Oil would be applied to the skin to allow the suction cup to slide. A massage is performed on the area to be treated to cause hyperemia and move the fluids. The purpose of this technique is to detoxify the body of toxins that circulate in the blood and lymph. For this technique the most used suction cup is the rubber pear.

• Technique of application and rapid extraction of the suction cup: This technique is used only on the back, and is to impinge on the lungs. The suction cup is applied, left for two or three seconds and separated from the skin with a quick movement to immediately apply it again at the next the process, thus covering the entire area to treated. This technique is specific for cases of much pulmonary congestion due to mucus. Helps excess mucus to come off through coughing. Glass suction cups are often u sed in this technique.

• Fixed dry suction cup: This technique consists of leaving the suction cup fixed on the skin, at points to treat the organic reflex areas of the body through its reflex on the back. It is also used in the treatment of so-called trigger points, that is, of maximum pain, generated by contractures and structural blockages.

• Suction cup bleeding: When there are very congested and inflamed areas at a certain point, a little blood can be drawn to lower the tension in that area. To do this, the skin is pricked with a lancet in that area and the fixed suction cup is placed. [t is the itself that drives out the amount of blood it needs to release, so that the area is decongested and improves more quickly release.

AROMATHERAPY

Aromatherapy, in alternative medicine, is the use of essential Oils extracted from plants. Essential Oils provide plants with their fragrance and their healing effects on the body and mind have been known since ancient times. The ancient Egyptians used them in cosmetics and medicine. They were also used to purify the air and as preservatives in mummification. Aromatic plants were also used medicinally in ancient Greece, Rome, China, India, and throughout until they were replaced by synthetic drugs in the late 19th century. Modern aromatherapy, along with the term itself, emerged in the 193 Os, from the work of the French chemist René-Maurice Gattefossé on the antimicrobial effects of essential Oils.

• Pepermint Oil: It is analgesic. It is used to calm the breath and as a digestive aid.

• Lavender Oil: An unmistakable aroma with therapeutic it is used for its calming and relaxing properties.

• Jasmine Oil: It can be sedating.

• Rosemary Oil: It has the ability to stimulate the nervous system.

• Thyme Oil: It has bactericidal properties.

• ESI Oils: They are natural organic that are not made from water, although they are soluble. They contain fatty or acidic liquids like those found in animal and vegetable Oils. The Oils range in colors from crystalline to deep blue.

• Oil do Terra: Lemon juice is from the to preserve its delicate nature, its are for topical use. Its aromatic and cleansing powers are known.

• Breathe: Contains Laurel, Peppermint, Eucalyptus, Lemon and Raven Sara leaves. [t is medicinal to the respiratory system and can be applied to the chest and back and feet. Its aroma is relaxing and allows a peaceful sleep.

• Deep Blue: This contains camphor, blue chamomile, Winter green, blue tassy, and osmanthus. They work together to soothe joint pain and sore muscles - their effects are deep and penetrating and their results are immediate.

• Drinking Oils: It is to help manage the between meals. Slim and Sassy contains grapefruit, lemon, mint, ginger, and cinnamon. Take 8 drops in 16 ounces of water, take to calm hunger, humor. It contains no sugar or caffeine and no artificial things and is 100 % therapeutic.

The essential Oils that are used most frequently in aromatherapy are lavender, suitable for headaches, stress states and insomnia and as a first aid in cuts, burns and insect bites; eucalyptus, used for colds and coughs; and mint, which is used as a stimulant and to combat nausea and dizziness. They are applied by means of massages, baths, compresses or inhalation. Because they are highly concentrated - for example, it takes 900 kg of roses to produce 1 kg of rose Oil - they are diluted in vegetable Oil for massages and in water for baths and inhalations. Some can administer internally, but with great caution and under professional supervision, as they can be if ingested.

Essential Oils are chemically complex - Oil can contain between 50 and 500 different chemicals - and they possess a large of medicinal They can dilate or constrict blood vessels, serve as sedatives or stimulants, and act on the adrenal glands, ovaries, thyroid, or in the process of digestion. Aromatherapy is considered especially useful in treating skin problems, such as wounds and burns;

breathing problems, such as colds, coughs, and sinusitis; muscle aches, arthritis, rheumatism, headaches, and migraine; and stress-related states such as insomnia, anxiety, and depression.

Essential and aromatic Oils have effects on the skin or skin organ. In situations of illness such as itching or itching, dryness and stress, we have many essences obtained from the distillation of herbs, flowers and nuts that provide LIS with permanent or temporary well-being from some discomforts caused by a immune system. Next we Will know some of these Oils:

• Almond Oil: It is obtained from a dried fruit that is very rich in nutrients, to which soothing properties are attributed to itching episodes caused by allergies, psoriasis, eczema and minor irritations on the skin of the Its aroma is similar to that of melted butter and not very greasy, which allows it to use as a sunscreen on days out on the home.

• Rosemary Oil: This Oil is used mainly to strengthen the scalp and hair, darkening it to a less light shade. It is also used in the field of aesthetics to apply anti-stress massages since it has a soft aroma similar to pine, so it should be used moderately in allergy sufferers. It is also considered according to recent discoveries that in Spain and France, countries Where it comes from, it is a rejuvenating Oil by preventing the appearance of wrinkles.

• Linase Oil: This oil is used mainly to massage areas with localized fat, such as the belly, forearms and thighs, as it has reducing properties. Strengthens the digestive system applied on the belly. It is extracted from the flax seed, and it is originally from Canada, one of its main producers in the World.

• Fafa Oil: This oil is used mainly for curly and dry hair, very among Asian, mixed race or black women. Applied frequently when combing, it frees up knots by smoothing out unruly hair strands. It is extracted from a purple flower, and is kept in dark, light-sensitive containers. Its intense aroma is another of the characteristics of this transparent Oil.

• Coconut Oil: Coconut was considered to have harmful for a time due to its saturated fats, but it is known that in some people it produces really beneficial effects. Sometimes used as an aphrodisiac with cinnamon, and Others in the kitchen as refried, desserts and salads as a substitute for olive. It produces energizing effects for those suffering from fatigue, weakness and muscle disorders.

Aromatherapy advocates that essential Oils can have a major effect on the and mind- The art and science of aromatherapy is to determine which oil or combination of oils is appropriate i n treating a specific condition and per son.

PERFUMERY. The use of fragrances given off by substances from nature has its origin since prehistoric times When men used the scent of animals to hunt. Later the European conquerors spread its use from the Waters of flowers to the moss. Man also offered the fruits of the earth to his divinities and found in the aromas of nature, resins and ointments the ability to drive away bad smells and make his life more pleasant. with the passage of time and with the improvement of the distillation techniques discovered by the alchemists, merchants and navigators found a "Perfume Route" that forced them to preserve the aromas as the Arabs did with musk, civet and water. of roses. The main perfumes of animal origin are musk, civet, ambergris and castoreum. Musk is obtained by drying the secretion of the preputial follicles of the musk deer. The musk ox, muskrat, and Florida alligator secrete similar substances. Civet is secreted by the civet cat, Viverra Sabetha, an animal of African origin. The substance is found in a double bag located under the tail, from which it is extracted from the caged animal two or three times a week Ambergris, a bile secretion from the whale sperm, is found floating in the sea: it is believed to be produced -as -of diseases.

The castoreum is a glandular secretion of the beaver. When it is fresh it is semi-liquid; he prepares himself for trade by drying him in the smoke. Animal are used to give greater permanence to vegetable aromas, which are more evanescent.

The Hebrews also knew how to the value of Oils such as Olive, the essences of myrrh and aloe as the verses of the Bible collect in facts such as the anointing of feet, the three Wise Men from the East in Bethlehem and the death of Jesus Christ. During the 15th and 16th centuries the center of this tradition of already established moved towards France and Italy. For a long time, the center of the natural perfume industry has in Grasse, France. The cultivation of flowers for perfumery is also carried out in Turkey, Bulgaria, India and Syria. Istanbul and Esmirne in Turkey are especially famous for the of rose essence.

In this period, however, hygiene is put aside and are used to "not smell like rams." It is as Common among ladies not to bathe as to wear scented under the armpits and between the thighs. As is evident, scabies was the order of the day both for the Common and among the rich and famous (one of the assistants of Juana I of Castilla and Aragon, also known as La Loca, wrote in one of her letters: "The queen's daughters gradually improve their scabies'). But the place of honor among the filthy is held by Henry IV of France: not only did he never wash himself, but he was not even in the habit of scenting himself. On their wedding night, his wife was about to faint and letters from her lovers' left testimonies of the nausea and dizziness they suffered when sharing her bed- But it seems that at least he bathed once. It was in the Seine, where before doing so, and in full View of all, he urinated profusely. And seeing that his son, the future Louis XIII, hesitated to get into the water, he told him a famous and paternal maxim that would make Saint Martin himself pale: «with confidence, bathe and do not be afraid that higher up the river others will have before that I".

This is how the cities of Florence and Venice were the capitals of When alchemy died after the birth of chemistry, the art of perfumery evolved notably by improving the distillation and quality of essences. Using oriental techniques, Venice the first blown glass jars, but many Italian glassmakers emigrated to Germany and Bohemia, finding quite hard quartz there that allowed them to carve, engrave, and decorate their containers. They put blowing aside and new techniques for packaging.

The sources of fragrance extraction are made from the smell of plants can be in the leaves (such as Sage, thyme or mint), in the bark (cinnamon), in the Wood (cedar, sandalwood, in the flower (Pink, purple), on the roots (lily) or on the fruit rind (Orange). It can also be secreted in the form of resinous gum (camphor, myrrh). The ancient art of fragrance extraction is based on four distillation techniques:

• Enfleurage. The extractive dissolution works for certain delicate flowers; using for Chis certain fatty substances that have the of absorbing on contact- If one proceeds at ordinary temperature, the operation is called enfleurage, as is the case with Jesse's rod and jasmine. It consists of impregnating the aromatic substances in fat and then extracting the fragrant oil with alcohol. Aromatic chemical are also used.

• Maceration. When by maceration, it is necessary to place the flowers in large kettles, keeping them submerged in order to release the smell.

• Squeeze. Another extractive procedure is expression; very suitable in citron, Orange and When the fruit is abundant, it is to collect the Oil.

• Distillation. This method is the most used especially for flowers, plants and herbs, such as lavender, roses, lavender, thyme, sandalwood, mimosa, etc. For this, a fairly large cavity alembic is used. The part of the vegetable that contains the essence, leaves, flowers, tree bark, etc.) is crushed and placed in the alembic. It is advisable not to put the material in direct contact with the boiler; for this reason it is placed in sacks or in a glass that is arranged in the center of the cucurbit. Sufficient water is added so that the material is completely bathed and after a few hours of maceration, distillation is carried out. Essential Oil is entrained by water vapor , although its boiling point is generally well above 100 a C. The distillation products are collected in a glass in which the water and the essence are easily separated. For the lighter essences, the so- called Florentine container is available. The essence goes to the top and accumulates in the container while the water escapes through a curved that rises from the base of the container. For the heavier essences, another of test tube is used in which the liquid is at the base and the water escapes in height. In all cases, the water that comes out carries a little of the essence in solution or in suspension.

This water returns to the alembic to take advantage of it in successive operations, so that the water, despite being waste, Will be aromatic.

MUD THERAPY

It is a very Old method, used for centuries. Already in the time of mud was used for miraculous purposes since the water and the minerals from the mud and clay act in a very healthy way on our although at first glance the treatment can be unpleasant due to the fact of having to cover ourselves with mud, the feeling of relaxation and well-being, is immediate. benefits. We can enjoy the anti-inflammatory, refreshing, absorbent, decongestant, healing and soothing properties that logotherapy offers us. It is recommended for oily or combination skin, as the clay eliminates acne blemishes and also reduces cellulite as it absorbs toxins accumulated under the skin. It should not be used on dry skin as it increases their dryness.

HOT STONES

One of the first therapies in spa is "Stone Massage", also known as Geothermal Therapy. It is described as massage therapy that incorporates volcanic hot stones or Cold river or sea Stones into its protocol, as well as crystals and semi-precious Stones. Its objective is to carry out an extremely relaxing and massage for the general It basically consists of the use of hot and Cold Stones for deep massages. It combines, through a modern technique, millenary knowledge Of Geotherapy, Thermotherapy and Mesotherapy, achieving, thanks to the synergy obtained, producing physiological and organic reactions of the highest benefit for the human Today, the "stone massage" is the most trend in the most prestigious spa's in the World. In them the therapy is complemented with a hydromassage bath, with an exfoliation with a mud wrap, with a sauna bath or with a shower as previous treatments. During the treatment essential Oils and music are used, the size, shape, weight and of the Stones are chosen individually to the and the effects that we intend to cause in the recipient.

The obsidian Stone massage is a therapy based on the energy from the Mexican volcanic lands to restore all its vitality to the body, eliminate toxins, stimulate its organic functions and combat stress and anxiety. Inspired by the ancestral wisdom of the peoples of Mesoamerica, the treatment recovers the benefits of Stones, applied to the body through pressure, massage and thermal stimuli. The effectiveness of the treatment has its origin in the combined action of the Stones with which different areas of the body are massaged and pressed. The exchange of energies, the temperature of the Stones and the therapist lead the patient to a deep State of relaxation and serenity.

Massage causes effects on the physical and psychological functions of the body producing mechanical, thermal and chemical stimuli. Effects on different parts of the body could be resulting from the skin. Helps the release of dead cells and the secretion of the superficial sweat and sebaceous glands. It acts on the secretory ducts, avoiding obstructions that could lead to Cysts, abscesses, etc. Increases by 2 or 3 C, when there are circulatory or neurovegetative disorders. Adipose tissue by intensifying local circulatory and metabolic activity and increasing blood flow favors the reabsorption of fatty tissue (although its total elimination is just from the stones Hot and Cold stones, black and White, alternate to massage the Basalt Stones are dark and dense volcanic rocks with a high iron content, the darker the Stones are, the longer they retain heat, which increases their magnetic power and therefore their Basalt has dark colors, Rhyolite, on the contrary, has light colors. Sedimentary Stones are effective due to their mineral nature, which accentuates their heat retention properties. Its texture should be smooth and Silky. Marble Stones are carbonate rocks that have undergone metamorphism and present a characteristic crystalline They are effective in balancing the temperature and produce stimulating effects.

This movement of energies takes place thanks to the bio-resonance of the Stones. Because the atmosphere is loaded with negative ions, the resonance neutralizes the increase in positive ions that takes place When we suffer stress or some alteration or chemical imbalance in our Therefore, the Stones amplify the energies by balancing the positive and negative ions.

In the East, the chakras are the seven energy centers of Our body. Each chakra develops a different function and is related to an organ or part of our body. Semi- precious Stones are used to balance these energy centers when there is a decompensation in the chakras. Through semi-precious Stones and their resonance, the chakras are activated, balanced to reduce stress and relieve tension, eliminating blockages, neutralizing emotions and promoting general well-being and harmony. When the chakras work well, the organs with which they are related receive the necessary energy and remain healthy, otherwise there are imbalances and blockages.

The application ofhot and cold stones act at two levels:

a). - Static: by exerting therapeutic pressure on specific

b) Dynamic: When performing well-defined massage maneuvers. Generally, during the massage, more than 60 volcanic rocks of different size, origin and Shape are used, they are heated in a professional to a temperature of 3 6 to 3 9 degrees Without burning or damaging the skin. Another technique combines 54 volcanic Stones and 18 marble, the former are heated and the latter cooled in a freezer or with ice. During the session, the therapist places Stones on the patient along the spine, forehead, eyes, hands, toes and energy points of the body, without forgetting the semi-precious Stones in the chakras.

Use some sensory movements:

1 Slow ascending and descending sliding with 2 stones.

2.- Upward rotary movement and downward sliding with 2 stones.

3.- Upward pressure and downward slide with 2 Stones.

4.- Upward kneading and downward sliding with 2 stones.

5.- Slow ascending sliding and descending vibrations with 2

6.- Slow ascending slide and descending waves with 2 stones.

7 Edge sliding with a Stone (knee, hands and feet).

8.- Circular edge pressures with a Stone (hands and feet).

9.- Undulating pressure with 4 Stones (abdomen).

10.- Slides with firm pressure upward with a stone. Hot Stone massage should only be performed by professionals and qualified massagers. The masseurs or therapists who wish to apply this therapy must have adequate training to learn how to place the stones, know what the energy are, how to adapt the Stones to the massage and the contraindications and what should not be done during the application. of the "stone massage". It is easy to learn, training is short-lived; but it is necessary to do it, since in addition to the basic principles of massage and a relaxation technique, this therapy works with energy, which is why it should not be taken lightly.

Wine Therapy and Chocotherapy

Wine therapy is a totally natural and healthy technique or treatment from which grapes are used, either the fruit itself with its seeds, or through jets of wine. Wine therapy is commonly used when cleaning and purifying the skin, thanks to the fact that externally the Wine helps to stimulate circulation.

USE of WINE-THERAPY. In therapy, a wine is done all over the body. This exfoliation is done from the feet to the head on both sides, after the exfoliation rests for a while. The patient Will go to the tub, a glass of wine Will be added, and there the patient will relax. And then the therapy is finished with a deep relaxing massage.

BENEFITS of WINE THERAPY. These beauty treatments have the ability, among others, to tone the breasts, firm the and soft, rejuvenate the muscles and the skin. It also serves for relaxation through massages with pulp, essential Oils and wines. Scientific studies in this regard have proven that the antioxidant action of wine acts more strongly than vitamins C and E, which has consolidated the use of this technique in few clinics, they have found a more effective way to stop the passage of time.

On the other hand, we have Chocotherapy. The use of for aesthetic purposes is obtained through the direct and application of this delicious food on the skin. Dark chocolate or "Dark chocolate" has antioxidant properties, both orally and subcutaneously. It consists of a "peeling" after which a massage is carried out, worked with hot chocolate. The result is highly toned, relaxed and hydrated skin. It is a de-stressing and energizing therapy. In addition to its external use and its flavor, its aroma has stimulating properties which stimulate good mood. Because of its high antioxidant content, cocoa attacks free radicals and cellular oxygenation. rich in it reduces inflammation of the blood vessels and improves circulation. Its seeds are rich in exantin and theobromine, which are tissue oxygenators, play a fundamental role in combating the signs of aging, stimulate the dermis and break thermal energy.

BENEFITS of CHOCOTHERAPY. The innovative massages and chocolate baths hydrate the skin and fight cellulite. It also eliminates tension, lack of vitality, tiredness and all the symptoms of stress. Recently, researchers discovered that is a powerful element for preserving beauty, due to its slimming, detoxifying and firming properties. Improves thanks to the production of endorphins, hormones that promote Our feeling of well- being and happiness. These hormones are generated Whenever a person is happy, when they activities that give pleasure, or when they find satisfaction in small daily activities.

USE of CHOCOTHERAPY. with the help of a brush, the is covered with a mixture containing cocoa, caffeine and various of essential Oils that enhance the reducing, stimulating and draining effects. The process of this peeling that is carried out with a massage in which the hot chocolate is rubbed on the skin, results in obtaining a toned, hydrated and relaxed skin.

TANNING LAMP

Another therapy that has very popular in Cold countries with few Sunny days, or even in Winter seasons, are tanning lamps. These are the main part of any tanning device that produces UV light for tanning. There are hundreds of different types of tanning lamps, most of which can be classified into two basic groups: low pressure and high pressure. Within the industry, it is Common to call high pressure unit "bulbs" and low pressure unit "lamps", although there are many exceptions and not all follow this example.

Both types require an oxygen-free environment inside the lamp. Fluorescent tanning lamps require an electrical ballast to limit the amount of current that passes through the lamp. While the resistance of a filament in incandescent lamps inherently limits the current within it, tanning lamps do not and instead have negative resistance.

They are plasmatic nerves devices, like a neon sign, and will pass as much current as the external circuit provides, even to the point of self- destruction. Therefore, a load is needed to regulate the current through them.

Tanning lamps are installed in tanning beds, tanning booths, tanning decks, or single lamp tanning units. The quality of the tan (or how similar it is to a natural sun tan) depends on the of light that is generated from such lamps.

SAND THERAPY

Did you know that depending on your skin type, on beach days you can take advantage of the properties of the sand placed on Your face? Well, for with Oily and shiny skin in areas of the body such as the face, the regenerative benefits of sand are already known to accelerate the exfoliation or removal of skin damaged by impurities such as blemishes, acne, scars and wrinkles.

Left for a maximum time of 10 up to 20 minutes it is enough to Start the skin regeneration process, shrink the skin and close the Wide open pores. On the other hand, in areas of the body with sensitive skin such as the shoulders, it is not recommended to place it since it increases hyper sensitivity and redness. Sand is the disaggregated and incoherent mass of mineral matter in a fine granular State, normally consisting of quartz (silica) with a small proportion of mica, feldspar, magnetite and other resistant minerals. It is the product of the chemical and mechanical disintegration of rocks under Weathering and abrasion-

When the particles have just formed, they are usually angular and pointed, smaller and rounded by friction caused by wind and water. It does not have to be precisely in Summer since the effects of ultraviolet rays affect us all year round, in addition to the fact that it has been shown that the care of tanned skin or skin to sunlight due to the type of work that is done, such as This is the case of sailors, builders, sellers, carriers and Others; It forces us to avoid extreme tanning by wearing hats and long-sleeved shirts in dark colors and not translucent. On Your next beach walk you take advantage of this natural beach sand facial and discover its wonderful.

ICE THERAPY

In Summer seasons, you may have heard of ice therapy to firm Your skin, well, this therapy also appears to be working to tone and Slim Your shape.

Why use cold to lose weight? As we have Said before, it seems that there are many taboos around cold, although it is very necessary for many things in life, for example and the most used, to alleviate pain in the mouth, throat, or some type of injury. We are going to focus more specifically on what to do when you intend to lose weight and you want to do it When cold, since some heat technique has not worked for you at all.

As we have seen above, there are multiple studies that reveal that the Cold reduces sizes and helps to tone more quickly than if you do it with heat, but think about the sensation that Your body has When leaving a of Cold water or a shower.

What is ice therapy? Ice therapy involves applying ice directly to parts of the body, such as the most flaccid parts or those Where you are more fat or overweight. What are the benefits of this treatment? There are many , among them:

Some of the are as follows. Firms the skin, preventing sagging of your body. Firms the tissues Improves and fights cellulite Reduce sizes Helps to stimulate blood circulation

What is the origin of ice therapy?

This technique appeared in Mexico and it is a Cold massage that combined with exercise and a healthy diet, denotes great positive effects on Your in addition to producing the generation of new. There are different ways to apply ice and to enjoy all its benefits, you can apply the ice directly, or to avoid burning you can apply gel bags, the latter you can buy at the pharmacy. There are some cities that have specialized centers for ice therapy, the technique is based on first placing a mud to prepare the skin, as well as exfoliating and purifying it by activating all the cells and also the blood supply, giving a light massage in the area activating it. This technique is Widely applied among the most famous and no side effects have yet been found, other than some of skin redness that fades over time

What audience is ice therapy intended for?

Ice therapy is used for anyone who wants to lose weight, firm and tone their muscles, it is not a technique designed only for the female sex, however, women are the ones who use it the most- Especially it is used in women who have children and from 40 years of age to reaffirm the most flaccid parts of their body, giving great results. It is also indicated for those who have followed a strict diet losing a lot of weight in a short time and cannot find an effective treatment. In addition, it is also recommended by cosmetic surgery doctors for patients with bags, dark circles or a fallen double chin to achieve greater tension in the areas. There are different types of ice in this therapy, for example one that includes essential Oils or herbs to improve the elasticity of the skin, it is also highly recommended to reduce stretch marks.

CARBOXYTHERAPY

A Renewing Ally in the Field of Aesthetics

In the dynamic world of aesthetics, the quest for beauty and rejuvenation has driven the development of innovative techniques that promise effective and long-lasting results. Among these alternatives, carboxytherapy has positioned itself as an attractive option for those who wish to improve the appearance of their skin and combat the signs of aging.

What is carboxytherapy?

Carboxytherapy is a non-invasive technique that involves the subcutaneous application of carbon dioxide (CO2) in a gaseous state through microinjections. This gas, naturally present in our bodies, acts as a cellular stimulant, triggering a series of benefits for the skin.

How does carboxytherapy work?

Carbon dioxide injected into the skin generates an effect similar to a micromassage that activates blood and lymphatic circulation. This, in turn, produces a series of benefits:

* **Increased oxygen and nutrients in the skin:** Increased blood flow promotes the delivery of oxygen and nutrients to cells, improving their metabolism and vitality.

* **Stimulation of collagen and elastin production:** CO2 activates fibroblasts, cells responsible for the production of collagen and elastin, proteins essential for skin firmness and elasticity.

* **Improved microcirculation:** Carboxytherapy stimulates blood and lymphatic circulation, eliminating toxins and improving the overall appearance of the skin.

* **Reduction of localized fat:** CO2 promotes lipolysis, a process that breaks down fat cells, helping to reduce accumulated fat in specific areas.

* **Tightening and firming effect:** The stimulation of collagen and elastin production, along with improved microcirculation, generates a tightening and firming effect on the skin.

Where can carboxytherapy be applied?

Carboxytherapy is a versatile technique that can be applied to various areas of the body, including:

* **Face:** To treat fine lines, wrinkles, sagging skin, dark circles, bags under the eyes, and improve skin tone and texture.

* **Neck and décolletage:** To combat sagging skin, improve texture, and prevent the appearance of wrinkles.

* **Buttocks, thighs, and abdomen:** To reduce localized fat, improve circulation, and combat cellulite.

What are the benefits of carboxytherapy?

Carboxytherapy offers several advantages that make it an attractive option in the field of aesthetics:

* **Non-invasive technique:** It requires no incisions or anesthesia, making it a safe and minimally invasive procedure.

* **Fast and visible results:** The results begin to be seen after the first sessions and intensify over time.
* **Minimal recovery:** No downtime required after treatment.

* **Long-lasting effects:** Results can last for several months, depending on the area treated and the patient's lifestyle.

* **Compatible with other treatments:** It can be combined with other aesthetic techniques for even more satisfying results.

Is carboxytherapy for everyone?

While carboxytherapy is a safe and effective technique for most people, it is important to consult with a specialist to determine if it is appropriate for your particular case. In some cases, it may be contraindicated for:

* Pregnant or breastfeeding women.

* People with heart or lung disease.

* People with uncontrolled diabetes.

* People with blood clotting disorders.

* People with active infections in the area to be treated.

How is a carboxytherapy treatment performed?

The carboxytherapy procedure is relatively simple and quick:

1. **Cleaning and preparation of the area:** The area to be treated is properly cleaned and disinfected.

2. **CO2 application:** Specialized equipment is used to inject CO2 into the skin through fine microinjections. The amount of CO2 injected will depend on the area to be treated and the patient's needs.

3. **Post-treatment massage:** A gentle massage is performed on the treated area to promote CO2 absorption and stimulate blood circulation.

How many carboxytherapy sessions are needed?

The number of sessions required will depend on the area to be treated, the treatment goal, and the patient's individual response.

CRYOLIPOLYSIS

A Cold Approach to Sculpting Your Body

In the dynamic world of aesthetics, the search for body harmony has driven the development of innovative techniques that go beyond traditional surgical interventions. Cryolipolysis, also known as fat freezing, has become one of the most popular alternatives for eliminating unwanted fat deposits and sculpting the body safely and effectively.

**What is it?

What is cryolipolysis?**

Cryolipolysis is a noninvasive technique that uses controlled cold temperatures to selectively eliminate fat cells. Unlike traditional liposuction, which involves surgery and fat extraction, cryolipolysis requires no incisions or anesthesia.

How does cryolipolysis work?

The cryolipolysis device applies extreme cold to the treated area, causing the fat cells to crystallize and subsequently die. These crystallized cells are then naturally eliminated by the body's lymphatic system, resulting in a gradual reduction of fat in the treated area.

Which areas of the body can cryolipolysis be applied to?

Cryolipolysis is a versatile technique that can be applied to various areas of the body with stubborn fat deposits, including:

* Abdomen

* Hips

* Flanks

* Back

* Arms

* Knees

* Double chin

What are the benefits of cryolipolysis?

Cryolipolysis offers several advantages compared to other fat removal methods:

* **Non-invasive:** It requires no incisions or anesthesia, minimizing the risk of complications and recovery time.

* **Effective:** It permanently eliminates fat cells, providing long-lasting results.

* **Safe:** It is a relatively safe technique with a low side effect profile.

* **Comfortable:** The procedure is painless and requires no special preparation.

* **Versatile:** It can be applied to various areas of the body.

Who are the ideal candidates for cryolipolysis?

Cryolipolysis is an excellent option for people who:

* Are in good overall health.

* Lead a healthy lifestyle with a balanced diet and regular exercise.

* Have localized fat deposits that do not respond to diet and exercise.

* Are looking for a non-invasive alternative to traditional liposuction.

What to expect during the procedure?

The cryolipolysis procedure typically lasts between 30 and 60 minutes per treated area. During the procedure:

* An applicator is placed on the treated area.

* The applicator administers extreme cold for a specified period.

* You may experience a sensation of intense cold or mild discomfort during the procedure.

* After the procedure, the treated area may temporarily redden or swell.

How many treatments are needed?

The results of cryolipolysis are not immediate. A gradual reduction in fat is observed in the weeks following treatment. In some cases, multiple treatments may be necessary to achieve the desired results.

What are the side effects of cryolipolysis?

The side effects of cryolipolysis are usually mild and temporary, and include:

* Redness

* Swelling

* Numbness

* Tenderness to touch

* Mild pain

In rare cases, more serious side effects may occur, such as:

* Hematoma

* Nerve injury

* Skin necrosis

How much does cryolipolysis cost?

The cost of cryolipolysis can vary depending on several factors, such as the doctor's experience, the clinic, and the number of areas treated. In general, the price per treated area ranges from $500 to $2,000.

In conclusion, cryolipolysis has become an attractive alternative for safely and effectively removing body fat. If you are considering this procedure, it is important to consult with an aesthetic physician to determine if it is the right option for you and to discuss your expectations and goals.**

It is important to note that the information provided in this article is of a general nature and does not substitute for professional medical advice. It is always advisable to consult with a qualified physician for specific and personalized information about cryolipolysis and its suitability for your particular case.**

PHLEBOLOGY

An Aesthetic and Medical Approach in Clinics

Navigating the Veins: An Approach to Phlebology

In the dynamic world of aesthetic medicine, phlebology has emerged as a crucial specialty, addressing venous and vascular conditions that affect both health and appearance. Beyond being a purely aesthetic field, phlebology focuses on the patient's holistic well-being, restoring vascular health and improving quality of life.

What is Phlebology?

Phlebology is a branch of medicine that specializes in the study, diagnosis, and treatment of diseases of the venous and lymphatic systems. It covers a wide range of conditions, from common varicose veins and spider veins to more complex disorders such as deep vein thrombosis and chronic venous insufficiency.

In the Field of Aesthetics:

In the field of aesthetics, phlebology plays a fundamental role in improving the appearance of the legs.

Varicose veins, those dilated, tortuous veins that swell and protrude from the skin's surface, are not only unsightly but can also cause discomfort and pain. Phlebology offers a variety of minimally invasive techniques to eliminate or treat these varicose veins, restoring the natural beauty of the legs and improving the patient's quality of life.

Aesthetic Phlebology Techniques:

* **Sclerotherapy:** This technique involves injecting a solution into the diseased veins to cause them to contract and disappear.

* **Thermocoagulation:** Heat is applied to the veins to destroy them and make them disappear.

* **Endovenous Laser:** A laser is used to destroy the veins from within.

* **Microsurgery:** In more severe cases, microsurgery can be used to eliminate varicose veins.

Benefits of Aesthetic Phlebology:

* **Improves the appearance of the legs:** Eliminates varicose veins and spider veins, giving the legs a smoother and more even appearance.

* **Relieves discomfort:** Reduces the feeling of heaviness, tiredness, and pain in the legs.

* **Improves circulation:** Eliminates clogged veins, allowing better blood flow.

* **Increases self-esteem:** Helps patients feel more confident and comfortable with their bodies.

Beyond Aesthetics: Phlebology as Preventive Medicine

While aesthetic phlebology focuses on improving appearance, its scope goes beyond that. The prevention of venous diseases is a crucial aspect of this specialty. Early detection and timely treatment of venous problems can prevent serious complications such as deep vein thrombosis and chronic venous insufficiency.

Importance of Consulting a Phlebologist:

If you are experiencing leg discomfort, such as varicose veins, spider veins, swelling, cramps, or pain, it is important to consult a phlebologist. An accurate diagnosis and a personalized treatment plan can help you regain your vascular health and improve your quality of life.

In conclusion, phlebology has become an essential specialty in the field of aesthetic medicine, offering effective solutions to improve the appearance and health of the legs. By combining minimally invasive techniques with a preventative approach, phlebology empowers patients to regain their well-being and enjoy a full life.

PRESSOTHERAPY

An Ally of Cosmetic Surgery for Recovery and Aesthetics

Cosmetic surgery has evolved by leaps and bounds in recent years, offering increasingly advanced solutions to improve physical appearance. However, once the surgical intervention is performed, the process does not end there. Postoperative recovery plays a fundamental role in achieving optimal and satisfactory results. In this scenario, pressotherapy emerges as a valuable ally for cosmetic surgery clinics, providing both functional and aesthetic benefits.

What is pressotherapy?

Pressotherapy, also known as pneumatic lymphatic drainage, is a non-invasive physical therapy technique that uses controlled air pressure to stimulate the lymphatic system. It is applied using a device consisting of inflatable boots, pants, or belts that fit the legs, abdomen, or arms, depending on the area being treated. The equipment generates sequential pressure that rhythmically increases and decreases, creating a drainage and compression effect on the tissues.

Benefits of pressotherapy in postoperative recovery

The application of pressotherapy after cosmetic surgery provides several advantages that promote patient recovery and optimize results:

* **Reduction of edema:** Fluid accumulation after surgery is a common phenomenon. Pressotherapy promotes lymphatic drainage, eliminating excess interstitial fluid that causes inflammation and swelling. This promotes cleaner healing and accelerates overall recovery.

* **Improved blood circulation:** The pressure exerted by pressotherapy also stimulates venous and arterial circulation. This promotes the transport of oxygen and nutrients to the tissues, which accelerates the healing and cell regeneration processes.

* **Reduced pain:** The accumulation of inflammatory fluids can cause discomfort and postoperative pain. Pressotherapy, by reducing edema, helps alleviate pain and improve the patient's sense of comfort.

* **Prevention of fibrosis:** Fibrosis is the excessive formation of fibrous tissue in the surgical area, which can cause skin irregularities. Pressotherapy helps prevent fibrosis by improving circulation and stimulating the elimination of inflammatory substances.

* **Muscle recovery:** In surgeries involving muscles, pressotherapy promotes the elimination of

Varicose veins, those dilated, tortuous veins that swell and protrude from the skin's surface, are not only unsightly but can also cause discomfort and pain. Phlebology offers a variety of minimally invasive techniques to eliminate or treat these varicose veins, restoring the natural beauty of the legs and improving the patient's quality of life.

Aesthetic Phlebology Techniques:

* **Sclerotherapy:** This technique involves injecting a solution into the diseased veins to cause them to contract and disappear.

* **Thermocoagulation:** Heat is applied to the veins to destroy them and make them disappear.

* **Endovenous Laser:** A laser is used to destroy the veins from within.

* **Microsurgery:** In more severe cases, microsurgery can be used to eliminate varicose veins.

Benefits of Aesthetic Phlebology:

* **Improves the appearance of the legs:** Eliminates varicose veins and spider veins, giving the legs a smoother and more even appearance.

* **Relieves discomfort:** Reduces the feeling of heaviness, tiredness, and pain in the legs.

* **Improves circulation:** Eliminates clogged veins, allowing better blood flow.

* **Increases self-esteem:** Helps patients feel more confident and comfortable with their bodies.

Beyond Aesthetics: Phlebology as Preventive Medicine

While aesthetic phlebology focuses on improving appearance, its scope goes beyond that. The prevention of venous diseases is a crucial aspect of this specialty. Early detection and timely treatment of venous problems can prevent serious complications such as deep vein thrombosis and chronic venous insufficiency.

Importance of Consulting a Phlebologist:

If you are experiencing leg discomfort, such as varicose veins, spider veins, swelling, cramps, or pain, it is important to consult a phlebologist. An accurate diagnosis and a personalized treatment plan can help you regain your vascular health and improve your quality of life.

In conclusion, phlebology has become an essential specialty in the field of aesthetic medicine, offering effective solutions to improve the appearance and health of the legs. By combining minimally invasive techniques with a preventative approach, phlebology empowers patients to regain their well-being and enjoy a full life.

PRESSOTHERAPY

An Ally of Cosmetic Surgery for Recovery and Aesthetics

Cosmetic surgery has evolved by leaps and bounds in recent years, offering increasingly advanced solutions to improve physical appearance. However, once the surgical intervention is performed, the process does not end there. Postoperative recovery plays a fundamental role in achieving optimal and satisfactory results. In this scenario, pressotherapy emerges as a valuable ally for cosmetic surgery clinics, providing both functional and aesthetic benefits.

What is pressotherapy?

Pressotherapy, also known as pneumatic lymphatic drainage, is a non-invasive physical therapy technique that uses controlled air pressure to stimulate the lymphatic system. It is applied using a device consisting of inflatable boots, pants, or belts that fit the legs, abdomen, or arms, depending on the area being treated. The equipment generates sequential pressure that rhythmically increases and decreases, creating a drainage and compression effect on the tissues.

Benefits of pressotherapy in postoperative recovery

The application of pressotherapy after cosmetic surgery provides several advantages that promote patient recovery and optimize results:

* **Reduction of edema:** Fluid accumulation after surgery is a common phenomenon. Pressotherapy promotes lymphatic drainage, eliminating excess interstitial fluid that causes inflammation and swelling. This promotes cleaner healing and accelerates overall recovery.

* **Improved blood circulation:** The pressure exerted by pressotherapy also stimulates venous and arterial circulation. This promotes the transport of oxygen and nutrients to the tissues, which accelerates the healing and cell regeneration processes.

* **Reduced pain:** The accumulation of inflammatory fluids can cause discomfort and postoperative pain. Pressotherapy, by reducing edema, helps alleviate pain and improve the patient's sense of comfort.

* **Prevention of fibrosis:** Fibrosis is the excessive formation of fibrous tissue in the surgical area, which can cause skin irregularities. Pressotherapy helps prevent fibrosis by improving circulation and stimulating the elimination of inflammatory substances.

* **Muscle recovery:** In surgeries involving muscles, pressotherapy promotes the elimination of

ELECTROTHERAPY

An ally in the pursuit of beauty in aesthetic clinics

In the dynamic world of aesthetics, the search for beauty and physical well-being has driven the development of innovative techniques that go beyond traditional methods. Electrotherapy is emerging as a promising alternative, offering a range of possibilities to improve skin health, combat the signs of aging, and noninvasively sculpt the body.

What is electrotherapy?

Electrotherapy is a branch of physiotherapy that uses electrical currents to stimulate body tissues for therapeutic and aesthetic purposes. These currents can be of different types, such as:

Galvanic: A low-intensity direct current that promotes hydration, healing, and the resorption of edema.

Faradic: A low-frequency alternating current that stimulates muscle contraction and improves blood circulation. * **High Frequency:** High-frequency currents generate heat and have bactericidal and anti-inflammatory effects.

Applications of Electrotherapy in Aesthetics

Electrotherapy offers a wide range of applications in the field of aesthetics, ranging from the treatment of **dermatological problems** to **body remodeling**:

1. Facial Treatment:

* **Facial Rejuvenation:** Electrotherapy stimulates the production of collagen and elastin, reducing fine lines and wrinkles and improving skin elasticity.

* **Photoaging:** Galvanic and high-frequency currents combat damage caused by sun exposure, such as dark spots and uneven pigmentation.

* **Acne:** Electrotherapy helps control sebum production, reduce inflammation, and eliminate bacteria, improving the appearance of acne-prone skin.

2. Body Treatment:

* **Fat Reduction:** Muscle electrostimulation helps burn calories and tone muscles, combating sagging skin and cellulite.

* **Lymphatic Drainage:** Galvanic currents stimulate lymphatic circulation, reducing swelling and improving fluid retention.

* **Electrolysis:** This technique uses electric current to permanently remove unwanted hair.

Advantages of Electrotherapy

Electrotherapy has become a popular tool in aesthetic clinics due to its many advantages:

* **Non-invasive and safe:** It requires no incisions or needles, making it a safe and comfortable option for patients.

* **Effective and visible results:** It offers visible and lasting results in a short period of time.

* **Versatile and adaptable:** It can be applied to a wide range of aesthetic needs, from the face to the body.

* **Combinable with other treatments:** It can be combined with other aesthetic techniques for even more optimal results.

* **Minimal side effects:** Side effects are generally mild and temporary.

Important considerations

Despite its benefits, it is important to keep in mind some considerations before opting for electrotherapy:

* **Consultation with a specialist:** It is essential to consult with a doctor or physical therapist specializing in electrotherapy to determine if it is an appropriate treatment and what is the best option for each individual case.

* **Preliminary evaluation:** A preliminary evaluation must be performed to rule out contraindications such as cardiac pacemakers, pregnancy, or dermatological conditions.

* **Application by trained professionals:** Electrotherapy must be applied by trained professionals to ensure its safety and effectiveness.

* **Hygiene and sterilization:** It is crucial to follow strict hygiene and sterilization protocols to prevent infection.

Conclusion

Electrotherapy is establishing itself as an effective and safe alternative in the field of aesthetics, offering a wide range of applications to improve skin health, combat the signs of aging, and sculpt the body. Its noninvasive approach, visible results, and adaptability to different needs make it a valuable tool for aesthetic clinics. However, it is essential to consult with a specialist and follow their recommendations to ensure a safe and effective experience.

OXIDERMOTHERAPY

A Renewing Breath for Your Skin

In the dynamic world of aesthetics, the pursuit of natural beauty and eternal youth drives constant innovation in treatments and techniques. Among the latest trends gaining prominence in aesthetic clinics is Oxidermotherapy, a non-invasive technique that promises rejuvenating and revitalizing results for the skin.

What is Oxidermotherapy?

Oxidermotherapy, also known as facial oxygen therapy, is an aesthetic treatment that uses pure oxygen to stimulate the skin and improve its appearance. Unlike other invasive methods, Oxidermotherapy does not require needles or incisions, making it an attractive option for those seeking a gentle and safe alternative.

How does Oxidermotherapy work?

The treatment is based on the application of pure oxygen through a diffuser specially designed for facial use. Oxygen, an essential element for skin health and vitality, is administered at different pressures and depths, penetrating the dermal and hypodermal layers.

Benefits of Oxidermotherapy:

Oxidermotherapy offers a wide range of benefits for the skin, including:

* **Improves cellular oxygenation:** The supply of pure oxygen stimulates cellular respiration, revitalizing cells and improving their metabolism.

* **Increases collagen and elastin production:** Oxygen activates fibroblasts, cells responsible for the production of collagen and elastin, proteins essential for skin firmness and elasticity.

* **Reduces fine lines and wrinkles:** Stimulating collagen and elastin production helps fill in fine lines and wrinkles, giving the skin a smoother, more youthful appearance.

* **Improves skin texture and radiance:** Oxygen promotes the elimination of toxins and blood circulation, resulting in softer, more radiant, and even skin.

* **Fights acne and blemishes:** Oxygen has anti-inflammatory and antiseptic properties that help fight acne, reduce inflammation, and prevent the appearance of new blemishes.

* **Deeply hydrates the skin:** Oxygen stimulates the skin's natural hydration, combating dryness and providing a healthier appearance.

* **Tones and firms the skin:** Cellular oxygenation improves skin tone and firmness, combating sagging and improving the facial contour.

Who is Oxidermotherapy indicated for?

Oxidermotherapy is a treatment suitable for all skin types, even sensitive skin. It is ideal for:

* People seeking a preventative treatment for premature aging.

* People with fine lines and wrinkles.

* People with dry or dehydrated skin.

* People with dull or lackluster skin.

* People with acne or blemish-prone skin.

* People looking to improve their skin's tone and elasticity.

How is an Oxidermotherapy treatment performed?

The treatment

Oxidermotherapy is simple and convenient:

1. **Facial cleansing:** The skin is deeply cleansed to remove any impurities or makeup.

2. **Oxygen application:** Pure oxygen is applied through a diffuser at different pressures and depths, adapting to the specific needs of each area of the face.

3. **Facial massage:** A gentle facial massage can be performed to stimulate blood circulation and oxygen absorption.

4. **Moisturizing:** A moisturizer is applied to retain moisture and protect the skin.

How many sessions are necessary?

The recommended number of sessions will depend on each patient's specific needs and treatment goals. In general, **10 sessions** are recommended, with a frequency of once a week or every two weeks.

What are the side effects?

Oxidermotherapy is a safe treatment and is well tolerated by most people. In some cases, mild side effects such as temporary redness or irritation may occur, which will disappear on their own within a few minutes.

Recommendations:

* It is important to choose a trusted aesthetic clinic with professionals trained in oxydermotherapy.

* A prior consultation is recommended to evaluate your specific skin needs and determine if oxydermotherapy is the right treatment.

* It is important to maintain good hydration and sun protection after treatment.

OZONE THERAPY

An Innovative Approach to Facial Aesthetics

In the dynamic world of facial aesthetics, the quest for natural beauty and prolonged youthfulness drives constant innovation in techniques and treatments. Among the alternatives that have emerged in recent years, ozone therapy is positioned as a promising option, captivating the attention of those seeking effective and long-lasting results.

What is ozone therapy?

Oxonotherapy is a minimally invasive aesthetic technique that uses **medical ozone** as the primary agent to rejuvenate and revitalize facial skin. Ozone, a molecule composed of three oxygen atoms, has unique therapeutic and aesthetic properties that make it an invaluable ally in skin care.

Benefits of Facial Oxonotherapy

The application of ozone to the face provides a wide range of benefits, both preventative and corrective:

1. Cell regeneration: Ozone stimulates the production of collagen and elastin, essential proteins for skin firmness and elasticity, combating sagging and wrinkles.

2. Deep oxygenation: Delivers oxygen to skin cells, improving blood circulation and revitalizing the appearance of the face.

3. Anti-inflammatory effect: Reduces inflammation, a key factor in premature aging and the appearance of various skin conditions.

4. Antibacterial and antiviral action: Eliminates bacteria and viruses present on the skin, preventing infections and improving overall skin health.

5. Dark spot lightening: Reduces uneven pigmentation, giving a more even and radiant skin tone.

6. Scar and stretch mark reduction: Promotes healing and reduces the visibility of scars and stretch marks.

7. Tightening effect: Provides a natural lifting effect, firming facial tissues and combating sagging.

8. Improves hydration: Stimulates the production of hyaluronic acid, retaining moisture in the skin and combating dryness.

9. Provides radiance: Revitalizes the face, giving it a radiant and healthy appearance.

How is Facial Oxonotherapy performed?

The facial oxonotherapy procedure is simple and minimally invasive:

1. Facial Cleansing: A deep facial cleansing is performed to remove impurities and prepare the skin for treatment.

2. Ozone Application: Ozone is applied in different forms, such as pure gas, ozonated water, or ozonated oil, using different techniques such as mesotherapy or subcutaneous infiltration.

3. Facial Mask Application: A facial mask with hydrating and soothing properties is applied to complement the treatment.

4. Moisturizing and Sun Protection: At the end of the procedure, the skin is moisturized and sunscreen is applied to protect it from UV rays.

How many sessions are necessary?

The number of sessions will depend on each patient's specific needs and treatment goals. In general, an initial course of **5 to 10 sessions** is recommended, performed weekly or biweekly, followed by monthly maintenance sessions.

Contraindications to Facial Oxonotherapy

Facial oxonotherapy is generally safe and well tolerated by most people. However, there are some contraindications to consider:

* **Pregnancy and breastfeeding:** Not recommended

Not recommended during pregnancy or breastfeeding.

* **Autoimmune diseases:** Consult your doctor if you suffer from autoimmune diseases.

* **Active skin infections:** Not recommended for active skin infections.

* **Ozone allergies:** It is important to perform an ozone sensitivity test before treatment.

Expected results. The results of facial oxonotherapy are visible gradually and progressively. Starting with the third or fourth session, an improvement in skin texture, greater luminosity, and a reduction in the appearance of fine lines and wrinkles can be observed. With a complete treatment, lasting results of up to one year can be achieved, depending on the patient's lifestyle and habits.

**Final considerations

Facial oxonotherapy is presented as a promising alternative in the field of facial aesthetics, offering a natural and effective approach to rejuvenate and revitalize the skin. While it is important to consult a medical specialist to determine if this treatment is appropriate for each case, oxone therapy is quite well-established.

HORMONAL THERAPY

In Aesthetics: A Balanced Approach to Beauty

The pursuit of beauty in the dynamic world of aesthetics and rejuvenation has led to the exploration of various techniques and treatments. Among them, hormonal therapy has gained ground in recent years, positioning itself as a promising alternative to address various aspects related to physical appearance and overall well-being.

What is Hormone Therapy?

Hormone therapy, also known as hormone replacement therapy (HRT), involves the administration of synthetic or bioidentical hormones to compensate for the natural decline in hormone production that occurs with age. In the aesthetic field, it is primarily used to address hormonal imbalances that affect the skin, hair, and other aspects of aging.

How does Hormone Therapy work in Aesthetics?

Hormones play a crucial role in various physiological processes, including growth, metabolism, sexual function, and skin health. As we age, the production of gender-assigned hormones such as estrogen, progesterone, and testosterone decreases.

This hormonal decline can manifest in the skin through various signs and symptoms:

* **Wrinkles and fine lines:** A lack of estrogen reduces the production of collagen and elastin, proteins essential for skin firmness and elasticity.

* **Dryness and loss of radiance:** The decrease in estrogen also affects hydration and blood flow in the skin.

* **Facial volume loss:** The reduction in human growth hormone (HGH) can lead to a decrease in volume in the cheekbones, temples, and other areas of the face.

* **Hair thinning and brittleness:** Hormonal changes can affect the hair growth cycle and its thickness.

Hormone therapy seeks to compensate for these hormonal deficiencies, restoring hormonal balance and, consequently, improving the appearance and health of the skin, hair, and other aspects of aging.

Benefits of Hormone Therapy in Aesthetics

The application of hormone therapy in aesthetics offers several potential benefits:

* **Improved skin texture and elasticity:** By increasing collagen and elastin production, the skin becomes firmer, smoother, and more radiant.

* **Reduction of wrinkles and fine lines:** Improved hydration and elasticity help blur fine lines and prevent the formation of new wrinkles.

* **Increased radiance and vitality:** Improved blood circulation gives the skin a healthier and more luminous appearance.

* **Hair strengthening and growth:** Hormonal regulation favors the hair growth cycle, reducing hair loss and improving hair thickness.

* **Reduction in hot flashes and other menopausal symptoms:** Hormone therapy can relieve bothersome menopausal symptoms, such as hot flashes, vaginal dryness, and mood swings.

Types of Hormone Therapy in Aesthetics

There are different types of hormone therapy that can be used in aesthetics:

* **Hormone Replacement Therapy (HRT):** This is the most common type of hormone therapy and is primarily used to treat menopausal symptoms in women. HRT can be administered in the form of pills, patches, gels, or implants.

* **Bioidentical Therapy:** This type of therapy uses synthetic hormones made with the same molecular structure as the hormones naturally produced by the body. It is considered a more natural option than traditional HRT.

* **DHEA Therapy:** DHEA is a precursor hormone that is transformed into estrogen and testosterone in the body. DHEA therapy may be beneficial

Suitable for men and women to improve energy, libido, and overall well-being.

Important Considerations About Hormone Therapy

Before considering hormone therapy for aesthetic purposes, it is essential to consult with a specialist to:

* **Evaluate your medical history:** It is important to know your medical history, allergies, and current medications to determine if hormone therapy is right for you.

* **Perform laboratory tests:** Blood tests may be performed to assess your hormone levels and determine the appropriate treatment dose.

* **Discuss risks and benefits:** It is important to understand the potential risks and benefits associated with hormone therapy to make an informed decision about treatment.

Conclusion Hormone therapy presents itself as a promising alternative to address various aspects of aging and improve self-acceptance.

BIBLIOGRAPHY

BOOKS :

• 12 Diets of Fullness, David Ruiz, Ebook 2016. Amazon

• Natural life and health. Dr. Josep Lluis Berdonces and Pedro Ródenas. Popular Medical Culture Editions.

• Aloe vera. Neil Stevens. Sirio Publishing House. 2nd edition 1998. Barcelona, Spam.

• American Inside Out. Sue Kay and Vaughan Jones. Discover the real you. Myers-Briggs Type indicator. Macmillan, 2007.

• The pleasure of eating well: foods to prevent and cure. Leme de Vidal, Eunice. South American Publishing House Association.

• The miracle of food. Jean

• Bertran Prieto, Pol (2019). "The four levels of Biosafety in . Retrieved September 19 , 2019.

ENCYCLOPEDIAS:

• Encarta Encyclopedia. Microsoft 2016. Microsoft.com

DICTIONARIES:

• Ocean Dictionary of Synonyms and Antonyms. Editorial. Barcelona, Spain.

• Spanish dictionary. Royal Spanish Academy. Twenty-first edition. Volume I and II. Madrid Spain. 1992.

PUBLISHERS

PROMONET
PUBLISHING

www.ingramcontent.com/pod-product-compliance
Lightning Source LLC
LaVergne TN
LVHW080025210926
848481LV00011B/3101